D0758683

Medicaid Politics

Selected Titles in the American Governance and Public Policy Series

Series Editors: Gerard W. Boychuk, Karen Mossberger, and Mark C. Rom

Brussels Versus the Beltway: Advocacy in the United States and the European Union
Christine Mahoney

City–County Consolidation: Promises Made, Promises Kept?
Suzanne M. Leland and Kurt Thurmaier, Editors

Collaborative Public Management: New Strategies for Local Governments
Robert Agranoff and Michael McGuire

Competitive Interests: Competition and Compromise in American Interest Group Politics
Thomas T. Holyoke

The Congressional Budget Office: Honest Numbers, Power, and Policymaking
Philip G. Joyce

Custodians of Place: Governing the Growth and Development of Cities
Paul G. Lewis and Max Neiman

The Government Taketh Away: The Politics of Pain in the United States and Canada
Leslie A. Pal and R. Kent Weaver, Editors

Healthy Voices, Unhealthy Silence: Advocacy and Health Policy for the Poor
Colleen M. Grogan and Michael K. Gusmano

Investing in the Disadvantaged: Assessing the Benefits and Costs of Social Policies
David L. Weimer and Aidan R. Vining, Editors

Lessons of Disaster: Policy Change after Catastrophic Events
Thomas Birkland

Managing the Fiscal Metropolis: The Financial Policies, Practices, and Health of Suburban Municipalities
Rebecca M. Hendrick

Medical Governance: Values, Expertise, and Interests in Organ Transplantation
David L. Weimer

National Health Insurance in the United States and Canada: Race, Territory, and the Roots of Difference
Gerard W. Boychuk

Out and Running: Gay and Lesbian Candidates, Elections, and Policy Representation
Donald P. Haider-Markel

The Politics of Ideas and the Spread of Enterprise Zones
Karen Mossberger

The Politics of Unfunded Mandates: Whither Federalism?
Paul L. Posner

Power, Knowledge, and Politics: Policy Analysis in the States
John A. Hird

Rethinking Health Care Policy: The New Politics of State Regulation
Robert B. Hackey

Scandalous Politics: Child Welfare Policy in the States
Juliet F. Gainsborough

Welfare Policymaking in the States: The Devil in Devolution
Pamela Winston

Medicaid Politics

Federalism, Policy Durability, and Health Reform

Frank J. Thompson

Georgetown University Press
Washington, DC

Library of Congress Cataloging-in-Publication Data

Thompson, Frank J.
Medicaid politics : federalism, policy durability, and health reform / Frank J. Thompson.
p. ; cm. — (American governance and public policy series)
Includes bibliographical references and index.
ISBN 978-1-58901-934-8 (pb : alk. paper)
I. Title. II. Series: American governance and public policy.
[DNLM: 1. Medicaid. 2. Health Policy—United States. 3. Politics—United States. W 250 AA1]

368.4'200973—dc23

2012003559

∞ This book is printed on acid-free paper meeting the requirements of the American National Standard for Permanence in Paper for Printed Library Materials.

15 14 13 12 9 8 7 6 5 4 3 2 First printing

In memory of my parents
Joseph and Alice Thompson

and to the future
Alice, Evelyn, Hugh, Molly, and Nora

Contents

Illustrations

Tables

Figures

Acknowledgments

In seeking to fathom the nature and origins of Medicaid durability from President Clinton to President Obama, I have benefited greatly from the assistance of others. I am deeply indebted to the Robert Wood Johnson Investigator Award Program for funding my research. The foundation's generous support expedited my efforts to gather and analyze pertinent data, paid for my site visits to interview key stakeholders, and allowed me to pare my teaching courseload so I could focus more intensively on the project. Additionally, the annual meetings of the Robert Wood Johnson award winners introduced me to a set of extraordinarily knowledgeable health care experts from a spectrum of disciplines. There was no better way to recharge my intellectual batteries for this project than listening to and interacting with these exemplars. As vital to this project as the investigator award program has been, it deserves emphasis that this volume's conclusions do not necessarily reflect those of the Robert Wood Johnson Foundation.

This book strives to speak to two audiences: those interested in health policy; and those who seek to hone their understanding of broader political, policy, and administrative dynamics. In targeting these groups, two individuals have, from the outset, provided me with invaluable advice, draft chapter by draft chapter. David Mechanic, who directs the investigator award program and is a premier medical sociologist at Rutgers, knows more about health care, broadly defined, than anyone else I have met. He unfailingly offered copious, timely, and insightful comments on the initial drafts. On the political science side, Tom Gais, director of the Rockefeller Institute of Government at the State University of New York–Albany, steered me in fruitful directions. It was Tom who first made me realize the importance of "executive federalism" and waivers as a policy tool. He also commented on each draft chapter, nudging me to extract the lessons of Medicaid for broader issues of American politics and governance.

With their emphases on "faculty governance," university cultures typically undervalue the role of leadership and management. But make no mistake; my progress on this book benefited greatly from two exemplary leaders. Marc Holzer, founding dean of the School of Public Affairs and Administration at Rutgers–Newark, has nurtured an organizational climate that supports and rewards scholarly research. He is the main reason I had the opportunity to join the Rutgers faculty in 2008. In turn, Joel Cantor, director of the Rutgers Center for State Health Policy, has helped create and sustain a thriving think tank that produces high-quality scholarly and applied work. I cannot imagine a more supportive setting in which to pursue my interests in Medicaid. Joel also read and commented on portions of my manuscript. He assigned one of the center's professional staff, Jennifer Farnham, to assist me with the project. Jennifer's contribution was stellar from beginning to end. She took the lead in assembling pertinent data, constructing tables, and performing statistical analyses. She also commented on each draft chapter and called my attention to Medicaid reports and updates that would have otherwise eluded me.

Others also stepped up to help. Bob Hackey, Leighton Ku, and Mark Rom read and commented on the entire manuscript. Bruce Vladeck proffered perceptive comments on chapter 2. David Rousseau of the Kaiser Commission on Medicaid and the Uninsured went well beyond the call in helping me assemble a Medicaid data set covering the 1992–2008 period. Dick Nathan helped incubate this project at an early stage and generally opened Medicaid doors to me during his close to two decades as director of the Rockefeller Institute of Government. At an early point, Don Kettl planted the seeds for this book in my mind. Barry Rabe read the manuscript and provided encouragement down the home stretch. Bram Poquette of the Center for State Health Policy always rose to the occasion when I asked for his assistance with the technical aspects of manuscript preparation.

I also owe much to the many public officials and other Medicaid stakeholders who took time out of their busy (often hectic) schedules to enlighten me about Medicaid. Their knowledge and insights were indispensable. Consultants helped me target my interviews in three states. My thanks go to Yvonne Bigos (Florida), Lynn Blewett (Minnesota), and Camille Miller (Texas) for steering me in such productive directions.

The staff of Georgetown University Press supported this book from beginning to end. I especially thank my editor Don Jacobs for his initial interest in the project as well as his encouragement and advice along the way.

Valuable as these individuals have been, none contributed as much as my wife, Benna. She brought the love, support, conversation, and humor to everyday life that helped me keep at it. Our shared interests in music, movies, theater, travel, and grandchildren kindled the periodic breaks that kept this project from being a grind.

All the above suggests that it "took a village" for me to write this book. Of course, I alone remain responsible for any defects that persist.

Frequently Used Abbreviations and Acronyms

ACA	Patient Protection and Affordable Care Act of 2010, or Affordable Care Act
CHIP	State Children's Health Insurance Program
CMS	Centers for Medicare and Medicaid Services
CBO	US Congressional Budget Office
GAO	US General Accounting Office until 2004; then US Government Accountability Office
GDP	gross domestic product
HCBS	home and community-based services
HCFA	Health Care Financing Administration
NGA	National Governors Association
OMB	US Office of Management and Budget

CHAPTER ONE

Medicaid and the Health Care Crucible

In early 2011 the House of Representatives' Budget Committee passed a resolution supported by its Republican members calling for "fundamental reform" of Medicaid—a federal grant program to the states. Led by the committee chairman, Paul Ryan (R-WI), the Republicans on the committee bemoaned that "skewed political incentives" had triggered Medicaid's unsustainable growth. To "transform and strengthen the Medicaid safety net," they called for devolving more authority to the states to unshackle them from "a misguided," federally imposed, "one-size-fits-all approach." They also proposed to slash the program's costs by converting it to a block grant that would place new constraints on the ability of states to obtain federal dollars to support their Medicaid initiatives. The Democrats on the committee denounced the proposal. In their minority report they asserted that "giving governors so-called flexibility is just a nice sounding way of giving them license to use federal taxpayer dollars . . . to pay for their pet initiatives without oversight and accountability." They averred that block granting and cutting Medicaid "in the name of reform is like saving a drowning person by throwing them an anchor."[1]

Given broader trends in health care and the huge stakes involved, political struggles over programs like Medicaid are hardly surprising. Among the many social policies that preoccupy the industrial democracies, none presents more excruciating challenges and choices than the provision of health care. Efforts to assure access to health care consume vast sums of money, mobilize a huge labor force, and spill over into economic, social, and political life in myriad ways. With medical science persistently yielding new and often expensive treatments and with the elderly growing as a proportion of the population, pressures to spend more on health care intensify. For these and other reasons, health insurance stands front and center in debates about the sustainability of the welfare state in the United States and abroad. Unlike the world's other advanced democracies, however, the United States faces this vortex of pressures without first having established a system for universal health insurance. Moreover, it confronts these forces in a political context marked by intense and basic ideological disagreement over government's proper role in a health insurance system.

As befits a fragmented political system with a culture leery of centralized authority, the United States depends on a messy, decentralized mix of public and private sources to provide health insurance. This system is shaped by a health insurance regime that features a dizzying array of federal and state policies—direct government subsidies, regulations, tax incentives, and more. This insurance system rests on three primary pillars. The first one targets coverage provided by employers and purchased directly by individuals. The second, Medicare, extends insurance to nearly everyone of age sixty-five and above, along with certain people with disabilities. Third, and of paramount concern to this book, Medicaid provides federal grants to the states to offer insurance to low-income citizens. Though Medicaid was initially seen by many as a poor second cousin to Medicare, Medicaid consumes $400 billion annually in federal and state funds and covers more people than Medicare—about 67 million (Yocom 2011, 1). It has become a pivotal component of the epic health reform law of 2010, which seeks to foster near-universal coverage in the United States.

Medicaid's prominence in the health care arena is in a sense surprising. Many astute observers have long claimed that "a program for the poor is a poor program" (Derthick 1979, 217). Means-tested programs are presumably prone to erosion because they serve a stigmatized, politically weak clientele. Some believe that the propensity toward deterioration becomes even stronger when the federal government relies on the states to implement a program. In part because of these views, health care reformers over the decades assumed that Medicaid would fade away as the country moved toward universal health insurance. Instead, Medicaid has in many respects been quite durable. It has resisted retrenchment, expanded, and become a platform for comprehensive health reform. This book seeks to fathom the sense in which Medicaid has proven durable and why. It does so by examining Medicaid's evolution during the presidential administrations of Bill Clinton, George W. Bush, and Barack Obama. For reasons I subsequently discuss, this period features a remarkable set of developments shaping Medicaid's durability. The period provides fertile ground for understanding the policy dynamics that strengthen the program and those factors that weaken it.

This chapter sets the stage for the more detailed inquiry that follows. It opens by placing Medicaid in the context of the broader health insurance system. Medicaid cannot be properly understood without fathoming its relationship to the policies that shape employer health insurance and Medicare. Having placed the program against this backdrop, I provide a primer on Medicaid, sketching briefly who gets what, when, and how from the program. The chapter then turns to the core concept that drives this volume: program durability. Drawing on insights from research focused on the sustainability of the welfare state, I clarify the definition of durability and assay the various markers that can be used to gauge it.

The chapter then illuminates factors likely to have an impact on Medicaid's durability. I consider two overarching forces that create a sense of fiscal strain and austerity for the entire health insurance system—the dynamics at play within the health care arena that drive up costs, and the political creation of scarcity via the antitax movement. The chapter then probes three factors thought to make Medicaid in particular a likely candidate for erosion—its status as welfare medicine, declining public trust in government, and interstate economic competition. Not all have been pessimistic about Medicaid's durability. In this vein, I assess a contending perspective that has more recently identified factors that bolster Medicaid in the health policy arena. Finally, the chapter clarifies the rationale for my focus on the 1993–2010 period, my methods, and the contribution to knowledge that I aspire to make. This volume fits squarely in the tradition of those who believe that it is important to study programs over time—to make "moving pictures" rather than take "snapshots" (Pierson 2004, 2). It pays particular attention to how policy shapes politics—how the feedback from policy and administrative choices fortifies or vitiates a program.

Medicaid and the Other Pillars

Medicaid politics intertwines with developments affecting the two other major pillars of the American health insurance system—employer coverage and Medicare. These developments have elevated Medicaid's importance. The proportion of Americans with employer or individual coverage declined by 7 percentage points from 1992 to 2010. This erosion has placed new pressures on Medicaid to extend coverage to low-income working people. Meanwhile, Medicare's enrollments have grown, but not as fast as Medicaid's. The share of the population covered by Medicare increased by about 2.5 percentage points in the 1992–2010 period, while Medicaid rose by more than 4 points. Medicaid has come to insure a slightly greater proportion of Americans than Medicare.[2]

Employer Insurance: Toward Erosion

Fifty-five percent of the populace receives health insurance through their employers, and about 9 percent purchases individual policies (US Census Bureau 2011). A vast spectrum of federal and state policies, principally tax incentives and regulations, constitute this "shadow" (Gottschalk 2000) or "private" health care regime (Hacker 2002). Tax subsidies for employment-related health insurance loom particularly large. Federal and state laws exempt employers' contributions to health insurance from being counted as employees' income subject to taxation; they also allow employees to deduct their premium contributions from their taxable incomes. The forgone revenue to the two levels of government as a result of these exemptions (i.e., tax expenditures) amounted to an estimated $209 billion in 2006, about two-thirds of the annual cost of Medicaid. Moreover, thanks to rapidly rising health insurance premiums and a growing workforce, this tax expenditure has risen by more than 150 percent during the past twenty years, controlling for inflation (Selden and Gray 2006).[3]

The government has also been involved in regulating insurance carriers. For many years the fifty states assumed center stage in shaping both the employer and individual insurance markets. They vary greatly in how stringently they regulate such factors as the standards for fiscal solvency of insurance companies, the services an insurer must cover, the rates they may charge, whether the companies must accept and renew those who want coverage (i.e., guaranteed issue), and whether they must offer policies in the three main markets—large employers, small employers, and individuals. Starting in 1974 with the Employee Retirement and Income Security Act, the federal government became increasingly involved in regulating insurance carriers. This law provided incentives for larger employers to self-insure, and the great majority of firms with five hundred or more employees do so (Swartz 2006). Under this arrangement, firms do not purchase employee coverage from health insurance companies. Instead, they directly absorb some portion of the financial risk for employee health expenditures. Typically, they pay a fee to an insurance company or other agent to process the claims from medical providers. Self-insurance allows firms to escape state regulation concerning services that must be covered and related matters.

During the 1990s many hoped that state regulatory reform would expand employer-based coverage and make health insurance more affordable. Although these initiatives galvanized progress in some states, they did not yield major breakthroughs. Nagging trade-offs afflicted these efforts. For instance, efforts by state regulators to prevent insurance companies from discriminating against high-risk individuals with more health problems typically drove up premium costs for everyone. This encouraged some smaller firms to drop insurance coverage for their employees and some (usually healthier) individuals not to sign up for insurance. In states with less stringent regulation, insurance companies in the small-employer and individual markets engaged in "cherry picking," whereby they avoided covering individuals with more serious, expensive health problems (Monheit and Cantor 2004; New York State Health Policy Research Center 2008; Swartz 2006). These and other problems helped trigger a major expansion of federal regulation of insurance under the health reform law of 2010.

As this experience suggests, the intricate system that shapes employer health insurance has not saved this pillar from erosion. The proportion of all employers offering health insurance slumped from 69 percent in 2000 to 60 percent in 2009 before rebounding some in 2010.[4] Employers have reduced or eliminated health insurance benefits for future retirees. The proportion of larger firms offering health benefits to active workers that also provided them to retirees dropped from 66 percent in 1988 to 31 percent in 2008 (Kaiser Family Foundation 2008, 30, 34, 192). Employers have also escaped the need to provide health insurance by relying more on contingent workers—that is, temporary employees or independent contractors (about 30 percent of the labor force) who usually receive no fringe benefits.[5] Given these developments, it is hardly surprising that the proportion of the population with employer-provided health insurance declined from slightly more than 65 percent in 2000 to 55 percent in 2010. This trend helped fuel an increase in uninsured Americans during this period, from 14 percent to more than 16 percent.[6]

The erosion of employer health insurance has also occurred through the thinning, rather than the complete withdrawal, of benefits. Thinning occurs when employer plans restrict the services covered, impose greater cost sharing, or limit the range of providers employees can access. The service packages covered by insurance vary considerably. Debates about service coverage at times revolve around whether insurers should subsidize access to some recently discovered medical treatment. But often the issue is even more fundamental—whether to pay for well-established, beneficial interventions. For example, deaths from colon cancer (more than 50,000 annually) can be reduced through early detection generated by periodic colonoscopies for people who reach the age of fifty years. Yet despite its benefits, the Government Accountability Office (GAO 2004b) reports that a significant minority of employer plans fail to cover such screening. Many employers have moved to limit the services covered under their insurance plans. A few have adopted mini–medical plans, which limit the number of doctor visits and expenses to be covered in a year (e.g., five doctor visits maxing out at $200 annually) (GAO 2007b, 10–18). Some states have altered their regulatory systems to permit employers to offer bare-bones coverage. In 2008, for instance, Governor Charlie Crist of Florida (R) persuaded the legislature to pass a bill that encourages insurance companies to offer policies with a low premium ($150 per month). In exchange, the law exempted these companies from state mandates that ordinarily require insurers to cover fifty-two specific services (Lemov 2008).

Thinning can also occur through increases in employee cost sharing. These costs come in several guises—including premiums, the amount those covered must pay to obtain insurance in the first place; deductibles, the sum the beneficiary pays providers out of pocket before insurance coverage kicks in; and copayments, the proportion of a given health care bill after any deductible that the individual pays. Employee cost sharing through these vehicles has increased markedly. Employers have, on average, expected their workers to share 27 percent of the costs of family health insurance; this rose to 30 percent in 2010. Driven by health care cost increases that have persistently outstripped the general inflation rate, the premium contribution of the average worker more than doubled from 2000 to 2010 (Kaiser Family Foundation 2010a, 1).[7] Those insured by their employers have also tended to pay larger deductibles and copayments. One analysis indicates that from 2001 through 2004, the out-of-pocket expense for health care grew by 16 percent, controlling for inflation. This trend significantly increased the proportion of people in high-burden families—that is, those that devoted at least 10 percent of their after-tax income to paying for premiums and health services (Banthin, Cunningham, and Bernard 2008, 189–90). Individuals who face high cost sharing more readily forgo recommended care and face serious problems paying their medical bills (Schoen et al. 2011).

Finally, thinning may occur by limiting the number of providers the insured may see. Many employers have long relied on managed care or preferred provider organizations, which strongly encourage their employees to use particular networks of providers. To contain premium increases, some carriers have moved to offer plans with much smaller networks than usual. Aetna, for instance, offered a plan with about half the doctors and two-thirds of the hospitals of its typical insurance policy (Abelson 2010).

The thinning of coverage and the declining number of employers offering health insurance have thrust Medicaid into the limelight as a possible vehicle for covering more low-income workers. At times, employees of large firms have turned to Medicaid. In early 2006, for instance, Pennsylvania officials released data showing that about one in six of Walmart's 48,000 employees in the state had signed up for Medicaid. Two other large employers in Pennsylvania, Giant Food Stores and Weis Markets, had comparable proportions of their workers in the program (Worden 2006). Data like these have prompted sporadic legislative initiatives to compel employers to expand health care coverage for workers rather than offload their costs to Medicaid. In 2006, for instance, Maryland lawmakers passed a bill aimed at Walmart that required employers with more than 10,000 workers to spend at least 8 percent of payroll on health benefits or contribute to a state fund for the uninsured. Subsequently, however, a US district court ruled that this state statute violated federal law (Appleby 2006).

Episodes such as these have generated concern that Medicaid contributes to the erosion of employer health insurance through crowding out. This displacement could occur in two ways. First, employers could decide not to offer any insurance or to provide less generous coverage because they know that at least some of their workers have access to Medicaid. Second, and independent of any employer consideration of Medicaid, workers may turn down the coverage offered by employers and sign up for Medicaid because it costs them less or covers more services. Existing data do not permit definitive calibration of the degree to which Medicaid displaces employer coverage, and estimates of the extent of crowding out vary. Some studies suggest that from 40 to 50 percent of new children enrolled in Medicaid during certain periods had access to insurance from their parents' employers.[8] But research using other methods yields much lower estimates of crowding out (Gruber 2003, 53). One overview of the evidence suggests that 15 percent of the decline in privately insured individuals can appropriately be attributed to expansions in Medicaid eligibility (Cutler and Gruber 1997). Other forces, such as rapidly rising health care costs, loom much larger than crowding out in vitiating employer-sponsored insurance.

As discussed in chapter 6, President Obama's health reform law of 2010 seeks to rejuvenate the private health insurance market by creating insurance exchanges, subsidizing the purchase of coverage, requiring people to obtain insurance, and enacting other steps. If this law survives to be fully implemented in 2014, it will help counter the forces of erosion that have afflicted this sector.

Medicare: A Bulwark under Stress

The fortunes of Medicaid also ebb and flow with policy developments related to Medicare. Being funded and directed by the federal government, Medicare as of 2010 provided benefits to some 47 million enrollees and cost the federal government about $500 billion. Approximately 85 percent of Medicare enrollees qualify by virtue of having reached the age of sixty-five. The remaining beneficiaries primarily consist of disabled individuals who have earned benefits under Social Security (e.g., through payroll taxes to the program for twenty of the past forty quarters). A small percentage of Medicare enrollees becomes eligible because they have end-stage renal disease (Kaiser Family Foundation 2010c).

At Medicare's birth in 1965, many health care reformers saw it as the steppingstone to national health insurance. Over time, they envisioned that it would cover new categories of people and extend additional benefits to its enrollees, and that Medicaid would likewise shrink in importance. But this has not happened. For instance, Medicare continues to offer limited subsidies for long-term care, either in nursing facilities or in home and community settings (Moon 2006, 184–85).[9] Instead, it relies on Medicaid to shoulder these costs.

On those occasions when federal policymakers have expanded Medicare, they have done little or nothing to divest Medicaid of its responsibilities. Consider, for example, the passage of the Medicare prescription drug bill in 2003. Before this law, state Medicaid programs had paid for prescription drugs for low-income Medicare enrollees. When federal policymakers expanded Medicare drug benefits, state officials hoped that it would reduce their Medicaid costs. But the final legislation included a provision known as the "clawback," which mandated that states rebate to the federal government a proportion of their current Medicaid drug costs for low-income Medicare enrollees. More specifically, the legislation called for states to pay 90 percent of these costs in 2006, with a gradual decline to 75 percent in 2015. The clawback increases for a state as the number of Medicare beneficiaries who also qualify for Medicaid rises (Moon 2006, 95). At least at the outset, the states were stuck with 15 percent of the tab for Medicare's new prescription drug benefit (US Department of Health and Human Services 2007b, 50).

In the years ahead the fiscal pressures on Medicare will mount. In addition to the multiple factors that generally fuel increases in health care costs, the aging of the population will expand the program's enrollees. Projections indicate that from 2000 to 2030 the population age sixty-five and over will double, from 35 million to 72 million, increasing from 12 percent to nearly 20 percent of the population. Meanwhile, the proportion of the population in the workforce paying taxes to support the program will shrink. Projections suggest that the number of workers for each older person will decline from five in 2000 to three in 2030 (US Census Bureau 2005, 12–13, 25).

Fiscal scoring devices embedded in Medicare exacerbate the sense that it may not be sustainable (Oberlander 2003, 9, 84–85). For example, Medicare relies on a trust fund derived from payroll taxes to cover hospital expenses for beneficiaries (i.e., Medicare Part A). When official reports on this fund indicate that projected expenditures will exceed the money available for benefits in the future, it triggers rhetoric in the media and elsewhere that Medicare will go "bankrupt." More recently, the Medicare Modernization Act of 2003 requires the program's trustees to issue a warning whenever the share of Medicare funded out of general revenues (as distinct from the trust fund supported by payroll taxes or by premiums) exceeds 45 percent of program spending. If this warning sounds in two consecutive years, the law requires the president and Congress to deal with the problem. Since the 2003 prescription drug program primarily relies on general revenues rather than other specially designated sources, Medicare spending seems sure to set off repeated fiscal alarms in the years ahead.[10]

Will rising expenditures and a sense of fiscal crisis unleash a brand of Medicare politics that leads to the program's retrenchment? The answer is unclear. Claims that the current program is "unsustainable" have become more numerous and pressing (e.g., Antos and Rivlin 2007). Some thinning of Medicare benefits may occur through greater cost sharing, lower provider reimbursement rates that diminish access, and other vehicles. Others have proposed to replace Medicare with a premium assistance program, which would essentially give enrollees vouchers to purchase coverage from insurance companies. For example, in 2011 and 2012, the House of Representatives passed budget resolutions that called for the eventual conversion of Medicare to a premium assistance program. On balance, however, Medicare continues to enjoy broad political support. Its enrollees constitute a growing proportion of the population and possess a strong incentive to defend it. Even if Medicare dodges appreciable retrenchment, however, fiscal pressures make it unlikely that the program will expand in ways that significantly diminish the need for Medicaid.

Medicaid: An Intergovernmental Colossus

The erosion of employer coverage and the drumbeat of budgetary pressures on Medicare heighten the significance of Medicaid as the third major pillar of America's health insurance system. Congress approved Medicaid in 1965 at the same time it enacted Medicare. Medicaid dominates the federal government's arsenal of grant programs. Intergovernmental grants are, of course, a major tool of federal policymakers and do much to define American federalism. The federal government funds nearly a thousand grant programs for states and localities,[11] and they make up more than 15 percent of the federal budget.[12] These programs target a spectrum of policy spheres—criminal justice, education, transportation, and environmental protection, to mention only a few. In historical terms, however, intergovernmental grants have increasingly become a story of health policy. At Medicaid's inception in 1965, health programs consumed 6 percent of all federal grants to state and local governments. By 2010 health accounted for 48 percent of all federal grants to these governments. Medicaid alone accounted for about 95 percent of all federal health grant dollars (OMB 2011).

The eminent political scientist Harold Lasswell (1958) described politics as those processes affecting who gets what, when, and how from the government. This perspective provides a useful lens for an initial snapshot of Medicaid during the 1993–2010 period.

The "Who" of Medicaid Politics

More than 65 million low-income people constitute the formally designated *who* of Medicaid, and they fall into four clusters.[13] Figure 1.1 gives an overview of the number of Medicaid enrollees in each cluster and the program expenditures on them. Able-bodied children make up about half of all enrollees and account for 20 percent of Medicaid expenditures. Nondisabled adults (mostly women) under the age of sixty-five years constitute about one-quarter of enrollees and absorb nearly 15 percent of Medicaid spending. Historically, most adults and children have qualified for Medicaid by virtue of being on the welfare rolls receiving cash assistance. During the past two decades, however, Medicaid has increasingly targeted low-income working families (especially their children) who lack insurance. Those with serious mental or physical disabilities under age sixty-five make up Medicaid's most expensive beneficiaries. Though they account for about 15 percent of enrollees, they garner from 40 to 45 percent of Medicaid spending. Many people with disabilities automatically qualify for the program when they become enrolled in and receive cash assistance from the federal government's Supplemental Security Income program. The members of this group rely on Medicaid not

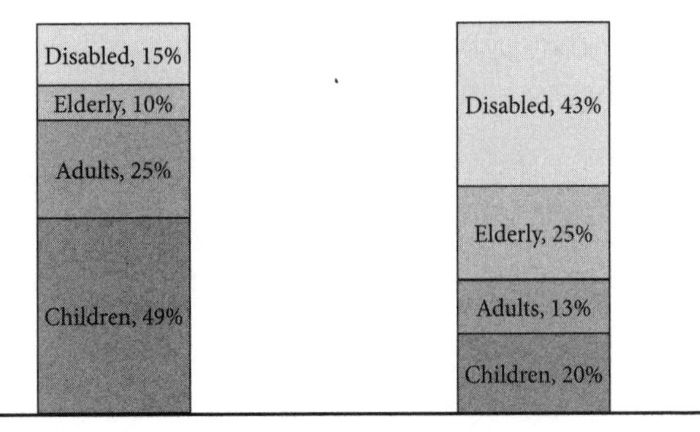

Figure 1.1 Medicaid Enrollees and Expenditures, Fiscal 2008

Source: Kaiser Slides, Henry J. Kaiser Foundation, November 2011. Reprinted with permission.

only to subsidize their medical costs but also to pay the expenses of long-term care, whether in institutions (e.g., nursing homes) or their homes and communities. The elderly constitute the smallest cluster of enrollees—10 percent of the total—but Medicaid spends one in every four program dollars on them.

Nearly all these elderly beneficiaries (along with some younger people with disabilities) are also enrolled in Medicare. Medicaid assists these "dual eligibles" by paying the substantial premiums, deductibles, and copayments that Medicare imposes. Roughly 60 percent of all Medicare recipients get help with these costs through retiree insurance provided by former employers or by purchasing coverage ("medigap" policies) from private insurance companies (Moon 2006, 6). But low-income enrollees cannot afford such supplemental coverage and seldom have retiree health benefits. Federal legislation approved in the late 1980s established the Qualified Medicare Beneficiary Program, which requires state Medicaid programs to cover the premiums and cost sharing of Medicare recipients with incomes below the poverty line. Other federal laws mandate that the states must pay part of the Medicare costs incurred by individuals with incomes up to 175 percent of the poverty line. Overall, the dual eligibles account for about 15 percent of Medicaid enrollees and 40 percent of the program's costs (Moon 2006, 6–9).

Understanding Medicaid requires an appreciation of the potential gaps between policy promise and program performance. National and state laws define eligibility for Medicaid in terms of such factors as income and assets. But the program's participation, or take-up, rates—that is, the proportion of those targeted by law for benefits who actually receive them—depend on effective administration. For instance, one study found that fewer than 65 percent of seniors living below the poverty line signed up for the Medicaid benefits to which they were entitled (Federman, Vladeck, and Siu 2005). The comparable take-up rate for seniors living at between 100 and 120 percent of the poverty line has been less than 20 percent (Moon 2006, 9). As chapter 3 shows, many children who are entitled to Medicaid have failed to get on the rolls or maintain their eligibility. These take-up issues anticipate a core theme of this book: that implementation and management matter greatly in shaping who benefits from Medicaid.

An astute assessment of who gets what from Medicaid must extend beyond the program's enrollees to the spectrum of stakeholders that derive psychic and material income from it. Of particular note, a vast complex of providers—nursing homes, hospitals, physicians, managed care organizations, home health agencies, drug companies, unions, and many more—depend substantially on the program for their income and jobs. As noted above, some employers also reap benefits when their low-income workers sign up for Medicaid.

The "What" of Medicaid Politics

At its core, Medicaid provides enrollees with a license to seek care subsidized by the national, state, and (to a limited degree) local governments. Medicaid coverage is in certain ways extraordinarily robust. The federal government requires states to cover a spectrum of traditional medical services (e.g., physician treatment, inpatient hospital care, laboratory services) and gives them the option of subsidizing many others (e.g., prescription drugs, dental care, eyeglasses). But this conventional benefit package does not begin to capture the vast and varied universe of Medicaid services—a universe that greatly exceeds that proffered by Medicare or employer health insurance.

Any effort to comprehend the "what" of Medicaid must quickly move beyond the medical model. Much of the long-term care that Medicaid subsidizes consists of personal assistance—helping enrollees cope with basic tasks of daily living, such as getting dressed and going to the toilet. (The federal government requires states to cover nursing home care and encourages home and community-based services, HCBS.) Yet even this observation only scratches the surface with respect to Medicaid services. In some states, for instance, Medicaid pays the workers who install a wheelchair ramp in a disabled person's home, the trainers who instruct family members on how to be effective caregivers, and the laborers who perform heavy household chores like washing floors and windows for homebound beneficiaries. A Medicaid fraud case in New York State in 2005 vividly illustrates the breadth of services the program subsidizes. The episode involved a Westchester County taxi company that stole more than $400,000 from Medicaid by billing hundreds of rides to doctor's offices and other medical facilities that either did not occur or were not authorized (Luo 2005).

Efforts are occasionally made to thin Medicaid's benefit package. In the early 2000s, for instance, the Bush administration signaled its willingness to support state waivers to extend insurance with limited benefits to new groups of low-income people. As discussed in chapter 5, a few states pursued this option. It also deserves note that some states cap the use of Medicaid services that are ostensibly part of the benefit package. A state might, for instance, offer a drug benefit but limit the number of prescriptions that an enrollee can obtain within a certain period.

In comparison with employer insurance and Medicare, Medicaid features far less cost sharing. This practice reflects the concern that such costs will more readily deter low-income beneficiaries from seeking needed care than would be true of more affluent individuals covered by Medicare or their employers. To be sure, Medicaid has not escaped some pressure to impose premiums, deductibles, and copayments on enrollees. The George W. Bush administration launched various initiatives in this regard, and some states obtained waivers to adopt this approach. But most states have not seriously pursued this option.

Although Medicaid is generally robust with respect to the services covered and the minimization of cost sharing, the program often emerges as strikingly thin (in some instances, emaciated) when it comes to assuring access to a broad range of providers. Medicaid payments to providers vary appreciably from state to state, but on the whole they lag behind those of Medicare and employer insurance. Payments to physicians, as distinct from institutions such as hospitals and nursing homes, are often especially meager (Thompson 1998). As a result some doctors will not see Medicaid enrollees or sharply limit the number they treat. Moreover, Medicaid enrollees at times lack knowledge about where to get care or face geographic barriers to obtaining it. Hence, the program has not fulfilled its original promise that it would assure access to "mainstream" health care.

This circumstance naturally raises the question of how much access to care Medicaid affords. Are Medicaid beneficiaries better off than those without insurance? After all, the uninsured are not shut out of the health care system entirely. Hospitals and emergency rooms typically cannot close their doors to them, and providers of all stripes deliver considerable uncompensated care—$35 billion annually, according to one estimate from the early 2000s (Institute of Medicine 2003, 5). On balance, however, a litany of studies attests to the important role of insurance in facilitating access.[14] In this vein, a careful analysis of 131 primary research studies by the Institute of Medicine (2002, 48, 57) concluded that those without insurance were less likely to receive preventive and screening services at all or on a timely basis. The analysis also found that uninsured people with chronic diseases—such as diabetes, cardiovascular disorders, and HIV infection—less readily received suitable care to manage their conditions.

Evidence indicates that the advantages of insurance apply to Medicaid coverage in particular. Medicaid enrollees have better access to care than the uninsured (e.g., Engel 2006; Federman, Vladeck, and Siu 2005; Kaiser Commission on Medicaid and the Uninsured 2009f). For example, children on Medicaid were found to receive more preventive care; they were 30 percent more likely to have ambulatory visits to a provider in a year. So, too, pregnant women on Medicaid receive more prenatal care during the first trimester than their uninsured counterparts (Lykens and Jargowsky 2002, 222; Gruber 2003, 56–57). An uncommonly rigorous study in Oregon reinforces these findings (Finkelstein et al. 2011). Researchers randomly assigned adult Medicaid applicants from the ages of nineteen to sixty-four to a cohort that became enrolled in the program and a control group that did not. One year later, the researchers found that the Medicaid enrollees had significantly greater health care utilization than the control group. Medicaid enrollees were, for instance, more likely to receive recommended preventive care—blood cholesterol checks, blood tests for diabetes, mammograms, and pap screening. Enrollees also had more outpatient visits and access to prescription drugs. Enrollees with heart disease had more hospital utilization than those in the control group.

Greater access does not, of course, automatically yield better health outcomes—less death, disease, disability, and discomfort. Robust insurance at times interacts with other factors to encourage people to seek treatment that produces no benefits and may even harm them (Mechanic 2006, 22). On balance, however, the health problems associated with a lack of insurance present more pressing issues than those flowing from "excessive coverage." The Institute of Medicine (2003, 13, 65, 107) has estimated that the uninsured adult population under age sixty-five suffers about 18,000 deaths annually that can reasonably be attributed to inadequate health insurance coverage. Overall, the uninsured face a 25 percent greater mortality risk. The institute also found that morbidity rates were greater for some 8 million uninsured individuals with chronic illnesses.

Medicaid presents a more mixed picture with respect to health outcomes. For instance, some evidence suggests that Medicaid enrollees with certain kinds of cancer fare no better than the uninsured (Institute of Medicine 2002, 53; Halpern et al. 2008). This pattern appears more pronounced among cancers where late diagnosis markedly reduces prospects for successful treatment, including melanoma and also breast, urinary, and colorectal cancers. Critics of Medicaid have also pointed to studies that suggest no better outcomes for Medicaid than the uninsured for coronary angioplasty (a procedure to open clogged heart arteries), lung transplants, and other surgical procedures (Gottlieb 2011). The quality of care extended to Medicaid recipients in nursing homes has also kindled concern. State inspectors annually visit all nursing homes that are certified to provide care to Medicare and Medicaid beneficiaries to note deficiencies that could adversely affect the health of the residents. Nursing homes with greater proportions of Medicaid enrollees (primarily larger, for-profit entities) have significantly more quality deficiencies than other nursing facilities (Amirkhanyan, Kim, and Lambright 2008, 338, 342, 347). This probably leads to poorer health outcomes for Medicaid enrollees relative to patients who pay privately.

Overall, however, the available studies indicate that those people who are enrolled in Medicaid have better health outcomes than those who are uninsured. For instance, white children on Medicaid were estimated to experience fewer acute health problems, to spend fewer sick days in bed or with restricted activity, and to have fewer absences from school due to illness (Lykens and Jargowsky 2002). Other studies credit Medicaid with reducing both infant mortality and deaths among older children (Gruber 2003, 57–58). A major problem with studies that seek to compare the health outcomes for Medicaid enrollees vis-à-vis the uninsured is that the two groups tend to differ appreciably in their characteristics. As one analysis notes, "Medicaid enrollees tend to be sicker than uninsured patients and to have lower socioeconomic status, poorer nutrition and fewer community and family resources" (Frakt et al. 2011, 364).[15] In this regard the Oregon study based on random assignment stands out because it controls more effectively than other studies for differences between Medicaid enrollees and the uninsured. This study found that after one year, Medicaid enrollees displayed significantly better outcomes on seven self-reported measures of health than the control group (Finkelstein et al. 2011, 27).

As for long-term care, any concerns about quality should not mask a more general point: Many elderly and disabled people would face dire health outcomes in the absence of the Medicaid safety net, however frayed its strands have become. For many who cannot pay, Medicaid assures access to long-term care services that would otherwise be unavailable.[16]

The "How" of Medicaid

Understanding the "how" of Medicaid is akin to mastering rocket science. The program's complexity partly derives from the degree to which it showcases federalism—a fundamental feature of the American political system. At its core Medicaid relies on a particular kind of intergovernmental grant to entice the states (not to mention the District of Columbia and US territories) to provide services to low-income people. Like other tools of government action (e.g., tax expenditures for employer insurance, Medicare payments to providers), federal grants have their own operating procedures, requirements, delivery mechanisms, and political dynamics (Salamon 2002).

Any policy tool gives some actors and perspectives more clout than others. Grants typically elevate the importance of the fifty states in determining who gets what from a program. This rings especially true in the case of Medicaid. Within the broad parameters set by federal law, each state possesses vast discretion to determine how generous its particular Medicaid program will be in terms of eligibility, payment rates to providers, services covered, and related matters. Of even greater significance, Medicaid puts states in the driver's seat concerning how much the federal government will spend on the program. Most federal grant programs are capped; that is, the federal government budgets a certain sum for states to use for some purpose beyond which it ceases to provide funding. In contrast, Medicaid, as an entitlement, requires the federal government to match at a specified rate whatever states choose to spend. So long as states do not stray from federal requirements concerning eligible populations, services covered, funding sources, and other matters, they receive a certain sum (the federal match) from the federal Treasury for every $1 they spend on Medicaid from their own sources. In the aggregate the federal government spends about $57 on Medicaid for every $43 the states commit. (The federal share will increase upon implementation of the health reform law in 2014.) The federal matching rate ranges from a low of 50 percent in more affluent states to a high of about 75 percent in poorer ones.

Grants as a policy tool also generate persistent questions about how much power the federal government should have in shaping Medicaid relative to the states. This issue constantly animates Medicaid politics. Advocates for the states push for the devolution of more authority to this level of the federal system on the grounds that it will spark innovation, galvanize policy learning, reduce red tape, and allow state policymakers to better reflect constituent preferences. States generally want the federal government to impose fewer mandates on them while funneling a steady stream of Medicaid dollars their way. Those wary of state discretion bemoan the geographic inequities in access to Medicaid services, with citizens in some states enjoying much more generous benefits. These centralizers favor more aggressive federal action to require state Medicaid programs to provide certain services to specific groups (e.g., all poor children).

In addition to the laws, regulations, and directives emanating from the federal government, the statutes produced by state legislatures shape Medicaid programs. The degree to which governors, advocacy groups, providers, public administrators, and others involve themselves in the politics of the legislative process varies greatly across the states. The ability of state legislatures to forge more precise Medicaid laws partly depends on their professionalism—for example, whether their members are paid enough to devote much time to their duties, are in session longer, and have ample staff support. But other factors also shape the degree to which state legislatures craft more detailed Medicaid statutes rather than delegate broad authority to the executive branch. For instance, the precision of Medicaid laws tends to increase if there is divided government, whereby different political parties control the governorship and at least one house of the legislature. Under this circumstance, legislators trust the executive branch less and typically do more to constrain its discretion through detailed statutes (Huber and Shipan 2003).

Even in states with more elaborate statutes, Medicaid administrators possess ample discretion to shape the program. They interpret the law, promulgate rules, issue directives, help set priorities among competing Medicaid objectives, and influence the standard operating procedures that guide the program's day-to-day conduct. They monitor operations and the task environment to detect problems and opportunities. Among the management challenges that Medicaid administrators face, three in particular stand out. First, they usually face the need to deal with multiple state agencies involved in implementing some facet of Medicaid. The federal government requires the states to designate a single state Medicaid agency to be responsible for the program. In fact, however, various state agencies often depend on Medicaid funding to serve their clienteles. In New York State, for instance, the Department of Health has primary responsibility for Medicaid. But a separate agency with its own commissioner, the Office of People with Developmental Disabilities, takes the lead in facilitating Medicaid services for many people with disabilities. Yet another New York agency focuses on Medicaid enrollees with substance abuse problems. The various state bureaucracies that participate in Medicaid often cooperate. But they also guard their turf and seek to advance the particular interests of their clients in state policy and budget processes.

Second, issues of intergovernmental management loom large for state administrators. They frequently consult, negotiate, and bargain with their federal counterparts over a range of matters. In many states they must also obtain the cooperation of county governments, which perform important functions such as the processing of applications and renewals for Medicaid applicants and enrollees. Federal and local administrators often bring priorities and commitments to the program that differ from those of state administrators. For instance, federal officials have been particularly aggressive about challenging states' use of certain funding sources for Medicaid (e.g., provider taxes and intergovernmental transfers) that they see as fiscal gimmicks designed to inflate the federal share of program costs. For their part county administrators have often been disinclined or ill equipped to conduct the kind of outreach and enrollment management that state administrators believe would assure higher take-up rates for children who are covered by Medicaid.

Third, state administrators face the challenge of overseeing complex networks of private firms and nonprofit organizations.[17] These networks primarily consist of the entities that deliver health care to Medicaid enrollees—hospitals, physicians, nursing homes, managed care organizations, home health agencies, community health centers, intermediate care facilities, and countless others. The top executives of these provider organizations along with their frontline staffs exercise discretion that significantly shapes the amount, cost, and quality of services delivered to Medicaid beneficiaries. The relationships of state bureaucracies to providers have assumed sundry forms. For much of the program's history, states served primarily as check writers paying the bills submitted to them by certified providers while monitoring for fraud and abuse. (Frequently, they contracted with private companies to conduct the routine aspects of claims processing.) As states increasingly moved to enroll Medicaid recipients in managed care plans in the 1990s, the relationship with providers changed. At this point, states faced the need to negotiate and monitor contracts with the large managed care organizations that serve Medicaid enrollees in certain geographic areas. More recently, some states, such as Florida, have used waivers to contract with private insurance companies to market various health care packages to Medicaid enrollees who can choose among competing plans. Each arrangement with providers presents state officials with a particular set of administrative challenges.

In sum, the state bureaucracies that receive grants from the federal government to operate Medicaid face formidable implementation issues. They need to be adroit at managing relationships with other state agencies, with other levels of government, and with a bevy of private businesses and nonprofits. States vary in the degree to which their administrators marshal the commitment, resources, skill, and guile to stimulate high levels of performance and accountability from these Medicaid networks. Although ostensibly quotidian, these implementation processes matter greatly. The "how" of Medicaid constantly circles back to affect the "who" and the "what" of the program.

The Concept of Program Durability

Given the fundamental features of the Medicaid program, how durable has it been during the Clinton, George W. Bush, and Obama years? To address this question, it is important at the outset to define and clarify the concept of program durability. "Durability," *Webster's* tells us, has to do with "lasting in spite of hard wear or frequent use"; it is about stability and above all "continuing to exist" (Guralnik 1982, 434). This definition provides a useful starting point. In the case of public programs, it connotes a political strength that allows them to resist retrenchment, erosion, or termination.[18] Construed broadly, the concept also characterizes the degree to which the program evinces accretion, growth, or enhanced effectiveness. Most any attempt to gauge durability is, of course, a balancing act. Over time, public programs tend to feature decline on some fronts and invigoration on others. This issue looms especially large in the case of grant programs because the federal government typically relies on the states to make critical policy and implementation decisions. At any given time, some states may be bolstering Medicaid while others are letting it erode. Beyond this the possibility exists that durability may characterize trends with respect to certain program beneficiaries (e.g., the elderly and people with disabilities) and not others (e.g., poor adults under sixty-five).

Efforts to gauge durability ideally track several markers over time. One cluster involves *formal legal specifications*. These include court rulings and changes in statutes approved by legislative bodies—decisions embedded in the high politics of policy that often attract considerable media attention. They also encompass less publicized formal decisions emanating from the executive branch of federal and state governments. These include administrative rules, state plans, waivers, executive orders, official letters, and more. Considerable research suggests the growing importance of executive action and implementation in American policy processes, in part as a response to the gridlock fueled by growing partisan polarization (e.g., Howell 2003; McCarty 2007). Some point to the rise of "executive federalism," where a "new intergovernmental dynamics" has taken hold that yield "significant changes in program management, coverage, and standards without new legislation" (Gais and Fossett 2005, 507).

In the case of Medicaid, struggles over formal legal issues frequently intersect with the program's status as an entitlement. Looking to the European model, legal scholars stress the importance of constitutional or statutory guarantees that all eligible citizens have an equal right to benefits. They view the courts as an important vehicle for upholding these rights (e.g., Jost 2003). As noted above, two key attributes define the Medicaid entitlement. First, the program features an open-ended funding commitment by the federal government, which matches at varying rates whatever the states spend. Second, Medicaid has historically been a service entitlement. Once a state determines eligibility, service packages, provider payment rates, and related design issues (subject to minimum federal requirements), it is legally obligated to offer them to all Medicaid enrollees within its borders. It cannot turn away or wait-list those who meet the eligibility criteria. From the Clinton to the Obama administrations, the politics of Medicaid as an entitlement has played out in efforts to convert the program to a block grant, in major executive branch actions (especially the growing use of waivers), and in court decisions.

Program resources constitute another important marker of durability. Expenditures loom especially large in this regard. To be sure, garnering more money does not guarantee success in building the administrative capacity (e.g., personnel, technology, facilities) needed to implement a program. Nor does it automatically augur well for program effectiveness, let alone the promotion of the general interest. Administrators can, for instance, make poor decisions that lead to high levels of waste and even corruption. But without the constant infusion of funds, prospects for program erosion increase greatly. Moreover, a program's ability to edge out its competitors in the budget process and attract even greater financial support typically speaks volumes about its political strength. At a cross-national level, studies of why welfare states persist or decline have often focused on trends in spending on social programs.[19] Analyses that target program retrenchment in the United States have done the same.[20] This analysis follows in this tradition by tracing trends in federal and state spending on Medicaid per poor person during the Clinton and George W. Bush administrations.

Program outputs and outcomes constitute the most important marker of durability. They have to do with the bottom line of social programs—the amount and quality of services (or resources) offered to some number of beneficiaries as well as the degree to which these outputs produce positive outcomes (e.g., less death, disease, disability, discomfort, and dissatisfaction in the case of health programs). Because they are typically difficult to measure, these durability indicators often suffer from neglect. In reviewing the literature on social policy retrenchment, for instance, the political scientist Jacob Hacker (2004, 243) contends than an excessive focus on "the highly visible politics of large-scale reform" has led observers to be too sanguine about the resilience of contemporary welfare states. Significant decline can occur in the absence of major legislative change through a subterranean, hidden politics involving street-level bureaucracies and everyday processes of government and administration. Hacker further notes that policy arenas "that rely substantially on public–private, or intergovernmental cooperation" are particularly susceptible to covert erosion. Hence, the politics of social policy retrenchment can be "invisible at the surface" and akin to "termites working on a foundation" (Pierson 2007, 33).

As noted above, Medicaid presents multiple concerns along these lines. For instance, convoluted enrollment procedures often prevent many qualified low-income people from joining and remaining on the Medicaid rolls. So, too, penurious payment rates at times impede access to health services for Medicaid enrollees. Throughout this book, I consider evidence related to these bottom-line indicators. In general, the available sources do not permit a highly calibrated tracking of output and outcome trends. Data are available, however, with respect to one key indicator: the number of enrollees. I use Medicaid enrollees per poor person as a pivotal measure of the program's durability.

General Pressures for Retrenchment

Observers have offered contending views of the forces shaping Medicaid's durability. Before examining these program-specific perspectives, however, two broad forces that pose a challenge not only to Medicaid but also to the broader health insurance system deserve attention. These forces fuel a sense of austerity, or scarcity, and they lead to claims that health care entitlements are unsustainable. One cluster emanates from the steady cost escalation in the health care sector; the other stems from the political creation of fiscal scarcity by policymakers.

The Relentless Rise of Health Care Costs

In simplest terms, the conviction in policy circles that the federal government's major health care entitlements cannot be sustained in their current form stems from the implications of a trend line. Unchecked, the projected growth in expenditures for Medicare and Medicaid will lead to some mix of three politically painful developments—less support for other vital government services, substantial tax increases, or excessive budget deficits and government debt.[21] To some degree the upward cost pressures on Medicaid and Medicare spring from the particular characteristics of these programs, such as their disproportionate role in assisting a growing elderly population. But to a large extent, their fiscal stress emanates from the forces driving up health care costs in all sectors of society. The medical care component of the Consumer Price Index rises year in and year out at a more rapid rate than the overall index.

Impressive advances in what medicine can do to help people stand front and center in stoking health care price increases. Research and development persistently yield new pharmaceuticals, devices, equipment, and knowledge that expand treatment options to enhance health. Nor is there an end in sight to the march of medical progress, however expensive. For instance, one assessment of eleven biomedical innovations likely to be widely adopted in the years ahead found that they would help combat cardiovascular disease, neurological disorders, cancer, and the biology of aging. Simultaneously, however, they would add appreciably to health care costs. The study concludes that "society faces its greatest spending risk not from demographic and health trends but rather from medical technologies" (Goldman et al. 2005, R-16). This realization has fanned the flames of concern about the country's "looming medical cost catastrophe" and the sustainability of current health care practices.[22]

Cost pressures also spring from inefficiency and waste in the American health care system. Many medical treatments do little or nothing to foster better health outcomes and all too frequently harm patients.[23] Policy analysts frequently cite the work of John Wennberg of Dartmouth Medical School in emphasizing that more care does not automatically equal better health. Working with Medicare data, Wennberg found great geographic variation across the country in the way that providers treat certain diseases. Of particular importance, higher-cost, intensive-service areas did not yield better health outcomes than lower-cost, less-intensive ones (GAO 2004c, 10).[24] Other evidence documents that much surgery is "needlessly extensive and commonly ineffective" (Mechanic 2006, 25).

Concerns about waste have helped kindle interest in "getting to no" in the health care system (Feder and Moran 2007, 186). Optimally, this involves developing the institutions and evidence that can reduce the many practices that do little or nothing to foster health. Proponents who seek to make medicine more evidence-based aptly note that many widely used treatments do not rest on data derived from randomized clinical trials or other sophisticated studies. They call for a great expansion in research to yield nuanced and credible practice guidelines that will foster cost-effective medical treatment. Conducting such research will be far from simple, however. Researchers will need to take into account the possibility that the benefits of a treatment may vary depending on the age, race, and gender of patients. The efficacy of an intervention may also depend on whether the patient has one health problem or multiple chronic conditions or ailments (Mechanic 2006, 118–19).

In addition to more research, reformers have endorsed the establishment of government institutions to promote practice guidelines. In this vein a special forum of health care experts and stakeholders convened by the GAO (2004a, 19) called for "an authoritative body of experts to develop and promulgate standards of practice. These standards, based on science and expert consensus, would guide clinical decision making and payers' determination about whether services claimed were medically necessary." But it will be extremely difficult to establish an institution with sufficient legitimacy and clout to play this role. Consider, for instance, the political fortunes of the federal Agency for Health Care Policy and Research in the early 1990s, when it issued evidence-based guidelines that pointed to the advantages of nonsurgical, less expensive treatments for people with acute back pain. In response, large numbers of orthopedic surgeons banded together to attack the agency as inept and biased. They vigorously lobbied Congress to cut the agency's budget. Sensing the political peril prompted by their efforts to fight waste, agency officials abandoned their attempts to develop practice guidelines (Mechanic 2006, 19–20). Subsequently, the Obama administration secured an appropriation for "comparative effectiveness" research to identify the most helpful medical approaches, only to see Republicans in Congress fight to defund it.

In sum, efforts to foster more cost-effective health care face formidable obstacles. To some degree, these difficulties emanate from the reluctance of the American public to accept limits on services they want whether imposed by a managed care organization or some other source. Opposition also comes from providers who value their professional autonomy and often see practice guidelines as "cookbook" medicine that serve patients poorly. And, of course, the economic interests at stake in the health care sector fuel resistance to paring waste. The twentieth-century reformer Upton Sinclair (1994, 109) once observed that "it is difficult to get a man to understand something, when his salary depends upon his not understanding it." In the health care system, one person's waste is another person's income. The surgeries that many experts deem unnecessary provide a livelihood for the doctors who perform them. The generic, less expensive drugs that many doctors recommend have less appeal to pharmaceutical companies than the profits obtained from marketing new, more expensive brands, even when they provide little additional health benefit. Ultimately, the institutional incapacity to restrict wasteful practices in the health care system combines with the propensity of science to yield new, valuable, and expensive treatments to boost health care costs. Although Medicaid has done more than most private insurance companies to contain costs, the program cannot escape the pressures for retrenchment that arise from the price escalation embedded in the broader health economy.

The Political Creation of Scarcity

Rising health care costs, the erosion of employer health insurance, shifting demographics, economic downturns, and related forces all fuel Medicaid's fiscal stress. But this stress also springs from major policy developments that ostensibly have nothing to do with health care. Since the 1980s a central strategic insight of the Republican Party has been to "starve the beast" (government) by sponsoring tax cuts that fuel deficits and debt. In justifying massive tax reductions in 1981, President Ronald Reagan captured the spirit of this strategy when he observed: "We can lecture our children about extravagance until we run out of voice and breath. Or we can cure their extravagance simply by reducing their allowance" (Brownlee 2004, 149). Budget deficits mounted rapidly during the Reagan years. Various tax increases, especially during the first year of the Clinton administration, ultimately helped restore a balanced budget. But the Clinton tax package was politically unpopular over the short term and contributed to the Republican takeover of Congress in 1995. In the eyes of many Republican leaders, this signaled that tax cuts with little attention to their revenue implications could be a successful strategy over time to shrink government.

President George W. Bush pushed the starve-the-beast strategy to new heights. Quoting his grandmother, he noted: "I've learned if you leave cookies out on a plate, they always get eaten" (Brownlee 2004, 221). Inheriting a $236 billion budget surplus from the Clinton administration, Bush persuaded Congress to approve a series of tax cuts that promised to drain the federal coffers of more than $4 trillion in revenues through 2013 (Hacker and Pierson 2007, 257). By fiscal 2008 the Clinton surplus had been transformed into an estimated deficit of $410 billion. The public debt had nearly doubled, growing from $5.6 trillion in 2000 to $9.7 trillion in 2008, from 58 percent of the gross domestic product (GDP) to an estimated 68 percent (OMB 2008, 26–27, 127–28). The global financial and economic crisis of 2008–9 and the resulting government expenditures to mitigate its effects increased the flow of red ink. Annual deficits rose to much more than $1 trillion.

Efforts to foster a climate of fiscal austerity in the states have also borne fruit. State governments have long had less fiscal flexibility than the federal government because nearly all of them face legal requirements to balance their budgets. Drawing primarily on the initiative and referendum, the antitax movement has sought to handcuff the states still further.[25] As the twenty-first century dawned, more than half the states had added tax or expenditure limitations to their constitutions or statutes. These provisions come in many guises. Some states impose strict caps on how much their expenditures can increase in a year. Other states require supermajorities in the legislature to approve any tax increases to fund state programs. Still other states require voters to approve any tax hikes that make it through the legislature and get signed by the governor. Whatever their precise manifestation, these restrictions have one thing in common: They make it harder for states to tap their wealth to pay for public programs like Medicaid.

The success of antitax forces at the state and federal levels has compounded the challenges of sustaining let alone enhancing Medicaid. They legitimate efforts to curb the program. To be sure, federal policymakers more than their state counterparts can dodge hard political choices by running deficits year after year. But at some point, tolerance for this approach will ebb. Those buying the nation's debt may become squeamish and trigger a sell-off of bonds with interest rates sharply rising. Key opinion leaders, policymakers, and members of the politically engaged public may increasingly stress the inequity of passing on costs to future generations and instead demand that the government put its fiscal house in order. To the degree that paring the debt gains a prominent position on the congressional agenda, the conservative bet that key policymakers will prefer the pain of cutting social programs to the pain incurred by raising taxes to support them will be put to the test (Hacker and Pierson 2007, 275–76). Medicaid will be at the center of this struggle, as the political developments in 2011 (discussed in chapter 7) vividly illustrate.

Contending Perspectives on Medicaid Durability

Surging health care costs and the success of the antitax movement have created a climate of austerity that makes health care programs in general vulnerable to retrenchment. Beyond these general forces, existing analyses point to factors about Medicaid in particular that could affect its political resilience. In this vein, pessimists zero in on at least three factors that heighten Medicaid's vulnerability: means-testing rather than universalism, declining trust in government, and interstate economic competition.

Advocates for universal entitlements, such as Medicare and Social Security, have taken a dim view of means-tested programs. As one observer underscores, "a program for the poor will always be politically vulnerable, underfunded and generally inadequate" (Jost 2003, 178). Low-income beneficiaries presumably lack the political clout to persuade policymakers to sustain programs like Medicaid. In contrast, universal entitlements provide benefits to people from all income strata and can count on broad, higher-status constituencies to defend them. In keeping with this theme, Medicaid has often seemed to play second fiddle to Medicare. The program usually pays health care providers at lower rates than Medicare, which results in Medicaid enrollees typically having less access to high-quality care than Medicare beneficiaries.

Others suggest that declining trust in government compounds the problem of programs for poor people. Political scientists have documented the growing tendency for people to see the federal government as looking out for special interests rather than people like themselves; Americans have also become more pessimistic about the competence of government to implement programs efficiently and effectively (e.g., Hetherington 2005). Diminished trust has especially undercut public support for programs that redistribute benefits from the better-off to the poor or otherwise call for people to sacrifice some benefit they currently enjoy. Evidence indicates that this lack of trust, rather than any increase in political conservatism, helped defeat President Clinton's comprehensive health reform proposal in 1994 and abetted the Republican takeover of Congress in 1995 (Hetherington 2005, 120–37). With all else remaining equal, limited trust makes Medicaid more vulnerable to cuts based on allegations that it features high levels of "fraud, waste, and abuse." The trust deficit heightens prospects for retrenchment to the degree that people see Medicaid as a redistributive vehicle for "welfare medicine."

A constraining model of federalism rooted in interstate economic competition could also threaten Medicaid's durability. For much longer than half a century, certain economists (including the seminal conservative thinker Friedrich von Hayek) have seen this competition as a check on government growth—as a barrier to the emergence of a "Leviathan state." In this view, states compete with one another to keep their tax burdens low in order to retain and attract businesses and the affluent. States that fail to keep the lid on taxes run the risk that these firms and individuals will vote with their feet by moving to states with lower taxes. This competition has prompted the prediction that countries featuring fiscal decentralization via federalism will, all else being equal, spend less on public services as a portion of their GDP than more unitary governments such as Great Britain. The dynamic appears more likely to apply when, as in the United States, Canada, and Switzerland, states have considerable autonomy over tax policy and do not depend heavily on the central government for revenues (Rodden 2003). State fears of becoming a welfare magnet also underpin this constraining model of interstate competition. This view holds that low-income citizens will gravitate toward states that offer more generous benefits. Hence states with more bountiful redistributive programs allegedly encourage needy people within their borders to remain while attracting low-income migrants from other states (e.g., Peterson and Rom 1990; Smith 2006).[26] Quite apart from whether people in fact vote with their feet in this way, state policymakers may perceive that magnet effects exist and respond by limiting Medicaid benefits.

Although these and related factors engender pessimism about Medicaid's durability, other analyses point in a more sanguine direction. This literature identifies four primary and interrelated factors that contribute to Medicaid's political resilience: a fragmented political system dependent on supermajorities, the middle-class nature of some Medicaid benefits, Medicaid's phalanx of supporting constituencies, and the dynamics of catalytic federalism.

Comparative analyses of the United States and Europe stress that the concentration of political authority, as in Great Britain, is a significant asset for those seeking major policy change (Pierson 2001). In contrast, the multiple veto points built into the American political system constitute a formidable obstacle course for those seeking to expand the federal government's role in providing health insurance. But this highly dispersed authority structure also serves as a brake on policy retrenchment. The need for legislation to obtain the approval of two houses of Congress and the president affords its opponents ample opportunities to block passage. The filibuster and other Senate practices further necessitate that retrenchment win the approval of supermajorities. The tendency of American elections to produce divided government where different parties control the various branches of government adds to the friction that reinforces the status quo. The dramatic rise in asymmetric partisan polarization among policy elites and the politically engaged during the past three decades has thrown additional sand into the gears of government. The ideological distance between Republican and Democratic representatives has increased, with the former moving sharply to the right and the latter trending somewhat less markedly to the left (Abramowitz 2010; Hacker and Pierson 2007, 264). Especially under conditions of divided government, this development makes it harder to forge compromise and assemble coalitions to pare the program.

Others stress that Medicaid is not just a program for the poor but also one for the middle class. The program's role in providing long-term care for the elderly has attracted particular attention. Focusing on nursing home benefits, for instance, one study notes that whereas Medicaid was "originally portrayed as a health care program of last resort for the marginalized," it has increasingly been framed "as a core entitlement for the mainstream aged" (Grogan and Patashnik 2003, 58; see also Grogan 2008). In this vein, the program provides health care security for middle-class families. Many elderly people start out paying for care in a nursing home but then deplete their assets and become eligible for Medicaid. In addition, the program protects the families of those in nursing homes from fiscal strain by excluding certain income and assets of spouses from consideration in eligibility decisions. Observers also note Medicaid's move toward the middle class on another front. In the wake of the welfare reform act of 1996, the emergence of the Children's Health Insurance Program in 1997, and related developments, Medicaid increasingly covered children and parents in working families with incomes well above the poverty line. This reach to the middle class enhances the public image of Medicaid and builds a supportive constituency with far more political assets than the welfare poor (Grogan 2008; Olson 2010).

Students of Medicaid have also pointed to the importance of providers in buttressing the program. As one analysis notes, "Medicaid's constituency has grown well beyond the nation's welfare poor." It includes a "sizable corps of physicians, hospitals, community health centers and public clinics," as well as nursing homes, home health care agencies, and managed care organizations, all of which have "tangible interests not only in what Medicaid pays but also in whom it covers" (Brown and Sparer 2003, 41–42). Hence, Medicaid's fortunes have become intertwined with political science theories that underscore the importance of supportive interest groups in shaping a program's evolution and survival. To a greater degree than many other redistributive programs, Medicaid can count on a coalition of politically potent providers to defend it.

Other analysts turn to "catalytic federalism" as the provenance for Medicaid's durability. This view directly challenges the constraining model of federalism focused on interstate competition for business and the affluent. Instead, it sees federalism as a boon to program growth as national and state officials "prompt and prod each other toward additional coverage expansions" (Sparer, France, and Clinton 2011, 41). The dynamics of fiscal federalism figure prominently in this model. Historically, the federal government has absorbed about 57 percent of the program's costs and states have paid the rest. This means that both levels of government leverage additional dollars when they expand the program. So, too, federal policymakers can support program expansions while shifting implementation burdens to the states. Meanwhile, Medicaid's retrenchment becomes more painful because states lose federal dollars when they cut. In these ways Medicaid provides ample opportunities for elected policymakers at both the national and state levels to claim political credit for expanding or protecting Medicaid beneficiaries without having to absorb the full costs of their choices (Brown and Sparer 2003, 42).

In general, the forces identified as bolstering Medicaid's durability point to the overall pertinence of theories of path dependence or "institutional stickiness" (Pierson 2004). In this view the initial policy framework and institutional design for a program like Medicaid spawn a set of networks and interests that benefit from the initiative and come to defend it. Positive feedback occurs. The original design tends to get locked in. Incremental change tends to prevail unless highly unusual political circumstances combine to open a policy window for major program transformation.

In assaying policy developments since 1993, this book considers the explanatory relevance of the propositions embedded in the contending perspectives on Medicaid's durability. Drawing on a qualitative case methodology, I cannot subject the propositions to rigorous empirical testing. But the evidence in this volume does permit informed assessment of their applicability. As will become apparent, my research reinforces and extends certain propositions while calling others into question. This analysis also suggests the need to round up other explanatory suspects to get to the bottom of the Medicaid puzzle. In the concluding chapter, I organize this exploration of explanatory factors around the competing constraining and catalytic models of federalism discussed above.

Focus, Methods, and Contribution

Four principal factors commend the 1993–2010 period as a springboard for assessing the forces shaping Medicaid's durability. First, the period features a range of political alignments at the national level—Democratic Party control of Congress and the presidency (1993–94, 2009–10), Republican control (2003–6), divided government with a Democratic president (1995–2000), and divided government with a Republican president (2001–2, 2007–8). Hence, Medicaid's fortunes can be assessed in different partisan and ideological contexts. It deserves note in this regard that 2003–6 was the only period since Medicaid's enactment in 1965 when the Republicans dominated both houses of Congress and the presidency. A focus on partisan dominance is especially important in light of the well-documented trend toward asymmetric partisan polarization. The ideological gap between Democrats and Republicans has grown both among policy elites and the politically engaged. This gap extends to health policy, where party affiliation predicts much about attitudes.

Second, the period encompasses both failed and successful legislative initiatives to modify Medicaid. Significant efforts to convert Medicaid into a block grant occurred in 1995 and 2003. The political dynamics surrounding these unsuccessful attempts at retrenchment shine bright light on Medicaid's durability. This period also featured an epic, albeit politically fragile, breakthrough—the passage of the Patient Protection and Affordable Care Act (also known as the Affordable Care Act, ACA) in 2010. This new law promised to extend health insurance to more than 30 million uninsured Americans. About half of them would gain this benefit via Medicaid. This major expansion of Medicaid under the banner of comprehensive health reform represents a remarkable reversal of fortune for the program. In the struggle for national health insurance since 1965, most reformers thought Medicaid would fade away as the country adopted national health insurance quite possibly modeled on Medicare. The factors that confounded these expectations and led to a larger role for Medicaid in the American health insurance system beg for attention.

Third, the period featured a remarkable surge in executive branch action to transform Medicaid, often with minimal legislative involvement. The Clinton and George W. Bush years featured the unprecedented use of waivers—a congressional delegation of authority to the executive branch to permit selective deviations from the law. Never in Medicaid's history had this policy tool been so prominent in the federal government's dealings with the states. In a significant departure from the past, states requested and received hundreds of waivers to reinvent their Medicaid programs. The proliferation of waivers raises myriad issues for Medicaid's durability. Is this development a manifestation of the hidden politics of policy retrenchment that some scholars have highlighted? Or, on balance, have waivers strengthened Medicaid?

Fourth, the period had years of both economic growth and downturn. Throughout much of the 1990s and 2000s, federal and state treasuries benefited from the revenues that a robust economy created. But the period also featured a mild economic slump in the early 2000s and the worst recession since the Great Depression toward the end of the decade. The ebbs and flows of the economy do not distinguish the 1993–2010 period from earlier Medicaid contexts. But it helps assure that the book's timeline permits consideration of Medicaid's fortunes in good times and bad.

This book relies primarily on a qualitative, case study methodology to tell the story of Medicaid's evolution during the Clinton, Bush, and early Obama years. In doing so, it taps various sources of evidence. A vast scholarly and professional literature on Medicaid, including works persistently produced by think tanks, provides the provenance for considerable insight. So does archival evidence on the program, such as executive branch documents, statutes, regulations, legislative hearings, waiver proposals, government Web pages, documents from private stakeholders (e.g., the National Governors Association), and the like. Major newspapers were also systematically scanned.[27] To attain trend data on Medicaid expenditures and enrollees that would facilitate state comparisons, I turned to the Kaiser Commission on Medicaid and the Uninsured.[28] The commission does a superb job in scrubbing the administrative data that states submit to the federal government. Its staff and consultants ferret out errors and inconsistencies in these data sets—no small task.

Finally, this study benefited from countless exchanges with Medicaid stakeholders. Some of these were informal. During the close to twenty years I lived in Albany, I came in contact with many people who had firsthand knowledge of New York State's capacious Medicaid program.[29] More recently, I became a resident of New Jersey, where I joined the Rutgers Center for State Health Policy. Here, too, contacts with officials, interest group advocates, and researchers sensitized me to the Medicaid issues in that state. Other contacts were more formal. This study draws on fifty-three open-ended, semistructured interviews with both public and private stakeholders in the Medicaid policy arena at the federal and state levels. I conducted more than half the interviews in site visits to three states—Florida, Minnesota, and Texas.[30]

Ultimately, this book aspires to make two contributions. For those interested in health care policy, it provides an overview of the growing role that Medicaid has played in America's health insurance system during the past two decades. It also anticipates future challenges that the program will face. This volume also speaks more generally to students of public policy, especially those interested in the sustainability of public programs or the welfare state more broadly. Scholars have stressed that the statutory enactment of a program or significant policy change represents only the first step in an ongoing political struggle. For four decades research on implementation has underscored the ways in which policy evolves after a bill becomes law (e.g., Pressman and Wildavsky 1973). So, too, studies of social policy and American political development have probed the conditions under which programs fuel policy feedback that leads them to thrive or erode (e.g., Hacker 2004). More recently, work has focused on the sustainability of "general interest" reforms comparing federal initiatives that endured with others that disappeared or deteriorated (Patashnik 2008). Those who have plumbed the forces that strengthen or vitiate programs over time have generated valuable insights and propositions.

But important research frontiers remain. For one thing, theory building would benefit from more explicit attention to how to conceptualize and measure the dependent variable over time—whether the program's "durability," "sustainability," or some other measure of vitality. For another, issues of durability related to federalism warrant greater attention. Intergovernmental grants like Medicaid not only necessitate careful attention to the commitment and capacity of the federal government in carrying out the program but also the fifty states. So, too, the political environments of government in multiple settings need to be probed. This study takes a step toward addressing these issues in the case of Medicaid.

Since my work on this volume commenced, three books have appeared that focus comprehensively on Medicaid. David Smith and Judith Moore (2008) have written a valuable history of Medicaid politics and policy at the national level from 1965 to 2007. So, too, Thomas Grannemann and Mark Pauly (2010) have crafted an insightful policy analysis of Medicaid. Much less focused on politics and policy evolution than this book, the authors deftly mine existing data on state variations in Medicaid and conceptualize the role the program can constructively play in broader health reform. The book offers a particularly compelling analysis of issues related to provider payment—long the Achilles' heel of Medicaid. Finally, Laura Katz Olson (2010) has assessed the politics of Medicaid, presenting much useful information about the program since its inception in 1965. Olson directs the lion's share of her attention to Medicaid's deficiencies in order to buttress her core theme that the program should be replaced with a single-payer, universal plan.

Although these volumes provide a useful knowledge base, this book goes beyond (or at least differs from) them in several ways. For instance, all three books were written before the big bang of federal health reform in 2010 and the unprecedented Medicaid expansion it mandated. Further, none of them takes the conceptual and empirical issue of trends in Medicaid durability during a defined period as its core organizing theme. This book also differs in the additional attention it devotes to waivers as a policy tool shaping the evolution of Medicaid. Moreover, my findings and normative assessments at times differ from those given in these volumes.[31] In sum, though my book covers some of the same terrain, it presents new perspectives and fresh evidence about Medicaid.

Plan of the Book

In exploring issues of Medicaid durability, this book proceeds as follows. Chapter 2 probes the failed efforts of House Speaker Newt Gingrich and President George W. Bush to retrench Medicaid by converting it from an entitlement to a block grant. It plumbs the political dynamics that led the federal government to increase its share of program costs during hard economic times. Having probed developments that saved Medicaid from significant erosion, the chapter then provides an overview of trends in Medicaid expenditures and enrollments during the Clinton and George W. Bush years. The patterns of growth embedded in these data provide a valuable backdrop for the examination of specific policy developments in subsequent chapters.

Chapter 3 assays the implications of two key developments with implications for Medicaid's durability: the passage of the welfare reform act in 1996, and the quest to expand coverage to children. Both helped distance Medicaid from its public image as "welfare medicine." The chapter also illuminates how relatively opaque implementation challenges can undercut policy promises of program growth. Chapter 4 shifts the spotlight to another major cluster of Medicaid enrollees: the elderly and people with disabilities. Here the story of Medicaid's durability intertwines with the quest to rebalance long-term care away from institutions toward home- and community-based services (HCBS). This initiative rested heavily on states' use of program waivers authorized under Section 1915c of the Social Security Act. This development affords an opportunity to address the more general question of whether waivers have fortified or vitiated Medicaid. Chapter 5 continues to explore this question by focusing on the outpouring of major demonstration waivers that many states used to reinvent their Medicaid programs during the 1990s and 2000s.

Chapter 6 then traces Medicaid's emergence as a key component of comprehensive health reform in 2010. The chapter links this development to the waiver processes that led the Massachusetts plan to become a template for national reform. It assays the bitter partisan debate over Medicaid's inclusion in the ACA, the implementation challenges the new law poses, and Republican efforts to repeal it. In conclusion, chapter 7 provides a summary assessment of the durability that Medicaid achieved from 1993 through 2010 and links the findings to contending models of federalism. More specifically, it points to six factors that help account for trends in Medicaid's durability during this period. The chapter then returns to the question of whether a climate of austerity brought on by rising health care costs and intensified political efforts to create scarcity for government will undermine Medicaid.

Notes

1. All the quotations here are from the US House of Representatives, Committee on the Budget (2011, 13, 99–100, 192).

2. These data are from the US Census Bureau (2010, 77). Before 1994 the bureau did not break out "private health insurance" in terms of whether it was provided by employers or purchased by individuals.

3. This tax break does not extend to people who buy individual health insurance policies on their own.

4. Larger employers with at least two hundred workers held steady with a 99 percent offer rate, but a growing proportion of smaller firms chose not to provide insurance. In 2010, however, a substantial increase in the offer rate among small firms with three to nine employees occurred. This caused the overall offer rate to rebound to 69 percent of all firms. The authors of the report, however, express skepticism about this uptick. They suggest that "non-offering firms were more likely to fail during the past year, and the attrition of non-offering firms led to a higher offer rate among surviving firms" (Kaiser Family Foundation 2010a, 4).

5. This is from GAO (2007b, 37). Firms with a high proportion of contract employees are also less likely to offer any health insurance to their workers. Firms where 35 percent of employees or more are part time have offer rates of 45 percent; in contrast, firms with fewer than 35 percent have rates of 67 percent. So, too, businesses employing more low-wage workers are less inclined to offer insurance to employees (Kaiser Family Foundation 2008, 36).

6. This is from US Census Bureau (2011). These numbers are supposed to represent the percentage of Americans who were without coverage for the entire year. In contrast, point-in-time estimates focus on those who lack health insurance at the moment they are interviewed (who may be temporarily without coverage). Some disagreement exists over the degree to which the Census Bureau is really presenting point-in-time numbers. For a general discussion of the validity of the Census Bureau figures, see CBO (2003).

7. In 2008 the average annual premium for employer-based family coverage was $12,680, more than double the cost of such a policy in 1999 (Kaiser Family Foundation 2008, 25, 32).

8. See, e.g., Blumberg, Dubay, Norton (2000); LoSasso and Buchmueller (2004).

9. E.g., Medicare generally limits rehabilitation in skilled nursing facilities to those who have been in a hospital for at least 3 days. This treatment is limited to 100 days per spell of illness.

10. See Moon (2006, 106). In 2008 the Medicare trustees reported for a third year in a row that Medicare expenditures from the general fund would exceed 45 percent. In response, the Bush administration submitted the Medicare Funding Warning Response Act of 2008, which called for a pay-for-performance system, among other things.

11. Estimates of the number of grant programs vary and depend on various definitions and assumptions; this figure comes from Dilger (2011, 6–7).

12. This is from Thompson (2008, S15). The stimulus package passed by Congress in 2009 at least temporarily elevated this proportion.

13. These estimates come from data furnished by the Kaiser Commission on Medicaid and the Uninsured.

14. Available studies typically link broad categories of insurance (e.g., employer, Medicare, Medicaid) to access and health outcomes. They seldom measure how robust the insur-

ance coverage is. If employer insurance thins in the coming years, with more restrictions on the type and amount of services covered and greater cost sharing for employees, the issue of "underinsurance" as distinct from "no insurance" becomes more salient (Blewett, Ward, and Beebe 2006). The strength of the correlations between insurance coverage treated as a dichotomous variable and both access to services and health outcomes could decline.

15. In noting this issue I do not mean to deny the possible validity of studies that point to Medicaid's limited benefits for acute maladies such as cancer or heart disease. In general, Medicaid does better at assuring access to primary as distinct from specialty care.

16. I am unaware of any study that systematically makes this comparison. In some cases the absence of Medicaid coverage might galvanize families or other social networks to provide such care. But for more acutely disabled and isolated individuals, Medicaid coverage seems sure to have benefits relative to being uninsured.

17. These networks also include some government providers, such as public hospitals and schools.

18. Students of public policy have devoted some attention to a theory of program termination. For a review of this literature, see Geva-May (2004). The general thrust of this research is that termination seldom occurs. Scholars seek to explain the relatively few cases where it has. This literature has some relevance for this book, in that it suggests forces that work to preserve Medicaid. But a focus on durability that incorporates a concern with "retrenchment" and "erosion" provides a better underpinning for the Medicaid story. No proposal to terminate Medicaid received serious consideration by policymakers during the period of this study. However, many national and state policymakers placed proposals to retrench the program on the policy agenda and occasionally prevailed. Moreover, as the implementation literature emphasizes, Medicaid, like other programs, faces the constant threat of drift and erosion.

19. E.g., Brooks and Manza (2006) track trends in such spending for cash benefits and services as a proportion of GDP in sixteen industrial democracies.

20. E.g., Gais (2009) assays retrenchment by tracking the decline in state and social welfare spending per poor person.

21. See Antos and Rivlin (2007). In contrast, Kronick and Rousseau (2007) argue that government revenues will grow enough to sustain Medicaid at current levels over the next forty years without great stress. From a political perspective, however, the key issue is whether major stakeholders perceive the growth in health care expenditures and entitlements to be unsustainable.

22. This quoted phrase comes from the title of a conference sponsored by the Brookings Institution in March 2008, www.brookings.edu/events/2008/0307-medicalcost.aspx.

23. Among other things, studies have documented substantial rates of medical error leading to injury and death (Mechanic 2006, 116).

24. Disagreement flourishes as to how much extra cost "excess services" generate. E.g., White (2011) assigns more importance to price as a driver of cost escalation relative to service intensity.

25. Matsusaka (2004) finds that, all else remaining equal, states with the initiative and referendum spend and tax less than states without these vehicles for voter participation.

26. More recently, concern has grown in some states that illegal immigrants from Latin America may deliberately move to their jurisdictions to seek health care, education, and other services.

27. These included the *New York Times*, the *Wall Street Journal*, and the *Washington Post.*

28. I am especially indebted to David Rousseau of the Kaiser Commission on Medicaid and the Uninsured, who graciously provided these data.

29. I especially benefited from the conferences, meetings, and projects of the Nelson A. Rockefeller Institute of Government in Albany.

30. I chose Minnesota because it has a reputation for good government and an innovative, progressive Medicaid program. I visited Florida and Texas because they lagged behind other states on my two main measures of Medicaid effort and because they have such large populations of uninsured residents. Florida had also garnered considerable attention because Governor Jeb Bush (R) had proposed a demonstration waiver. The interviews were confidential and typically lasted an hour. I conducted the great majority of them in person and the rest on the telephone.

31. For example, Olson (2010, 152) tends to be more critical of the use of waivers to foster home and community-based services than I am. She also assigns greater explanatory significance to a "Medicaid medical industrial complex" than this study does (p. 182).

CHAPTER TWO

Dodging the Block Grant Bullet and Other Signs of Resilience

This chapter follows three significant developments for Medicaid's durability in the 1993–2010 period. All three testify to the program's political resilience. The first is the premise that one can learn much about the sources of a program's strength by assessing failed legislative efforts at retrenchment. In this regard I focus on the abortive attempts to convert Medicaid from an entitlement to a block grant in 1995 and 2003. Both initiatives—one led by the House of Representatives' majority leader, Newt Gingrich, in concert with Republican governors; and the other led by the George W. Bush administration, working with Governor Jeb Bush (R) of Florida—constituted serious (albeit quite different) efforts to retrench Medicaid.

Second, the willingness of federal policymakers to rescue Medicaid during difficult financial times receives attention. This development is less important than Medicaid's ability to evade conversion to a block grant. But it traces incremental action to deal with Medicaid's structural weakness as a countercyclical program. Unlike the federal government, states are required to balance their budgets. This places them in a quandary when recessions occur and unemployment rates rise. Just at the time when more people need Medicaid and can qualify for it, falling tax revenues mean that states can less easily serve them. This has prompted Medicaid stakeholders to wage a political fight for an enhanced federal contribution during tough economic times. Three times since 1992—once in 2003 over the opposition of President Bush, and then again in 2009 and 2010, with President Obama's support—Congress responded to economic downturns by temporarily increasing the federal government's share of Medicaid costs. The politics that prompted Congress to throw the states a life preserver (an exercise in what I call "compensatory federalism") casts light on the program's durability.

Third, the expenditure and enrollment data for Medicaid for the period from 1993 to 2008 come under the microscope. Given that the two efforts to convert Medicaid into a block grant failed, how much did the program grow? Did it gain ground in all fifty states, or did its fortunes vary sharply from one state to the next? In general, the data trends reinforce the impression of Medicaid's expansion and strength during the Clinton and Bush years.

Clinton Stymies a Block Grant

During the Clinton and Bush years, Medicaid witnessed two major trials by fire in the legislative arena. Both threatened to vitiate Medicaid's status as a financial entitlement to the states and as a program guaranteeing benefits to enrollees. The most direct challenge to Medicaid occurred after the Republicans' stunning congressional triumph in the 1994 election. When the dust cleared in early November, the Republicans controlled both houses of Congress for the first time since 1954. They held 230 seats in the House of Representatives and, with the switch of 2 Democrats to the Republicans, 52 in the Senate. The party had also scored significant gains at the state level. When Congress convened in January 1995, Republicans controlled 30 governorships; by 1996 this figure had edged upward to 31. The shock and awe of the Republican victory fueled demoralization and uncertainty among Democrats. The historian David Smith (2002, 40) has noted that in the face of the Republican triumph and subsequent policy offensive, "Democrats were uncertain whether to fight, strike a deal, or run for cover." Although a Democrat continued in the White House, it was far from certain that he would be willing and able to shield Medicaid from significant retrenchment.

To probe the implications of the 1995–96 period for Medicaid's durability, I assay key developments through three phases. The first featured an alliance between the Republican governors and House speaker Newt Gingrich that led to congressional approval of a Medicaid block grant in November 1995. The second ran from mid-November to early January, when the Republicans shut down the government in an effort to compel the president to accept significant Medicaid retrenchment. The third, starting in January 1996, amounted to a last ditch effort by the National Governors Association (NGA) to rescue Medicaid "reform" from the ashes.

Passage: Republican Governors and Speaker Gingrich

Under the leadership of the House of Representatives' speaker, Newt Gingrich, the Republicans in Congress devoted most of their first one hundred days to launching key provisions of their Contract with America. During the election, Gingrich had touted this contract as a kind of platform that Republicans would pursue once they assumed office. Medicaid was not mentioned in the document. Nor is there evidence that Gingrich had specific plans for the program. The contract had, however, endorsed significant tax cuts and a balanced budget. This meant that the Republicans would need to seek considerable savings in federal entitlement programs.

Although Medicaid was not Gingrich's top priority, it was much on the minds of key Republican governors. They felt frustrated with federal constraints on their ability to shape the program and its relentless pressure on their budgets. Soon after the election, John Engler of Michigan, Tommy Thompson of Wisconsin, and several other governors urged Gingrich and the Senate majority leader, Robert Dole of Kansas, to convert both the welfare and Medicaid entitlements to block grants. Gingrich liked the idea and promptly reached out to the governors. By late January 1995 a group of ten Republican governors (including Engler and Thompson) had formed to work with two key committee chairs in the Senate and two in the House to develop plans for restructuring Medicaid (Smith 2002, 47, 67). Working under the banner of a Republican Governors' Association Task Force on Medicaid, Governor Engler announced in March 1995 that Gingrich had assured him the program would be transformed into a block grant. An influential Senate Republican, Bob Packwood of Oregon, also indicated that he had an "open mind" on the conversion (Havemann 1995b).

The involvement of Republican governors would be a signature feature of efforts to retrench Medicaid during the next year and a half. To understand the policy process that unfolded, their involvement needs to be placed against the backdrop of what political scientists call "representational federalism." This concept focuses on the degree to and ways in which state officials influence federal policy processes. With the growing activism of the federal government in the 1960s, concern mounted in some quarters that state governments were losing a meaningful role in the American system of federalism. In the late 1970s, however, the Harvard political scientist Samuel Beer (1978, 9) challenged this view. While acknowledging "a large and sudden surge upward in the growth of the public sector, largely under the impetus of the central government," he did not see this development as massively shifting power to the national level. Instead, he stressed "the emergence of new arenas of mutual influence among levels of government" that "is adding to our national system of representation." He identified two arenas for state representation that political scientists had neglected. One involved the power that accrues to states in their role as administrative agents of the federal government. In implementing federal grant programs, such as Medicaid, states possess vast discretion to shape who gets what, when, and how (a central theme of this book). A second arena featured the rise of the intergovernmental lobby, which works to shape legislative outcomes in Congress. This lobby not only consisted of associations representing such major state and local players as governors, legislators, mayors, county executives, and city managers; it also included organizations focused on specific functional areas (e.g., the Association of State Medicaid Directors).

Within the intergovernmental lobby, governors are especially important. Governors rely on individual, partisan, and bipartisan vehicles to shape federal policy. As individuals, governors frequently seek to influence national policymakers in ways that benefit their particular states. In this regard thirty-five governors representing more than 85 percent of the nation's population have offices in Washington (Nugent 2009, 116). Governors also turn at times to partisan organizations or coalitions to present their views to Congress and the president. Thus the Republican Governors Association, established in 1963, not only seeks to elect more governors from that party but also works to leave its ideological stamp on public policy issues affecting the states. The Democratic Governors Association, founded in 1983, pursues similar goals from its side of the partisan divide. Governors also work through bipartisan organizations. Some of these are regional associations such as the Southern Governors' Association. By far the most important, however, is the NGA. It was created in 1908 when the governors met with President Theodore Roosevelt to discuss environmental issues, and it became the National Governors' Conference in 1965 before evolving into the NGA in 1977.

The NGA has several standing committees, including one on health policy, and a staff of about a hundred. The governors typically convene at winter and summer meetings at which two-thirds of those present and voting can approve an NGA policy position. It also has an executive committee that can adopt interim positions by a two-thirds vote between meetings of the governors to guide the NGA's lobbying efforts. The executive director of the NGA frequently testifies before Congress on health policy issues. The association also employs lobbyists to work Congress. Although these lobbyists feel a need for restraint in claiming to speak for the governors, they engage in considerable "underground work" with congressional staff members to obtain information and share general NGA concerns.[1]

The degree to which governors tread individual, partisan, or bipartisan paths to influence federal policymakers varies with the issue and context. For instance, in the intensely polarized circumstances of 1995, Republican governors pursued a partisan approach to Medicaid. The Democratic governors and the NGA played little role in the initial drive to pass a Medicaid block grant. Only after the initial Republican initiative to revamp Medicaid died in January 1996 did Congress turn to the NGA in an effort to salvage some vestige of restructuring. Throughout 1995 the Republican governors, led by John Engler, aggressively worked with Speaker Gingrich to keep the block grant legislation on track. Engler was so involved that the most detailed study of the period refers to him as "omnipresent" and as "a sort of fourth branch of government" (Drew 1996, 350, 359).

As the Medicaid legislation moved through the policy process, key Republican governors sought to fend off attempts to weaken or derail the block grant. Among other things, they resisted efforts by Republican moderates in the Senate to soften the legislation. In October 1995, for instance, Majority Leader Dole indicated that he would support an attempt by Senator John Chafee of Rhode Island (R) to preserve the Medicaid entitlement. This announcement prompted a burst of angry phone calls from the Republican governors, and Dole (at the urging of his presidential campaign staff) soon retreated (Drew 1996, 313).[2] Engler and other Republican leaders also had to manage tensions within their ranks over the design of a new Medicaid formula to apportion funds among states. In September 1995 draft legislation circulated by congressional staff recommended a formula for allocating the block grant that would benefit states with higher population growth in the South and West. High-growth states with certain other characteristics (e.g., greater poverty rates) could garner 9 percent annual increases in their grants. In contrast, many states in the Northeast and Midwest with stable populations would not receive much more than the minimal 2 percent. Distribution of the proposal triggered immediate complaints from several Republican governors, with those from Connecticut, Minnesota, New Jersey, New York, and Pennsylvania criticizing the plan. Governor Arne Carlson of Minnesota called the proposal "unfair, harmful, and completely unacceptable" and claimed that it would force cuts in his state that would be "political suicide" (Havemann 1995a; Havemann and Goldstein 1995; Pear 1995c). Adjustments to the final legislation (discussed below) eased some of the pain for states with little population growth, but only marginally. Despite the acute stress emanating from decisions concerning the allocation formula, twenty-five of thirty Republican governors endorsed the Medicaid block grant (Havemann and Rich 1995).

The dogged advocacy of a Medicaid block grant by Engler and other Republican governors greatly enhanced prospects for the proposal's passage. But their efforts would have gone for naught without the leadership of House speaker Gingrich. His charismatic, transformative leadership rested on a formidable intellect, big ideas, and a keen (if at times overweening) sense of his role in history. He also possessed tactical and strategic insights largely born of his participation in a no-holds-barred Republican insurgency in the House of Representatives throughout much of the 1980s. His leadership qualities allowed him to surmount many of the veto points in the American policy process. Upon becoming speaker in 1995, for instance, he moved quickly to weaken committees in the House and to set up structures that would allow him to dominate the policy agenda in that body (Zelizer 2007). He quickly grasped that key Republican governors could be valuable allies in helping Congress transform Medicaid. These and other insights helped him persuade the Senate, which had no fervent and abiding interest in a Medicaid block grant, to go along with the idea. Finally, and less successfully, his vision led him to believe that Congress' control over appropriations would enable him to trump the president's veto power and win major cuts in Medicaid and other entitlements.

The twists and turns of congressional politics leading to the approval of a Medicaid block grant as part of the Balanced Budget Act of 1995 have received attention elsewhere (e.g., Drew 1996; Smith 2002). Suffice it to note for present purposes that the Medicaid block grant approved by Congress in November 1995 promised severe retrenchment. Above all, it terminated Medicaid as a financial entitlement by capping the funds states could receive under the program annually. Up to the cap, states could count on a federal match for the money they spent on

Medicaid from their own coffers. Expenditures over the limit would come exclusively from state (and in some local cases) resources. The new legislation also cut future federal outlays to the program. The original budget resolution passed by Congress called for a Medicaid retrenchment of $182 billion over a period of seven years. The final legislation endorsed by Congress showed only slight slippage, with the cut set at $163 billion (*Congressional Quarterly* 1996, 7–19).

The new law assured states that they would get at least a 3.5 percent increase in federal dollars in 1997, 3 percent in 1998, 2.5 percent in 1999, and 2 percent thereafter. States with more poor residents, Medicaid case loads with more serious health problems, and higher health care prices could get increases in federal support up to a growth rate of 9 percent in 1997 and slightly more than 5 percent thereafter. Moreover, ten states that up to this point had the lowest Medicaid spending per poor person would be allowed to grow at a maximum rate of 7 percent in later years. Congress reduced states' maximum financial match from 50 to 40 percent and gave them some discretion to choose among formulas to optimize their federal subsidy (*Congressional Quarterly* 1996, 7–19).[3]

In addition to capping the federal government's financial obligation to Medicaid, the block grant curbed other aspects of the entitlement. The law gutted the right of Medicaid applicants, beneficiaries, and providers to sue states for failure to comply with federal law. Instead, these stakeholders would need to be content with filing a complaint against the state with the secretary of health and human services. Beyond this, the law provided states with vastly more discretion to shape program specifics. To be sure, the law continued to impose some requirements. For instance, states had to continue to insure low-income pregnant women and children under the age of thirteen years. Federal regulations requiring states to monitor the quality of nursing home care for enrollees remained in place, despite the efforts of key Republican governors to have them deleted. The law also insisted that Medicaid continue to help the elderly pay their Medicare Part B premiums. But under the banner of "federalism not paternalism," the legislation devolved vast new authority to the states to determine whom they would cover, the benefits they would offer, and how much they would pay providers.[4]

A Focusing Event and Public Opinion Turns

Congress approved the Medicaid block grant as part of a broader reconciliation bill incorporating tax cuts and a balanced budget on November 17, 1995. With the benefit of hindsight, the Republican proposal to retrench Medicaid and other entitlements might seem like a fool's errand. After all, President Clinton had vowed to veto the measure, which he did on December 6. Congressional Republicans knew it would be nearly impossible to muster the two-thirds vote to override this veto. In November 1995, however, it was far from obvious that Medicaid would emerge unscathed. Although Republicans would not get all of what they wanted, they might well win significant concessions from Clinton. After all, the president had promised welfare reform, and the Republicans hoped to link his ability to achieve that goal with his willingness to also accept a Medicaid block grant. They knew that, as governor of Arkansas, Clinton had frequently expressed frustration with Medicaid mandates. Moreover, the president intended to seek reelection in 1996. If the Republicans put him on the defensive in the court of public opinion, his will to defend Medicaid might wilt. And the Republicans were not alone in thinking that Clinton might compromise. A top official in the Department of Health and Human Services at that time said that he was uncertain until mid-February 1996 whether the president would ultimately accede to some version of a block grant. Clinton, in his view, was "finely tuned to short-term political stuff." He might well make significant concessions if polls indicated that his resistance to the Republican initiatives was hurting his reelection prospects.[5]

During the next two months, Republican congressional leaders engaged in a struggle with the White House to persuade President Clinton to accept their plan. To bring the president to the bargaining table, the Republicans employed a government shutdown. Their ability to use this tool flowed from the fact that they had embedded the Medicaid block grant in the Balanced Budget Act of 1995. If the president vetoed the measure, he still needed Congress to appropriate funds to run the government. Typically, Congress would do so by passing a continuing resolution that would appropriate funds for a short period. Brief shutdowns had occurred in the past during times of impasse between the president and Congress. But Gingrich was the first to see the tactic as a major weapon to extract concessions from the White House. In his view, "if we don't provide the money, in the end they run out of options" (Drew 1996, 336). Republican leaders understood that a shutdown would be a major focusing event that would attract concerted media attention and elevate the importance of public opinion in the policy process. Several of them optimistically recalled that much of the public had blamed President George H. W. Bush when the government closed briefly in 1990 (Drew 1996, 324).

The Republicans first tested the utility of a shutdown in mid-November by passing a continuing resolution loaded with provisions that Clinton found unacceptable. The president vetoed the measure, and the government closed for six days. During negotiations, the Republicans pried a commitment from the president that he would submit a proposal to balance the budget in seven years (the time frame for their plan). When Clinton agreed, Congress approved a continuing resolution to keep the government running until December 15. By agreeing to a balanced budget, the White House had now placed itself in a position where it had to examine how much money could be wrung from Medicaid and other entitlements. For the Republican leaders, the task became to compel the president to submit his balanced budget proposal promptly, to get him to use realistic numbers (i.e., those endorsed by the Congressional Budget Office), and to make major concessions to them. To keep the heat on the president, the Republican leaders vowed that they would pass no more continuing resolutions. Another impasse between the two parties soon occurred, and the federal government closed for a record twenty-one days from mid-December until early January 1996.[6]

During this prolonged shutdown, intense and often bitter negotiations occurred between congressional leaders and President Clinton concerning the Medicaid block grant, cuts to Medicare, and other measures. In general President Clinton adhered to the position that Medicaid needed to continue as an entitlement. But he did make concessions to the Republicans. At one point he agreed to a proposal that would yield Medicaid savings of $54 billion over a period of seven years. Of far greater importance, he endorsed a per capita cap on Medicaid. By so doing, he accepted the Republican argument that the federal government's financial commitment to Medicaid should not be completely open ended. Under his plan, states that enrolled more people in Medicaid could count on federal dollars to cover them at the specified match rate. But the plan allowed the federal government to limit the amount it would spend per Medicaid enrollee. The cap would vary by type of beneficiary because some Medicaid enrollees cost much more to serve than others (e.g., children with developmental disabilities). If states exceeded the level of expenditures allowed per beneficiary of a certain type, the state would have to pay the additional sum without the federal match. Although much less dramatic than the Republican proposal, the potential of a per capita cap to retrench Medicaid should not be underestimated. The Clinton administration would probably have recommended relatively generous caps per enrollee. But later conservative presidents could have used the mechanism to press the states to spend less on Medicaid. Faced with lower caps, states might well curb services to beneficiaries or cut provider payments, thereby threatening access to care. If these approaches to cost containment proved inadequate, states might limit enrollment.

Although the Clinton proposal was a significant concession, the Republican leaders saw it as insufficient. Governor John Engler, who did much to shape Republican views on Medicaid and who participated with congressional leaders in many of the White House negotiating sessions, strongly opposed the per capita cap, telling the press: "It was thought to be virtually impossible to make the Medicaid program worse. But the president has found a way" (Havemann 1995c).

Ultimately, however, Medicaid's fortunes depended less on the negotiating skills of participants in the White House sessions than on public opinion trends by late 1995. The quest to gauge public opinion has increasingly preoccupied policymakers during the last half century. They now operate in a political environment saturated with polling. Major organizations, such as Gallup, conduct surveys on their own or in conjunction with news organizations. The president, national party organizations, and other elected officials commission polls on countless policy matters. These surveys help shape policy outcomes. The failure of President Clinton's comprehensive health reform in 1994, for instance, partly reflected sagging support for his proposal in the polls. Opinion surveys tend to weigh more heavily in policy processes when highly visible debates occur. To the degree that policymakers can keep discussions technical and out of the limelight, public opinion become less significant.[7]

Clinton administration officials at times expressed concern that the Republican plans for Medicaid and Medicare would linger in a technical realm. In early October, for example, the secretary of health and human services, Donna Shalala, complained that congressional action on Medicaid was creating a "human tragedy in seemingly technical votes" (Havemann and Rich 1995). The prolonged government shutdowns served as a focusing event for the public, helping to assure that the debate on Medicaid and Medicare would not remain the province of political insiders.[8] Ultimately, two trends in public opinion strengthened President Clinton's resolve not to compromise with Republican leaders.

One featured mounting public concern about cuts to the federal government's health programs. The efforts of the Clinton administration and various advocacy groups to alert the public to Republican plans for Medicaid had gotten off to a slow start. By midyear, however, groups representing Medicaid providers began to voice alarm. The American Health Care Association, a trade group for some 11,000 nursing homes, started buying newspaper ads predicting that the proposed Medicaid cuts would hurt the elderly and disabled (Pear 1995a). By May the American Hospital Association had begun running commercials that criticized the Republican plans.

As summer ebbed and the Republican commitment to a block grant became clearer, President Clinton also joined the effort. In doing so, the welfare mothers and their children who made up the great majority of Medicaid beneficiaries received little attention. Instead, the president stressed the implications of Republican plans for the elderly—a more middle-class and politically active group. For instance, in mid-September 1995 Clinton appeared at the Home for the Aged of the Little Sisters of the Poor in Denver to warn that the Republican proposal would prevent 1.3 million Americans from receiving long-term care under Medicaid (Pear 1995a). In his weekly radio address on September 30, he asserted that the Republican proposal would allow states to impoverish a husband or wife who needed Medicaid to place a spouse in a nursing home. He declared: "I don't think it should be a precondition that if a husband has to go into a nursing home, his wife has to go into the poorhouse" (Havemann and Rich 1995). The White House also orchestrated a series of TV ads that warned of the dire consequences for the elderly if the Republicans had their way (Clinton 2004, 682). During the shutdown, the Clinton administration continued its public defense of Medicaid and encouraged outside groups to intensify their efforts. In December, for instance, advocates for the elderly and people with disabilities lined up fifty wheelchairs on the lawn of the Capitol with signs showing the number in each state who would lose Medicaid benefits under the block grant.[9]

For their part the Republican congressional leaders denounced the "scare tactics" of the Democrats and advocacy groups. They also turned to the Republican governors to legitimize their plans. In early December, for example, the congressional leaders invited eight of them (including Governor George W. Bush of Texas) to come to Washington to voice support for the Medicaid block grant (Vobejda and Havemann 1995).

Polls conducted by the Democrats increasingly signaled their success in generating public concern about the Republicans' plans for Medicare and Medicaid. A substantial majority of the public indicated that the proposed spending cuts went too far (Drew 1996, 324, 364). The behavior of the Republican congressional leaders in White House negotiating sessions provided additional signs of vulnerability. According to President Clinton (2004, 682), both Speaker Gingrich and Republican House majority leader Dick Armey vehemently complained to him that the Democratic television advertisements attacking Republican proposals for Medicare and Medicaid were needlessly frightening the elderly (in Armey's case, scaring his mother-in-law).

In addition to fueling concerns among the elderly about their health benefits, Democrats drew succor from other polls not directly related to health care. In November Speaker Gingrich's rating with the public stood at 25 percent favorable and 56 percent unfavorable. In contrast, President Clinton's approval rating had crept up to its highest level in eighteen months, 52 percent (Drew 1996, 324). As the second shutdown persisted into January, the pollster for the Democratic National Committee advised Clinton that his combative stance in dealing with the Republican congressional leaders was contributing to his rise in the polls. Surveys also persistently showed that the public blamed the Republicans for the shutdown by a margin of about two to one; a majority wanted the two sides to stop bickering and work out some agreement (Drew 1996, 334, 358, 365). Given these trends, the White House had less and less incentive to make major concessions to the Republican negotiators. As the second shutdown dragged into its third week in early January with no agreement in sight, Gingrich reluctantly acknowledged the need for another continuing resolution. In reviewing matters, he admitted to a miscalculation. He had expected that poll numbers for Republicans might suffer over the short term in the wake of the shutdown, but he noted: "We didn't calculate that a surge in Clinton's numbers would cause him to dig in even more" (Drew 1996, 360). Congress soon appropriated operating funds for the entire federal government.

The NGA Attempts a Rescue

The demise of Republican efforts to cut Medicaid funding substantially did not immediately quell the quest for a block grant. Again, governors played a central role in providing life support to the concept. Throughout 1995 key Republican governors, led by John Engler, had been front and center in the push for a Medicaid block grant. They had shaped and defended the proposal. Engler himself had participated in negotiating sessions at the White House and had provided tactical advice to Gingrich to keep the pressure on the president through a second government shutdown. Engler also counseled Gingrich to disregard the bad poll numbers—noting that, as governor of Michigan, he had encountered a similar problem early in his term but had then won reelection by a commanding margin (Drew 1996, 350, 359). Now, however, Engler and other Republican governors faced the fact that this partisan approach had failed. They therefore turned to the NGA in search of a bipartisan deal on Medicaid.

Efforts within the NGA to reshape Medicaid intensified in January. After a hundred hours of negotiation, a six-member bipartisan committee of governors (cochaired by Republican Tommy Thompson of Wisconsin and Democrat Bob Miller of Nevada) endorsed a proposal for reforming Medicaid. Though Thompson noted that the proposal represented a "very, very fragile compromise," it began to pick up steam (Havemann 1996). The governors attending the NGA's annual winter meeting unanimously endorsed it in early February 1996. Speaker Gingrich praised the initiative, as did Senate majority leader Dole and President Clinton (Purdum 1996). Republican leaders in Congress promptly scheduled five days of hearings on the NGA proposal in late February and early March.

The six-page NGA plan revamped the financial and benefit provisions of the Medicaid entitlement (US House Committee on Commerce 1996d, 22–25). The governors essentially accepted Clinton's concept of a per capita cap on Medicaid that would grow annually by an inflation factor. But they also supported an "insurance umbrella," whereby states could get additional federal dollars if they faced unexpected fiscal pressures. Their proposal shifted a greater proportion of Medicaid's costs to the federal government, declaring that its minimum match rate would be 60 percent rather than 50 percent. The proposal devolved new authority to the states on many fronts. For instance, while continuing to require that states cover pregnant women and low-income children through age twelve, it repealed the mandate that states phase in Medicaid coverage for all uninsured poor children from thirteen through eighteen. The proposal vastly expanded the states' discretion to determine eligibility, giving them the option of covering people living at up to 275 percent of the poverty line. In terms of benefits, the governors proposed to preserve Medicaid's current list of required services but gave the states "complete flexibility" in defining "the amount, duration, and scope of services." The proposal also stripped Medicaid providers and beneficiaries of the right to sue state officials in federal court. In sum, the NGA plan no longer envisioned the massive financial cuts to Medicaid embedded in the block grant legislation that Congress had approved in November. But, like that legislation, it devolved substantial new authority to the states and weakened the Medicaid entitlement.

While praising the governors for their initiative, the Clinton administration and key Democrats in Congress soon voiced reservations. Appearing at congressional hearings, the secretary of health and human services, Donna Shalala, detailed the administration's objections. For instance, she decried the termination of the Medicaid entitlement for all poor children from age thirteen through eighteen. She objected to eliminating the ability of beneficiaries to sue in the federal courts to enforce their rights. She expressed concern that lowering the maximum state contribution to 40 percent (rather than 50 percent) would burden the federal Treasury. She also cautioned that the NGA's proposal did not explicitly assure that the assets of spouses and adult children would be protected when an elderly family member needed nursing home care (US House Committee on Commerce 1996d, 91–96).

In addition to questioning the substance of the proposal, its Democratic opponents worked to undercut the credibility of the NGA's endorsement. In this vein, Senator Jay Rockefeller (D-WV) observed at one hearing (US Senate Committee on Finance 1996, 70): "I have been a governor; I know exactly how those NGA things work. Somebody says we have a bipartisan agreement because the main Republican and the main Democrat agreed, so they vote it right through, and everybody says it is unanimous. Well, it is not unanimous. It is not unanimous at all. Most of them have not looked at it."

The Democratic governors increasingly realized that their endorsement of the NGA's proposal put them in conflict with the White House and their party colleagues in Congress. President Clinton invited several Democratic governors to the White House to express his reservations (Havemann 1996).

Ultimately, the NGA's initiative foundered during the bill-drafting process. The Republican congressional leaders had directed the staffs of key congressional committees to work closely with the NGA in converting the six-page proposal into law. But the draft legislation that emerged could not surmount simmering partisan tensions. In late May 1996 the Democratic governors on the bipartisan committee abandoned their support for the proposal, complaining that Republicans had transformed the agreement into partisan legislation that would undermine health care for the poor. Although the Republican leaders claimed that the draft contained much more than 75 percent of what the NGA had endorsed, Governor Lawton Chiles (D) of Florida called it a "bait and switch" (Havemann and Harris 1996). The collapse of the NGA's initiative ended any prospect for a Medicaid block grant for the rest of Clinton's term. When the president tentatively raised the issue of a per capita cap on Medicaid in 1997, the NGA released a letter signed by forty-one governors (including Engler and Thompson) opposing any kind of federally imposed limit on Medicaid spending (US House Committee on Energy and Commerce 2003a, 97).

In retrospect, the events of 1995 and 1996 emerge as a watershed in Medicaid politics—as an occasion for substantial learning by policymakers and advocates on both sides of the partisan divide. Democrats more firmly grasped the political popularity of defending Medicaid against retrenchment. In turn, Republican leaders came away with a new sense of the political risks of frontal attacks on the program. Although many of them continued to support the concept of a block grant and of paring Medicaid funding, they concluded that a more covert, nuanced approach would probably be necessary to achieve retrenchment, at least during the next few years. (It was not until the rise of the Tea Party in Congress in 2011 that a clarion call to block grant and severely cut Medicaid again surfaced.) As is discussed in chapter 3, the approval of a welfare reform bill in 1996 altered the terrain for Medicaid politics by allowing Medicaid to distance itself further from the image of "welfare medicine." Finally, the events of 1995 and 1996 imparted an institutional lesson about American politics. Until the rise of the Tea Party in 2011, it discredited the Gingrich hypothesis that the ability of Congress to withhold funding and shut down the government could be a potent tool in extracting concessions from a recalcitrant president. It led the Republicans to conclude that prospects for major Medicaid retrenchment depended on their ability to gain control of both houses of Congress and the White House. By 2003 the Republicans had achieved this partisan dominance.

A Republican Government Fails to Enact a Block Grant

Republican efforts to cap Medicaid expenditures and substantially devolve the program resurfaced again in 2003. Ostensibly, the political odds seemed aligned in their favor. For the first time in Medicaid's history, the Republicans controlled the House (229 to 204), the Senate (51 to 48), and the presidency. Moreover, they held twenty-seven governorships, nearly as many as in 1996. Former governor Tommy Thompson, a key player in the 1996 efforts to convert Medicaid into a block grant, had become secretary of health and human services.

The Republican experience in 1995 and 1996 had left its mark. From the outset the White House shunned any effort to cast Medicaid reform as part of a broad visionary effort to empower the states to innovate, to recast the federal government's role in society, or to balance the federal budget while pursuing tax cuts. Instead, the George W. Bush administration portrayed its proposal as a relatively minor change that would not threaten the Medicaid entitlement. It asked Thompson, as secretary of health and human services, to take the lead in advancing the plan. The administration's proposal emphasized that the states' participation in a new capped grant would be voluntary; they could stick with the regular entitlement if they preferred. Moreover, the capped grant would not apply to Medicaid's "mandatory" populations (e.g., poor children and low-income pregnant women) and services (e.g., hospital care). Instead, it would target optional benefits (e.g., dental services) and enrollees (e.g., certain people with disabilities who had incomes above the poverty line). Medicaid would fund the optional element of the program through a capped grant. States selecting the option would receive two allotments—one for acute care and the other for long-term care. After several years, these allotments would in all probability grow at a lower rate than increases in the Medicaid entitlement. The states that chose the capped grant for optional enrollees and services would have much greater flexibility to shape program benefits. These states could, for instance, target enrollees in particular geographic areas rather than face the requirement to offer services statewide. The proposal featured a modest "signing bonus" for the states that selected the capped grant. The participating states would receive an additional $12.7 billion in federal funds during the early years—a step that would help them cope with the weak economy and revenue shortfalls of the early 2000s. The proposal was budget neutral, however; after seven years, the upfront bonus would be subtracted from federal allocations to the states for three years (Pear 2003c).

Although this proposal was voluntary and was introduced with much less fanfare than the Gingrich initiative of the mid-1990s, its potential impact was substantial. First, the capped grant applied to most Medicaid spending. Mandatory enrollees and services accounted for only 35 percent of program costs. Optional services for mandatory groups absorbed another 20 percent. The remaining 45 percent of Medicaid dollars funded optional services and enrollees—primarily the elderly and people with disabilities (Swartz 2003, 3). Second, the proposal might subsequently open the door to a political strategy based on divide and rule. Voluntary acceptance of the capped grant by enough states could well ease efforts to retrench the program in the future. The interests of states with capped grants would over time diverge from those remaining in the regular entitlement program. A subsequent conservative administration that wanted to convert the entire program to a block grant would probably face a less unified coalition of governors braced to defend the program.

"Block" (as in Grant) Becomes a Dirty Word

The Bush administration's strategy for promoting the proposal involved two basic steps: Shun the label of block grant, and build support among the governors. In the language of intergovernmental relations, the term " block" generally applies to federal grants that devolve substantial discretion to the states to set priorities and choose approaches to deal with some problem (e.g., children's health). Many specialists in public administration have seen block grants as an antidote to the propensity of American policy processes to proliferate ever more categorical programs, each relatively narrow in scope with its own specific federal requirements. The multiplication of these categorical "silos," "pickets," or "stove pipes" often thwarts the integration of social service delivery. Although originally touted as vehicles for unshackling the states to achieve more creative and effective public management, block grants in the 1980s and 1990s increasingly morphed into tools for cutting the federal government's costs (Stenberg 2008). In the context of Medicaid, initiatives under President Reagan in the early 1980s and Speaker Gingrich in the mid-1990s linked block grants to efforts to cap federal funding for the program while devolving more authority to the states.

Rather than deal with the symbolic baggage of espousing another version of a block grant, Republicans repeatedly denied that the term applied to their Medicaid proposal. In turn, Democratic leaders in Congress saw this gambit as an exercise in linguistic legerdemain and worked assiduously to pin the block grant label on the president's plan. This tension over labeling surged to the fore at a congressional hearing in February 2003. In his opening statement, Secretary Tommy Thompson underscored that the Medicaid proposal "is not—this is not a block grant" and that "the Medicaid entitlement will be unchanged." In response, Democrat after Democrat at the hearing disagreed. For instance, Representative Henry Waxman of California observed that "if there is a cap on federal funds, . . . if there are few requirements on how the program is run, and there are no enforceable rights, that is the earmark of a block grant." But emphasizing again that funding for mandatory clients and services would still function as an open-ended entitlement, Thompson responded that "the proposal is not a block grant." Again and again, this pattern of "no it's not" / "yes it is" characterized the hearing. At one point, Representative Sherrod Brown (D-OH) characterized the presentation of the proposal and Thompson's defense as "Orwellian" (US House Committee on Energy and Commerce 2003b, 26, 33–34, 36, 45).[10]

The Effort to Rally the NGA

In promoting its Medicaid plan, the Bush administration explicitly targeted the NGA. By mid-February 2003 Tommy Thompson announced that he had presented the administration's proposal to the NGA's Executive Committee and reached out on a "bipartisan basis" to thirty governors. He openly expressed interest in arranging a special meeting with the Democratic governors (US House Committee on Energy and Commerce 2003b, 26). Simultaneously, the White House arranged for three Republican governors—Jeb Bush of Florida (the president's brother), Bill Owens of Colorado, and John Rowland of Connecticut—to lead the charge within the NGA.

The three governors partly worked through the NGA's regular channels to advance the White House's interests. In this regard they set the table for the president's proposal by urging the NGA's executive committee not to lobby for a temporary increase in the federal Medicaid match. During much of 2002 both Republican and Democratic governors had backed the NGA's efforts to persuade Congress and the president to increase this match to help states cope with the economic downturn of 2001 and 2002. In mid-January 2003, however, the three Republican governors broke ranks with this position. Instead, they affirmed that any short-term fiscal relief ought to be contingent on significant Medicaid reform. According to Jeb Bush, seeking temporary relief without fundamental reform "was partisan. It was the position of big government" at a time when the federal government "can't just keep printing money" (Tannner 2003).

The trio of governors also pursued a much more aggressive strategy to prevent the NGA from standing in the way of the president's Medicaid initiative. In doing so, they acted as agents of certain White House staff members (including Karl Rove) who believed that the NGA had generally failed to support the president's policy priorities.[11] The NGA's executive director (the holder of a PhD in economics who had previously worked for the nonpartisan Congressional Budget Office) prided himself on providing the governors with thorough, objective information on the implications of federal policy proposals. This information often shaped the governors' views and at times their lobbying agenda. Working in this tradition, the NGA staff had sought to clarify the details of the Bush administration's skeletal Medicaid proposal by sending Secretary Thompson a list of sixty questions (Pear 2003a). Key White House staff members interpreted these and related NGA activities as impediments to advancing the president's agenda. Responsive to their concerns, governors Bush, Owens, and Rowland attacked the NGA on several fronts in early 2003. In late February Owens publicly complained that the NGA staff was biased toward the Democratic Party (Tanner 2003). The three governors simultaneously worked behind the scenes to mobilize support to fire the NGA's executive director. They suggested that their fellow Republican governors protest the NGA's partisan bias by withholding their dues from the association. The three governors noted that elimination of the NGA might well allow the governors to work more effectively through their own partisan organizations. Ultimately, the three Republican governors failed to rally enough support from other governors to disrupt the NGA. But their activities strongly signaled to the NGA staff that it should bend over backward in giving the president's Medicaid plan "fair" treatment.

With pressure coming from the Bush administration and the three Republican governors, the NGA established a ten-member task force in an attempt to forge a bipartisan agreement on Medicaid reform. Governors Jeb Bush and Tom Vilsak (D-IA) served as cochairs. Despite sharp partisan differences, the task force inched toward a fragile agreement among eight of its ten members in early June 2003. Drafts from the task force supported aspects of the Bush administration proposal, albeit with looser spending caps. But the task force added a provision that alarmed the administration: shifting state costs for those simultaneously enrolled in Medicare and Medicaid (the dual eligibles) to the federal government. Because estimates at the time put these costs at $40 billion per year, this would impose a significant new fiscal burden on the federal government (Goldstein 2003). Within ten days, this tentative bipartisan agreement collapsed when the Democratic governors announced they could no longer support the proposal. This withdrawal may in part have reflected their sense that the Bush administration would never agree to absorb the costs of the dual eligibles. But it also responded to pressure from Democratic congressional leaders who wished to preserve the Medicaid entitlement. In this regard Senator Edward Kennedy (D-MA) personally persuaded Governor Vilsak to abandon the draft proposal. He also phoned several other governors to urge opposition to the bipartisan agreement and asked other members of Congress to rally governors from their home states to reject the measure (Connolly 2003).

After the demise of the bipartisan effort, the five Republican governors on the task force expressed hope that they could strike a separate deal with the administration on Medicaid reform. But given other presidential priorities, such as securing passage of a new drug benefit for Medicare enrollees, the failure to obtain some semblance of bipartisan backing discouraged the Bush administration from pressing ahead. As in 1995 and 1996 the effort to block grant Medicaid aborted (Connolly 2003).

The NGA's response to the Bush administration's Medicaid initiative illuminates certain dynamics of representational federalism. Political scientists have aptly noted how the NGA helps governors make their views heard by federal policymakers. But lobbying efforts do not flow in one direction; elected policymakers also seek to shape interest group behavior. Having been assigned an important role in restructuring Medicaid, the Democrats in the NGA came under intense pressure from their fellow party members in Congress to reject a bipartisan approach that would weaken the Medicaid entitlement. In this way the deep partisan polarization in Congress spilled into an organization that was less intrinsically inclined in that direction. For its part, the Bush administration also pressured the NGA. Having developed a Medicaid proposal with little input from the governors, the White House recruited three loyal Republicans to advance their plan within the NGA. The attention directed at the NGA by the White House and Congress testifies to the importance of the association. Once the governors reach substantial agreement, federal policymakers find it politically awkward to oppose their recommendations. But the 2003 episode also points to the ability of federal policymakers to shape the preferences of governors and make it impossible for the NGA to be a potent advocate on a particular issue.

More Federal Dollars in Tough Times

Medicaid not only demonstrated its durability by eluding efforts to convert it to a block grant; it also evinced political strength by advancing one variant of compensatory federalism: the principle that the federal government ought to increase its share of Medicaid costs during economic downturns. As noted above, Medicaid suffers from the problem that just when the economy slows and state revenues decline, the demand for Medicaid services grows. Specific elements of the Medicaid formula compound the problem for those states most severely afflicted by a sagging economy. The per capita income figures that determine the federal match significantly lag current economic conditions. For instance, the deep recession of 2008 and 2009 affected Nevada more adversely than most states. Under ordinary circumstances, however, the state's federal matching rate for fiscal 2010 would be based on personal income data from 2005 through 2007, when its economy was booming (Peters 2008, 6). These realities have prompted governors to lobby federal policymakers for an increase in the federal Medicaid match in times of economic distress. Their efforts succeeded in 2003, 2009, and 2010.

The 2003 episode presents the more intriguing case because the Bush administration opposed a temporary bailout for the states unless its Medicaid proposal won congressional approval. In that event states opting for the new block grant would receive a temporary increase in federal dollars. In the absence of reform, the president vowed to reject any request for additional federal assistance. Ultimately, however, the president could not induce sufficient party discipline in Congress to deliver on this commitment. An early sign of trouble emerged when the governors held their winter meeting in February 2003. Although the president stressed the link between temporary fiscal help and his block grant proposal at a White House reception for the governors, Senate majority leader Bill Frist (R-TN) was more equivocal. He told the governors that he preferred tying short-term relief to basic reform, but he would not rule out offering temporary assistance to the states without it (Pear 2003b, 2003c). Early in 2003 key Republicans and Democrats in Congress joined hands to sponsor legislation that was more generous to the states 2003b, c, than the president's Medicaid proposal (US House Committee on Energy and Commerce 2003a, 33). Senators Ben Nelson (D-NE) and Susan Collins (R-ME) played a lead role. By mid-2003 congressional supporters had managed to insert temporary Medicaid relief for the states into the Jobs and Growth Tax Relief Reconciliation Act of 2003. Though chafing at the end run around Medicaid reform by the governors, President Bush signed the bill into law because it contained additional tax cuts that he strongly favored. The bill provided $10 billion in additional Medicaid funds for five fiscal quarters through an increase in the federal match for each state of just under 3 percentage points. To receive the new funds, the states had to agree not to lower their Medicaid eligibility thresholds for the duration of the enhanced match.[12]

In 2009 Medicaid relief for the states came expeditiously and with little need for vigorous lobbying by the governors. The Democrats controlled both houses of Congress by wide margins as well as the presidency. Moreover, key policymakers believed that the country faced its worst fiscal crisis since the Great Depression. In this context, Medicaid spending possessed appeal not only as a lifeline for low-income people but also as a vehicle for economic stimulus. Federal dollars would flow into the economy without delay as the states protected their Medicaid programs from massive cuts. For their part, all but a handful of congressional Republicans opposed the stimulus package. Many of them strongly preferred tax cuts rather than increased federal spending to galvanize the economy. Yet despite Republican opposition, Congress approved the American Recovery and Reinvestment Act in mid-February 2009.

This law appropriated $87 billion (more than 10 percent of the total stimulus package) to increase the Medicaid match rate for states from October 1, 2008, through December 2010. The law froze a state's current match under the regular Medicaid program to provide a floor for additional federal assistance. (Ordinarily, the Medicaid formula adjusts this match annually based on a state's relative standing among states in per capita income.) Given this floor, the statute promised each state a minimum increase in the federal match of 6.2 percentage points. States experiencing particularly significant unemployment became eligible for still more federal dollars. Given these terms, states such as California saw their federal match rate grow from 50 to nearly 62 percent. In exchange for more federal support, states had to refrain from making their eligibility standards and procedures more restrictive than they were on July 1, 2008, comply with federal requirements to pay providers promptly, and meet various other stipulations (GAO 2009d).[13] With states continuing to experience considerable fiscal stress, the Obama administration persuaded Congress to continue the enhanced match at a somewhat reduced rate through June 2011. But faced with mounting federal deficits and debt, Congress demonstrated no interest in continuing the enhancement beyond that point.

The Growth of Medicaid Expenditures and Enrollments

Medicaid's success in winning additional federal support in hard times and in dodging block grant initiatives testifies to its durability. But these legislative developments leave open the question of whether various input and output measures also paint a picture of program resilience. In this regard, trends in Medicaid expenditures and enrollments during the Clinton and George W. Bush administrations deserve attention.

From 1992 to 2008, national and state expenditures on Medicaid nearly tripled, rising from $116 billion to $339 billion.[14] As figure 2.1 depicts, Medicaid grew by 90 percent in inflation-adjusted dollars. (See table A.1 in appendix A for

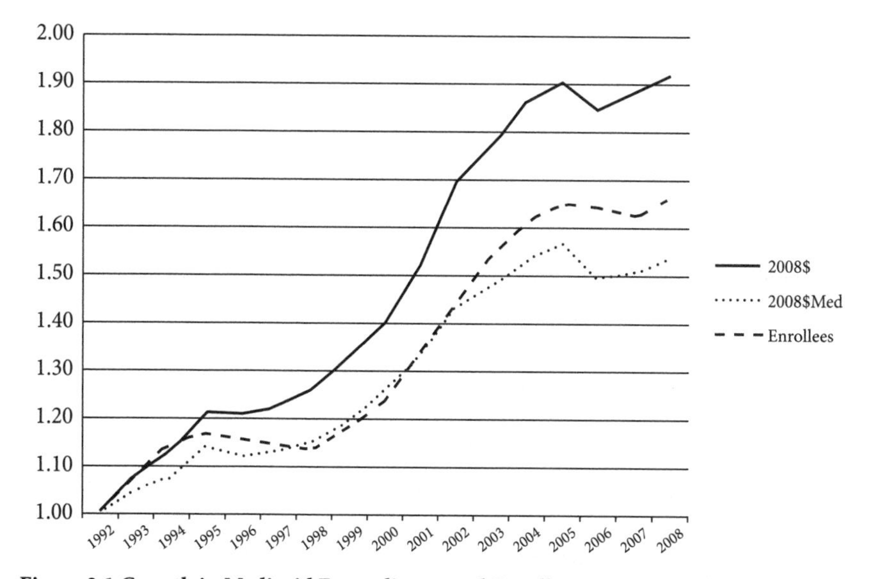

Figure 2.1 Growth in Medicaid Expenditures and Enrollees, 1992–2008 (no 1999 enrollment data)

Source: Kaiser Commission on Medicaid and the Uninsured; a more detailed description of the source appears in table A.1.

more detail.) The upward march of expenditures continued year after year. In only two of sixteen years, 1996 and 2006, did Medicaid outlays in constant dollars dip. Medicaid, of course, shares a pressing challenge with other types of health insurance—the tendency for the medical care component of the Consumer Price Index (CPI) to outpace the general inflation rate year in and year out. States run the risk that their enhanced Medicaid effort will be Sisyphean—that despite pouring more dollars into the program, they will lose ground because of rising health prices. Figure 2.1 shows that when one examines Medicaid expenditure trends in constant medical dollars, the increases from 1992 to 2008 diminish. Still, Medicaid spending grew by a robust 53 percent during the period. Again, declines occurred in only two years. (See table A.2 in appendix A.)

Other expenditure data also point to Medicaid's durability. The program's outlays as a proportion of all national health expenditures edged upward, from 12.7 percent in 1992 to 14.7 percent in 2008.[15] Moreover, both the states and the federal government committed higher percentages of their budgets to the program. Medicaid rose from 17 percent of state spending in 1992 to 22 percent in 2008. About 80 percent of the states saw an increase in Medicaid outlays as a percentage of their total budgets (including intergovernmental grants).[16] So, too, Medicaid's share of federal outlays grew from approximately 5 percent in 1992 to 7 percent in 2008 (OMB 2010).

The increases in Medicaid spending partly reflected surging enrollments (also depicted in figure 2.1). The number of Medicaid beneficiaries grew by 66 percent from 1992 to 2008, from 36 to 59 million. (The data refer to the number of different individuals enrolled in Medicaid at some point during a year. Because many people gain eligibility only to lose it after a brief time, these figures exceed the numbers signed up for Medicaid at a given point.) By and large the increases were steady, with enrollment slightly declining in five of fifteen years. (See table B.1 in appendix B.)

Aggregate expenditure and enrollment trends testify to Medicaid's political strength. But they do not illuminate Medicaid's effort relative to the size of the population in need. One way to probe this issue is to examine Medicaid spending and beneficiaries per poor person. Although far from a perfect measure of effort in relation to need, Medicaid scholars have found the indicator to be reasonable and convenient.[17] Figure 2.2 tracks trends in Medicaid spending in constant dollars (the overall CPI plus the medical care component) and enrollees per poor person. The percentage increases in the three measures generally mirror those discussed above for overall spending and enrollment. In this regard Medicaid outlays per poor person in 2008 constant dollars nearly doubled, from $4,700 to $8,500; in constant health care dollars, the hike approached 50 percent. In turn, Medicaid enrollees per poor person grew by two-thirds, from 0.9 to 1.5. Increases in these ratios tended to occur annually—in twelve of sixteen years for constant dollars, in eleven years for medical dollars, and in thirteen years for enrollees. The last three years of the Bush administration, however, present some cause for concern. Medicaid spending per poor person receded in each year, culminating in a drop of nearly 5 percent in 2008. After declining in 2007, enrollees per poor person also endured a shrinkage of 5 percent in 2008. (See tables A.1, A.2, and B.1 in appendixes A and B.) This erosion primarily reflected a swelling of the ranks of poor people, from 36.5 million in 2006, to 37.3 million in 2007, and to 39.8 million in 2008.

Overall enrollment and expenditure trends could, of course, obscure substantial gains for some groups and erosion for others. Did some cohorts of Medicaid enrollees evince more growth than others? Did, for instance, more middle-class Medicaid beneficiaries (the elderly and people with disabilities) benefit at the expense of low-income children and their families? Or did the growing number of mandates imposed on the states to cover children combine with the creation of the Children's Health Insurance Program (CHIP) to put this cohort at the head of the line? To probe these possibilities, I examined enrollment and expenditure trends for the four main categories of beneficiaries—children up to eighteen, nondisabled adults under sixty-five, the elderly and people with disabilities under sixty-five.

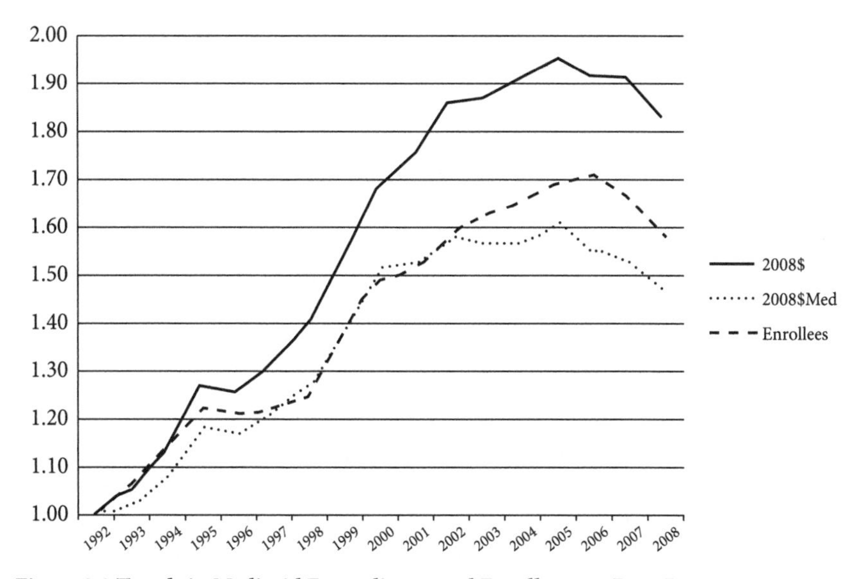

Figure 2.2 Trends in Medicaid Expenditures and Enrollees per Poor Person, 1992–2008 (no 1999 enrollment data)

Sources: Expenditure and enrollment data come from the Kaiser Commission on Medicaid and the Uninsured, and poverty data are from the US Census Bureau; a more detailed description of the sources appears in table A.1.

With one exception, there do not appear to have been significant shifts in the share of Medicaid benefits garnered by the four clusters of enrollees. The four cohorts have, with slight annual variations, held their own as a portion of Medicaid beneficiaries. Children consistently made up about 50 percent of all enrollees;[18] nondisabled adults, about 25 percent; people with disabilities, 15 percent; and the elderly, 10 percent.[19] Substantial stability also characterized Medicaid expenditures on each of the four clusters. However, some change has occurred in the monies spent on the elderly compared with people with disabilities. From 1992 through 2008 Medicaid outlays on the elderly declined from 33 to 25 percent of program expenditures. In contrast, expenditures on people with disabilities increased from 37 to 43 percent. The exact dynamics leading to this shift are unclear. This finding is, however, consistent with a thesis I develop in chapter 4—that people with disabilities and their providers may well be the most politically potent of Medicaid's four cohorts.

Finally, the data provide some clues concerning the implications of economic downturns for Medicaid expenditures and enrollments. Given that states face mandates to balance their budgets, do they contract their Medicaid programs when recessions precipitate declining revenues? Or do heightened needs for assistance prompt Medicaid expansion? The 1992–2008 period does not permit a definitive answer to these questions. Nonetheless, it deserves note that considerable Medicaid expansion occurred in the leanest economic years. One stressful time for the states occurred from 2001 to 2002, when the GDP grew at annual rates of 0.8 and 1.6 percent, respectively, and unemployment edged upward. During these two years Medicaid expenditures increased by 8 and 12 percent, compared with an average of slightly more than 3 percent for the other more affluent years depicted in table 2.1. Increases in spending per poor person averaged 5 percent per annually—about the same as for the other years.[20] So, too, Medicaid enrollment increases in 2001 and 2002 clocked in at 6 and 9 percent, whereas the other years featured an average growth rate of about 4 percent (see table 2.3 below). Turning to enrollees per poor person, however, the average increase in 2001 and 2002 was 3 percent, whereas the mean for the other years in the table was about 3.5 percent. The onset of the Great Recession in late 2007 yielded somewhat different patterns. In 2008 the GDP shrank by 0.3 percent and in 2009 by 3.5 percent. For those two years, Medicaid expenditures in constant dollars grew by about 2 and 9 percent, respectively. But Medicaid spending per poor person declined by nearly 5 percent in 2008 and just under 1 percent in 2009. Data on enrollments for 2008 mirror this finding.[21] The number of Medicaid enrollees grew by 2 percent from 2007 to 2008 but did not keep up with a 7 percent jump in the population living in poverty. The overall image is, then, one of greater Medicaid expansion in lean times but not necessarily at a rate that keeps up with the greater need brought on by economic downturns.

Peering Below the Surface: State Variation

Surveying national trends with respect to Medicaid expenditures and enrollments can, of course, mask vast differences in the program's fortunes in particular states. Indeed, some of the pessimism about Medicaid's durability comes from the failure of widely publicized Medicaid expansions in states such as Oregon and Tennessee (Oberlander 2007; Hurley 2006). Have some states aggressively expanded Medicaid while others have allowed it to wither? Before examining this change, however, the substantial variation among states in their current Medicaid effort warrants attention.

Variation in States' Commitment to Medicaid

The policymakers who designed Medicaid in 1965 understood that states differed greatly in their capacity to fund the program. To cope with this disparity, they relied on a funding formula that takes into account the per capita income of each

Table 2.1 State Quartiles in Medicaid Expenditures and Enrollees per Poor Person, 2008

States by Expenditures	*States by Enrollment*
Top quartile	
(range: $11,852–$17,697; mean: $14,452)	(range 1.65–3.05; mean: 2.03)
Vermont	Vermont
New York	Delaware
Connecticut	Maine
Alaska	Alaska
Massachusetts	Massachusetts
Maine	Connecticut
Rhode Island	California
New Hampshire	Wisconsin
Minnesota	New York
Delaware	Washington
Pennsylvania	Hawaii
New Jersey	Iowa
Maryland	Pennsylvania
Second quartile	
(range: $7,908–$9,979; mean: $8,813)	(range: 1.41–1.63; mean: 1.55)
Iowa	Arkansas
Hawaii	New Hampshire
Washington	Maryland
Wisconsin	Tennessee
Wyoming	Minnesota
Missouri	Illinois
West Virginia	Michigan
Nebraska	West Virginia
Ohio	Oklahoma
New Mexico	Rhode Island
Oregon	Wyoming
North Carolina	Utah
Third quartile	
(range: $6,827–$7,767; mean: $7,374)	(range: 1.27–1.40; mean: 1.33)
Tennessee	Mississippi
Michigan	Louisiana
Louisiana	South Carolina
Arkansas	Alabama
Illinois	New Mexico
Oklahoma	Ohio
Mississippi	North Carolina
Utah	Arizona
California	Missouri
North Dakota	Oregon
South Carolina	Nebraska
Indiana	Florida

(*Continued*)

Table 2.1 State Quartiles in Medicaid Expenditures and Enrollees per Poor Person, 2008

States by Expenditures	*States by Enrollment*
Last quartile	
(range: $4,738–$6,738; mean: $6,061)	(range: 0.88–1.24; mean: 1.09)
Virginia	New Jersey
Kentucky	Indiana
Kansas	South Dakota
Idaho	Kentucky
Arizona	Idaho
South Dakota	Georgia
Montana	Texas
Florida	Virginia
Alabama	Colorado
Colorado	Kansas
Texas	North Dakota
Georgia	Nevada
Nevada	Montana
US average: $8,506	US average: 1.49

Sources: Data on 2008 expenditures are from the Kaiser Commission on Medicaid and the Uninsured and Urban Institute's analysis of HCFA/CMS-64, www.statehealthfacts.org/comparemaptable .jsp?ind=177&cat=4. Data on 2008 enrollment are Urban Institute estimates based on data from the Medicaid Statistical Information System, www.statehealthfacts.org/comparemaptable .jsp?ind=198&cat=4. Persons in poverty data are from the US Census Bureau, www.census.gov/hhes/ www/poverty/histpov/hstpov2.xls.

state relative to the national average. Although the law stipulated that the federal government should pay at least half of a state's Medicaid costs, poorer states were to get more. This formula has persisted over the decades and yields considerable variation in federal support. In fiscal 2009, for instance, thirteen states with higher per capita incomes got the minimum match of 50 percent (e.g., Connecticut, New Jersey, and New York). Most states enjoyed federal match rates of 60 percent or higher with nine poorer states (e.g., Arkansas, Mississippi, and West Virginia) receiving matches ranging from 70 to 76 percent of their Medicaid costs (Kaiser Commission on Medicaid and the Uninsured 2009e).

Over the decades, the Medicaid funding formula has drawn considerable fire. The GAO (2003b), for instance, issued a series of reports claiming that the formula fails to target states that need help the most (see also Peters 2008). In its view, per capita income suffers from many defects as an indicator of state need for federal assistance and should be replaced with more timely, sensitive measures (specifically, total taxable resources adjusted for poverty rates and the price of health care in a state). The GAO also favored eliminating the 50 percent floor on the federal match, which tends to benefit richer states with fewer poor people. Whatever the merits of these ideas, they have gained little traction in Congress. States that benefit from the current Medicaid formula stand ready to block any such change.

The federal formula has not eliminated disparities among states in their commitment to Medicaid. Table 2.1 illuminates some of these differences by dividing states into quartiles based, respectively, on their expenditures and enrollments per poor person. States appear in rank order of their Medicaid effort. Program spending per poor person ranged from $17,700 in Vermont to $4,700 in Nevada. The mean expenditure in the top quartile was more than double that in the bottom cohort. All but two states in the top group (Alaska and Minnesota) are in the Northeast or Mid-Atlantic regions. States in the bottom quartile disproportionately come from the Southeast, though certain Plains and Mountain states also appear.

In considering differences in state expenditures, it deserves note that the quartile ranking of states does not simply reflect variations in health care prices. For instance, at least half the states in the top quartile of Medicaid expenditures per poor person do not have health care costs above the national average.[22] Moreover, other studies find that adjustments for geographic cost variation only marginally reduce differences among the states in their Medicaid spending (Grannemann and Pauly 2010, 64–65).

Table 2.1 also indicates that Medicaid enrollments per poor person varied considerably, ranging from 3.1 in Vermont to 0.9 in Montana. In general, the states that spend more on Medicaid relative to the population living in poverty also enroll more people. A separate analysis found the correlation between the expenditure and enrollment measures to be 0.72 (Pearson *r*). To be sure, there are some outliers. California, for instance, ranked in the third quartile on the expenditure measure and in the first on enrollment. New Jersey scored in the top group on expenditures but in the bottom quartile on enrollees. Factors that create these incongruities in the two rankings include (1) state differences in the breadth and amount of services they offer beneficiaries, (2) provider payment rates, and (3) enrollee case mix (with the elderly and people with disabilities costing more to insure).

In considering differences in table 2.1, it deserves note that higher federal match rates do not prompt states with lower per capita incomes to keep up with more affluent jurisdictions. Twelve of the thirteen states in the top quartile on the expenditure measure had match rates of less than 60 percent, whereas only five states in the bottom quartile did. As for enrollees per poor person, eleven of the thirteen states in the top group had federal matches below 60 percent; only five states in the bottom quartile did. If the federal funding formula effectively equalized the capacity and inclination among states to spend on Medicaid, there would be zero correlation between the match rate and expenditures per poor person. Instead, the correlation between the rate and the indicator is −0.42. The correlation between this rate and enrollees per poor person is −0.27 (these correlations are based on 2008 data). The Medicaid allocation formula has been criticized for failing to do more to equalize state effort (e.g., Grannemann and Pauly 2009). But these correlations do not necessarily mean that the federal funding formula inadequately compensates less affluent states for their Medicaid investments. Beyond wealth, states differ in their political ideologies and cultures—in their willingness to tax available resources to provide programs for the disadvantaged.

Trends among the States: Expenditures

Data on state variation at a point in time provide one lens through which to assay Medicaid's durability in different states. Trends provide another. Table 2.2 divides the states into four quartiles based on their percentage increase in spending per poor person from 1992 through 2008.[23] The increases appear first in constant 2008 dollars and then with an adjustment for growth in the medical care component of the CPI. With respect to the general inflation rate, a central finding stands out: *All fifty states participated in the trend toward greater commitment to Medicaid on this measure.* To be sure, growth rates varied considerably among the states, with New Mexico leading the way at 258 percent and Indiana bringing up the rear at 18 percent. Turning to constant medical dollars, the increases appear less robust. Nonetheless, a picture of Medicaid growth still emerges. Forty-seven states evinced increases, with only Colorado, New Hampshire, and Indiana manifesting declines. Growth in constant medical dollars ranged from 187 percent in New Mexico to –5 percent in Indiana, with a median increase of 54 percent.

A table based on trends at two points in time (1992 and 2008) could, of course, obscure volatility among the states in their growth and quartile rankings. Do data covering shorter time frames suggest a steady ratcheting upward in expenditures per poor person? Or do states behave more like accordions, increasing sharply in certain years and then shrinking in others? To address this issue, I examined Medicaid expenditure trends per poor person in constant dollars for the fifty states during eight two-year time spans in the 1992–2008 period.[24] In general, states moved steadily upward and did not seesaw dramatically between growth and contraction. In this regard 80 percent of the states increased in most of the periods (at least five of eight); and 50 percent of the states increased in at least six time spans. Only two states increased in only three of the eight periods.

Not surprisingly, the markedly different growth rates among the states precipitate shifts over time in their quartile rankings with respect to Medicaid spending per poor person. The asterisks in table 2.2 indicate states that either gained or declined in quartile placement. States fall into three general categories: climbers, sustainers, and backsliders. Fourteen states qualified as climbers by increasing their quartile from 1992 through 2008. Not surprisingly, eleven of the states in the top quartile fit this description. In some cases, such as New Mexico, states grew at a sufficiently dramatic rate to move up two quartiles. Twenty-four states quali-

Table 2.2 State Growth Rates in Medicaid Expenditures per Poor Person, 1992–2008

States Ranked by Percentage Increase in Expenditures per Poor Person (2008 dollars)	*Percentage Increase in Expenditures per Poor Person (2008 dollars)*	*Percentage Increase in Expenditures per Poor Person (2008 medical care dollars)*	*Expenditures in dollars per Poor Person, 2008*
Top quartile			
New Mexico	258.1	186.8	7,993**
Alaska	204.1	143.6	16,185**
Mississippi	193.8	135.3	7,261**
Vermont	187.9	130.6	17,697
Oklahoma	177.8	122.5	7,312**
Hawaii	167.0	113.9	9,654**
Idaho	164.3	111.7	6,526
Minnesota	160.5	108.7	13,790**
Wyoming	142.3	94.1	9,124**
West Virginia	140.6	92.7	8,760**
Maryland	138.9	91.4	11,852**
Iowa	136.8	89.7	9,979**
Arkansas	130.2	84.4	7,627**
Second quartile			
North Carolina	125.0	80.2	7,908**
Oregon	124.6	79.9	7,991**
Delaware	124.1	79.5	13,441
Arizona	123.4	78.9	6,405
Illinois	110.0	68.2	7,418
South Carolina	108.9	67.3	7,110**
Florida	108.8	67.3	6,199
Maine	108.0	66.6	14,261
California	106.4	65.3	7,251
Missouri	101.4	61.3	9,090
Nebraska	94.3	55.6	8,448
Utah	93.6	55.0	7,258
Third quartile			
Alabama	91.9	53.7	6,042
Texas	91.7	53.6	5,598
Pennsylvania	89.6	51.8	12,210
South Dakota	82.9	46.5	6,303
Tennessee	78.4	42.9	7,766*
New York	77.8	42.4	17,417
Montana	77.3	42.0	6,209*
Kentucky	73.4	38.9	6,642*
Washington	71.6	37.5	9,254*
Michigan	69.7	35.9	7,735*
Virginia	67.9	34.5	6,738*
Wisconsin	66.9	33.7	9,171*

(Continued)

Table 2.2 State Growth Rates in Medicaid Expenditures per Poor Person, 1992–2008

States Ranked by Percentage Increase in Expenditures per Poor Person (2008 dollars)	*Percentage Increase in Expenditures per Poor Person (2008 dollars)*	*Percentage Increase in Expenditures per Poor Person (2008 medical care dollars)*	*Expenditures in dollars per Poor Person, 2008*
Last quartile			
Nevada	65.8	32.8	4,738
Connecticut	63.5	31.0	16,462
Ohio	59.1	27.4	8,384
Louisiana	58.3	26.8	7,700*
Georgia	53.7	23.1	4,968
New Jersey	50.4	20.5	11,976
Kansas	50.0	20.2	6,573*
North Dakota	39.9	12.0	7,222*
Rhode Island	38.2	10.7	13,896
Massachusetts	33.9	7.3	14,885
Colorado	22.5	−1.9	5,858*
New Hampshire	20.8	−3.2	13,808
Indiana	18.2	−5.3	6,827*
US average	83.1	46.7	8,506

**States that increased their quartile ranking.

*States that saw their quartile ranking decline.

Sources: Data on 2008 expenditure are from the Kaiser Commission on Medicaid and the Uninsured and Urban Institute's analysis of HCFA/CMS-64 data, www.statehealthfacts.org/comparemaptable.jsp?ind=177&cat=4. Data on 1992 expenditures are from the Kaiser Commission on Medicaid and the Uninsured and Urban Institute's analysis of HCFA/CMS-64 data. The inflation adjustment is based on the consumer price index calculator at www.bls.gov/data/inflation_calculator.htm; the medical care inflation adjustment is based on the Bureau of Labor Statistics' series CUUR0000SAM. Data on persons living in poverty are from the US Census Bureau, www.census.gov/hhes/www/poverty/histpov/hstpov2.xls.

fied as sustainers by growing at a rate that allowed them to maintain their quartile ranking in spending per poor person. States such as Massachusetts and New York clustered in this group. Although both states grew at rates below the median, this largely reflected the high base from which they started in 1992. Both were in the top quartile in Medicaid spending per poor person in 1992 and remained there in 2008. Twelve states emerged as backsliders by declining in their quartile rankings.

The different growth rates among states in their Medicaid expenditures per poor person naturally prompt the question of whether states are becoming more alike. To address this issue I examined the coefficient of variation among states in Medicaid outlays per poor person in 1992, 2000, and 2008. Overall, the data suggest highly incremental convergence. The coefficient of variation declined from 0.46 in 1992 to 0.40 in 2000 and to 0.37 in 2008. State variation remained considerable.

It deserves note that the first year of the Obama administration featured the largest decline in GDP experienced during the 1993–2010 period. In response forty-nine states spent more on Medicaid (constant dollars) in 2009 than they did in 2008. Increases ranged from 35 percent in Wisconsin to a low of –4 percent in Indiana. But state spending tended to lag increases in the population living in poverty. Medicaid spending per poor person declined in twenty-seven states. States ranged from –18 percent in the case of Alaska to an increase of more than 33 percent in Louisiana.

Trends among the States: Enrollment

Table 2.3 rank orders states in terms of their percent increases in Medicaid enrollees per poor person. In general the data mirror the findings on program expansion suggested by expenditure trends. *Enrollees per poor person increased in all fifty states from 1992 through 2008.* Growth rates on this measure ranged from 126 percent in Oklahoma to 8 percent in Virginia. In 1992 thirty-two states had fewer Medicaid enrollees than residents living in poverty, whereas in 2008 only two states (Montana and North Dakota) did.

As with expenditures, considerable fluidity marks the relative rankings of the states on the enrollment measure (see the states marked by an asterisk). Twenty-six states grew at rates that caused them to either gain or lose in their quartile rankings on enrollees per poor person. Thirteen increased at a sufficient rate to qualify as climbers. In some cases, such as Arkansas and New Mexico, states moved from being well back in the pack on the enrollment indicator to being close to the front. Because they began from a higher enrollment base, states with more generous programs in 1992, such as Massachusetts and Pennsylvania, tend not to be in the top growth cohort in table 2.3. Vermont and Maine are exceptions, however. Both are in the top growth cluster, even though they had been in the first quartile of states on beneficiaries per poor person in 1992. Thirteen states were enrollment backsliders in the 1992–2008 window, and the remaining twenty-four were sustainers.

As with expenditures, enrollment growth in most states during eight periods between 1992 and 2008 tended to be steady. Nearly 40 percent of states increased in at least six of eight periods; 75 percent of the states grew in a majority of time frames. Seesaw effects of greater than 10 percent tended to be the exception rather than the rule.[25] In contrast to expenditures per poor person, however, the enrollment indicator did not show movement toward convergence. The coefficient for enrollees rose from 0.20 in 1992 to 0.27 in 2000 and again in 2008. Still, it deserves note that the coefficient of variation among states in enrollees per poor person is about two-thirds that for expenditures.

Table 2.3 State Growth Rates in Medicaid Enrollees per Poor Person, 1992–2008

States Ranked by Percentage Increase, Enrollees per Poor Person	*Enrollees per Poor Person, 1992*	*Enrollees per Poor Person, 2008*	*Percentage Increase, Enrollees per Poor Person*
Top quartile			
Oklahoma	0.681	1.541**	126.16
Vermont	1.412	3.045	115.61
Hawaii	0.832	1.733**	108.36
South Carolina	0.681	1.376**	101.94
New Hampshire	0.811	1.621**	99.92
Louisiana	0.705	1.393**	97.67
Maine	1.129	2.216	96.25
Arkansas	0.836	1.628**	94.66
New Mexico	0.692	1.343**	94.18
Connecticut	1.035	2.000**	93.25
Idaho	0.605	1.137	87.78
Delaware	1.250	2.346	87.69
Nevada	0.499	0.933	87.17
Second quartile			
Iowa	0.929	1.693**	82.32
Alabama	0.749	1.345**	79.71
Minnesota	0.892	1.595**	78.78
Maryland	0.916	1.617	76.47
Illinois	0.881	1.553**	76.20
Mississippi	0.801	1.403**	75.16
New York	1.038	1.806	73.92
Alaska	1.240	2.142	72.71
Wisconsin	1.100	1.889	71.74
California	1.166	1.995	71.06
South Dakota	0.707	1.189	68.33
West Virginia	0.936	1.543	64.92
Third quartile			
Massachusetts	1.275	2.093	64.18
North Carolina	0.817	1.327	62.48
Missouri	0.814	1.311	61.12
Texas	0.704	1.115	58.53
Tennessee	1.032	1.607	55.79
Pennsylvania	1.083	1.646	52.03
Florida	0.843	1.275	51.20
Indiana	0.809	1.201	48.44
Washington	1.169	1.735	48.33
Arizona	0.908	1.313*	44.57
Michigan	1.071	1.545*	44.27
Wyoming	1.004	1.433	42.70
Last quartile			
Rhode Island	1.044	1.474*	41.20
Utah	1.018	1.410	38.52

States Ranked by Percentage Increase, Enrollees per Poor Person	*Enrollees per Poor Person, 1992*	*Enrollees per Poor Person, 2008*	*Percentage Increase, Enrollees per Poor Person*
Georgia	0.822	1.136*	38.14
Kentucky	0.871	1.173*	34.69
Nebraska	0.966	1.288*	33.30
Oregon	0.968	1.290*	33.25
New Jersey	0.984	1.240*	26.01
Colorado	0.878	1.033*	17.70
Kansas	0.883	1.024*	15.96
Ohio	1.158	1.334*	15.18
Montana	0.781	0.876	12.11
North Dakota	0.887	0.962*	8.44
Virginia	1.027	1.108*	7.82

**States that increased their quartile ranking.

*States that saw their quartile ranking decline.

Sources: Data for 1992 are Kaiser Commission on Medicaid and the Uninsured and Urban Institute estimates based on data from HCFA-2082 reports. Data for 2008 are Urban Institute estimates based on data from the Medicaid Statistical Information System, www.statehealthfacts.org/comparemaptable.jsp?ind=198&cat=4. Data on persons living in poverty are from the US Census Bureau, www.census.gov/hhes/www/poverty/data/historical/hstpov2.xls.

Conclusion

Two central propositions emerge from this chapter. *First, Medicaid demonstrated substantial political strength from 1993 to 2010 by resisting two major efforts to convert it to a block grant, establishing a beachhead for compensatory federalism, and manifesting growth in expenditures and enrollments per poor person.* The failure of Speaker Gingrich and the Republican governors to turn Medicaid into a block grant and dramatically cut it in 1995 became a political watershed. This episode did not appreciably sap the desire of the Republican leaders to retrench the program. But when they acquired control of Congress and the White House in 2003, it led them to shun an open, frontal strategy for curbing Medicaid. The Bush administration's more nuanced, "voluntary" approach to weakening the Medicaid entitlement via a block grant failed to gain traction among the governors and in Congress. Meanwhile, the dawn of the new millennium witnessed successful initiatives by the governors to breathe life into the principle of compensatory federalism—the concept that the federal government should pay a larger share of Medicaid costs during economic downturns. These policy developments along with myriad other factors (many of which receive attention in later chapters) provided fertile soil for Medicaid's expansion. Every state increased its Medicaid expenditures per poor person (in constant dollars) from 1992 through 2008, with more than half more than doubling their effort. So, too, every state saw increases in its enrollees per poor person. The ACA of 2010 could fuel further dramatic increases in these expenditure and enrollment indicators.

These developments should not, of course be construed as a Panglossian claim for Medicaid's vitality and impregnability. Data on expenditures and enrollments obviously convey little about the quality of services delivered to beneficiaries, let alone the implications for their health. When one controls Medicaid expenditures for increases in the medical care component of the CPI, the magnitude of the program's growth lessens. During economic downturns, Medicaid effort tends to lag increases in the number of poor people. Moreover, states vary greatly in Medicaid spending and enrollees per poor person. Thus the impressive pattern of Medicaid expansion suggested by the data needs to be kept in perspective.

Nor should the failure of block grant initiatives and the triumph of compensatory federalism be read as a predictor of future developments. In this regard a case can readily be made that President Bush might well have been able to terminate the Medicaid entitlement if he had placed a priority on doing so. The Bush administration cared more about preserving its political capital to pass a Medicare drug benefit, obtain additional tax cuts, and transform Social Security than about capping Medicaid. The monetary enticement the Bush proposal offered the governors to support a block grant was anemic (essentially a small, short-term loan that the states had to repay). A more focused, aggressive approach by a Republican president operating with majorities in Congress might well lead to success in converting Medicaid to a block grant. The rise of the Tea Party and Republican gains in the 2010 election again thrust proposals to convert Medicaid into a block grant into the limelight. They terminated support for compensatory federalism, at least over the near term. These developments receive more attention in chapter 7.

This chapter also highlights a second proposition: *The road to significant changes in federal Medicaid law goes through the governors.* This is not to suggest that governors can place Medicaid on the policy agenda of Congress. Nor does it mean that federal policymakers invariably cede to the wishes of governors. But once significant Medicaid legislation does make it onto the congressional agenda, national policymakers view the governors as an important component of a winning coalition. Several factors buttress this proclivity. First, governors have a reputation (usually well-deserved) for having substantial insights concerning how Medicaid works and its impact on their states. Hence, their views on whether and how to change the program naturally have considerable weight in federal policy deliberations. In some instances, as in 1995 with Governors Engler and Thompson, it allows governors to shape the particular policy changes pursued in Congress. Beyond Medicaid, governors also have credibility as "experts" on the states' interests in the federal system and as major players (in some cases "rising stars") in American politics.

Second, governors provide political cover and legitimacy for policymakers in Washington. Without the endorsement or at least acquiescence of a number of governors, the White House and Congress can less easily avoid being blamed for retrenchment by Medicaid providers and beneficiaries. Optimally, those seeking to constrain Medicaid prefer to find political cover in a bipartisan resolution from the NGA. But such bipartisan support is very hard to achieve on major proposals. Hence, congressional leaders may resort to a more partisan strategy, as in 1995, when Republican governors joined with them in support of a block grant. Third, governors have resources to sustain vigorous lobbying on Medicaid if they choose to do so. The success of Republican governors in pressuring Majority Leader Dole to resist the efforts of Senate moderates to preserve the Medicaid entitlement comes quickly to mind. Governors can also play a role in communicating the benefits of a proposed Medicaid restructuring to key stakeholders and the public. Few, if any, advocates command as much attention from the media as governors. Fourth, governors at times have sufficient political clout in electoral politics within a state to earn deference from federal policymakers. The willingness of Dole to defer to an alliance of Republican governors and Speaker Gingrich in part reflected his desire to win their acceptance when he ran in the 1996 presidential primaries.

From the vantage point of Medicaid durability, governors emerge as valuable but fickle allies. Although governors have often abetted Medicaid expansion, its growth can also create a sense that it is out of control. As a top staff member for one governor put it, "No amount of money was ever enough. Yet there were constant complaints about the program."[26] In normal times, governors work through the NGA to protect Medicaid as a fiscal entitlement to the states, to fend off unwanted mandates, and to gain more discretion to shape the program. But when major Medicaid reform appears more prominently on the congressional agenda, governors have often supported steps that would weaken the program.

Ideology and party matter in this regard. Republican governors led the way in championing the Medicaid block grant initiative in 1995. Certain of them also became advocates for the Bush administration's proposal to restructure Medicaid in 2003. For their part, Democratic governors have shown occasional receptivity to Republican-led block grant initiatives. On balance, however, they have more readily defended the program from nationally instigated retrenchment. When working through the NGA on bipartisan task forces, they frequently insist on provisions that conservatives in Congress find unacceptable (e.g., having the federal government assume all costs for the dual eligibles). Moreover, their inclination to work in a bipartisan way through the NGA often runs into opposition from Democratic partisans at the national level. In 1996 Democratic governors working on an NGA compromise received signals from the Clinton administration to back off from a tentative agreement with their Republican colleagues. Congressional Democrats applied similar pressures when an NGA committee attempted to forge a bipartisan proposal in 2003. This pattern jibes with the more general political science finding that party leaders in central governments under federalism often have substantial leverage over the policy positions of their copartisans at other levels of government.[27]

Notes

1. Interview 6, September 2, 2010.

2. Senator Chafee focused particular attention on preserving the entitlement for people with disabilities. The Republican governors did not prevail on all issues. Chafee succeeded in saving Medicaid provisions that protected spouses from impoverishment if a husband or wife went into a nursing home (Smith 1998, 249).

3. A state could choose to use either its total taxable resources or per capita income as a basis for determining its federal match.

4. Representative Michael Bilirakis, Republican chair of the House Commerce Committee's Subcommittee on Health, used the phrase "federalism not paternalism" as he praised the massive repeal of Medicaid mandates (Havemann and Goldstein 1995).

5. Interview 1, July 15, 2009.

6. Congress had approved certain appropriations bills, so only some federal departments suspended operations.

7. See Brodie and Blendon (2008). In making the case that public opinion about a focusing event loomed large in this case, I make no general claim that public preferences generally drive policy. For example, Shapiro and Jacobs (2011) contend that policy elites have done much to shape the views of mass publics in an era of partisan polarization.

8. Drawing on Birkland (1997, 22), a focusing event can be defined as a "sudden, relatively rare" occurrence widely understood as harmful that is known to the public and policymakers virtually simultaneously. Birkland explores the circumstances under which these events galvanize changes in policy but also notes that they can have a "blocking effect" (p. 142).

9. This is from Havemann (1995a). Grogan and Patashnik (2003) provide an overview of how Democrats increasingly framed Medicaid as an indispensable benefit for the middle-class elderly.

10. I am not alone in referring to the Bush initiative as a kind of block grant. See also Swartz (2003) and Stenberg (2008).

11. Before 2003 tensions between the NGA and White House staff had developed over the testing provisions of the president's No Child Left Behind initiative (interview 2, July 24, 2009).

12. States also received an additional $10 billion in federal grants for more general purposes.

13. Among other things, the increased Federal Medical Assistance Percentages could not apply to payments for eligibility expansions implemented after June 30, 2008, or to Disproportionate Share Hospital (DSH) payments (Kaiser Commission on Medicaid and the Uninsured 2009a, 2).

14. As of 2006 the Kaiser Commission on Medicaid and the Uninsured reported the following breakout of Medicaid spending by function: hospital inpatient services, 14 percent; other acute care, 39 percent; long-term care, 36 percent; drugs, 6 percent; and DSH pay-

ments, 6 percent. (DSH monies flow to institutions that treat larger numbers of Medicaid enrollees and the uninsured.)

15. These data were furnished by the National Health Statistics Group, Office of the Actuary, Centers for Medicare and Medicaid Services.

16. National Association of State Budget Officers (1993, 2009). States vary in the ways they portray their budgets to the media and public. New York State, for instance, reports all expenditures—those from its own sources and from federal grants. New Jersey, in contrast, presents its public budget in terms of what it spends from state sources. The National Association of State Budget Officers adopts New York's approach in providing comparative data.

17. In this regard Grannemann and Pauly (2010, 54–55) note that spending per poor person "depends on the extent and mix of services covered and the prices paid for these services. Not all benefits go to persons actually below the poverty level, and not all persons below the poverty level receive benefits." Still, they conclude that the metric "provides a reasonable and convenient indicator of the overall level of resources a state devotes annually to meeting the needs of a typical low-income person."

18. The number of children with public health insurance rose more dramatically than this figure suggests because of the birth of CHIP in 1997. Most states, however, chose to create separate CHIP programs. Only children covered under CHIP Medicaid expansions show up in the enrollment data.

19. If implemented in 2014, the ACA promises to greatly increase the proportion of Medicaid enrollees who are nondisabled adults under the age of sixty-five years.

20. The average is based on all years in the table other than 2008, when GDP declined.

21. State-specific enrollment data for 2009 were not available at the time of this writing.

22. This calculation is based on two indicators—a cost index derived by the GAO (2003b, 40–41) and an estimate of Medicare spending per enrollee in different geographic areas (Dartmouth University 2008).

23. Expressing change as a percentage can, of course, provided an inflated picture of increased Medicaid effort when a state starts from a very low base. To some extent one can compensate for this problem by also examining whether a state has improved its quartile ranking.

24. The data points are 1992, 1994, 1996, 1998, 2000, 2002, 2004, 2006, and 2008.

25. The data intervals are every two years. A minority of states experienced sharp declines in enrollees per poor person for brief periods. Colorado, for instance, increased by 25 percent on the enrollment indicator in the 1992–94 period followed by a 20 percent drop from 1994 to 1996 before continuing its upward trajectory.

26. Interview 23, December 14, 2010.

27. See Rodden (2006, 119–120). Governors seek assistance from Congress on many policy matters. Pushing too hard on Medicaid may aggravate their relationships with their party colleagues in ways that impair their ability to achieve other policy concessions. Harmony within the party's ranks may also bolster its electoral prospects.

CHAPTER THREE

Beyond Welfare Medicine

The Take-Up Challenge

In the decades leading up to 1993, many portrayed Medicaid as "welfare medicine." This phrase had several connotations. In a general sense, it implied that Medicaid was second-class care that gave less access to high-quality services than others received through their insurance. But in the case of children and non-disabled adults below sixty-five years of age, it also implied that Medicaid served people on welfare. Those receiving cash assistance under Aid to Families with Dependent Children (AFDC), a federal grant program to the states, automatically became eligible for Medicaid. This link to AFDC did much to brand and stigmatize Medicaid as welfare medicine. Policy developments in the 1990s and 2000s, however, weakened this link. In essence, Medicaid shifted its primary focus from serving welfare recipients to helping low-income working families.

This chapter plumbs two key policy developments that abetted this delinkage: the passage of the welfare reform act in 1996, and a multipronged initiative to provide health insurance to low-income children. First, I briefly shine the spotlight on welfare reform, a seminal moment in the history of American social policy. This law abolished AFDC and replaced it with a program called Temporary Assistance to Needy Families (TANF). In the wake of the new law, income rather than welfare status became a key criterion among adults for Medicaid eligibility. After considering the politics of welfare reform, I turn to the primary focus of this chapter: the quest to insure children independent of the welfare status of their families. This initiative had commenced in the 1980s with a series of Medicaid mandates directing states to cover poor children and pregnant women. It took a giant step forward with the passage of CHIP in 1997.[1] CHIP provided additional monies to the states at an enhanced federal matching rate to insure children with incomes up to (and ultimately above) 200 percent of the poverty line. It gave states the option of implementing CHIP by expanding their Medicaid programs.

The chapter then turns to the challenge of implementing the Medicaid mandates and CHIP. This analysis compels us to return to a core theme of chapter 1: the possibility that subterranean administrative processes can function as termites in the foundation of Medicaid and thus widen the gap between policy promise and program performance. In this case, the *take-up challenge* loomed large. Many low-income children who could qualify for Medicaid or CHIP remained uninsured. This chapter focuses on the sources of the take-up problem and the efforts of top policymakers and other stakeholders to counter it. It assays how the perennial concern to combat government waste along with rising political antagonisms toward illegal immigrants led to policies that complicated take-up efforts. It also probes efforts of the George W. Bush administration to use "unsatisfactory" take-up rates for Medicaid as a weapon against CHIP eligibility expansions. I then examine the bottom line—the degree to which states tried to foster higher participation rates and succeeded. After a review of efforts during the Obama years to expand CHIP and enhance take-up, I consider the implications of the case for American federalism and Medicaid durability.

The Welfare Reform Act of 1996

From its inception in 1965, Medicaid had been joined at the hip to AFDC, a Depression-era welfare program. Though AFDC had originally been seen as a means for providing pensions to widowed mothers, it had morphed into a program under which great numbers of recipients had children out of wedlock and never married. Although most people used AFDC as a temporary crutch to get through an economic rough patch, it appeared that the program had become a way of life for others. A sizable contingent of adults remained on welfare for eight years or more.[2] Many of their children subsequently became unwed mothers on the AFDC rolls.

Since the 1960s the social construction of AFDC recipients had increasingly turned negative, with substantial numbers of Americans viewing them as indolent, promiscuous, and undeserving. The fact that black Americans made up disproportionate numbers on the rolls added a racial overlay to this perception. For their part, politicians often reinforced adverse stereotypes. For instance, while Ronald Reagan was campaigning to be the Republican nominee for president in 1976, he introduced the public to a "welfare queen" in Chicago who had allegedly bilked AFDC and other social programs out of some $150,000 and drove around in a new white Cadillac. The fact that this and other claims played fast and loose with the facts did little to limit their role in buttressing negative sentiments toward welfare (Hetherington 2005, 78–79). The low status of welfare recipients meant that close ties to AFDC were a political liability for Medicaid. So long as AFDC recipients made up a large proportion of its enrollees, Medicaid's status as "welfare medicine" would be front and center. Some conservatives went so far as to blame Medicaid for encouraging a culture of dependency. In this view poor single women were more willing to have children because they knew that they could turn to Medicaid. Whatever the empirical validity of this claim, some evidence in fact suggested that welfare recipients were reluctant to take low-wage jobs and leave the rolls because it meant giving up their health insurance (Starr 2011, 49). From the perspective of enhancing Medicaid's political durability, efforts to delink it from welfare had much to offer. The welfare reform act of 1996 moved in this direction.

By the time Bill Clinton ran for president in 1992, many Democratic Party leaders believed that welfare policy had become an ace in the hole for Republicans at election time. However, Clinton was determined not to be outflanked, so he made welfare reform one of his signature initiatives during the campaign. And once he had become president, after extensive negotiations with the Republicans who controlled Congress, he delivered on his promise by signing into law the welfare reform act—the Personal Responsibility and Work Opportunity Reconciliation Act—in August 1996. This law replaced the AFDC entitlement with TANF and above all stressed that welfare recipients should work. It also imposed a five-year time limit on how long they could remain on TANF.

On the surface the welfare reform act looked like a baby step toward delinkage. After all, those on TANF would continue to qualify for Medicaid. But two developments elevated the significance of the law. The first involved a decision by congressional Republicans to establish a new Medicaid eligibility category for non-TANF adults. Very late in the negotiations over welfare reform, two Republicans, Senator John Chafee (RI) and Representative Nancy Johnson (CT), insisted that no person eligible for Medicaid under current AFDC eligibility standards should lose their health insurance. To accommodate them, the Republican leadership proposed to freeze in place a state's eligibility criteria for AFDC as of July 16, 1996 (adjusted subsequently for inflation), for purposes of Medicaid enrollment. This assured that individuals who met these criteria would be entitled to Medicaid even if they no longer qualified for a state's new TANF program. The effort of the Republican leadership to accommodate Chafee and Johnson infuriated Republican governor John Engler (MI), who had done much to represent the views of the Republican governors in negotiations over the bill. He thought forcing states to create two eligibility pathways to Medicaid (TANF and the old AFDC criteria) would impose a needless and costly administrative burden on them. And he felt so strongly about the matter that he threatened to hold a press conference opposing the welfare reform bill if the provision remained. To head off this possibility and to placate the governors, the Republican congressional leadership added funding to the bill to compensate states for the costs of implementing a dual-eligibility system (Haskins 2006, 318–24).

A second major and unexpected development unfolded in the wake of the passage of the welfare reform act. The number of welfare recipients plummeted, while many states simultaneously sought ways to expand Medicaid to new categories of nondisabled adults. From 1996 to 2006 the TANF rolls dropped by more than 60 percent, from 12.3 million to 4.6 million (US House Committee on Ways and

Means 2008, 7–27). Meanwhile, many states worked to assure that those who had left TANF but still met the old AFDC criteria remained covered by Medicaid. Even more important, several states pursued significant coverage expansions for adults primarily through demonstration waivers. (For the role of these waivers, see chapter 5.) These expansions helped offset the decline in those eligible for Medicaid by virtue of receiving cash assistance. Partly as a result, nondisabled adults preserved their share of Medicaid enrollments at about 25 percent in the aftermath of welfare reform. The fact that adults held their own in enrollment should not obscure the relatively small dent Medicaid made in helping them obtain coverage. As of 2008 more than 17 million adults living at or below 133 percent of the poverty line lacked health insurance, with childless adults making up nearly 70 percent of this group (Schwartz and Damico 2010). This group eventually became the primary target for the Medicaid expansions authorized by the ACA of 2010.

In sum, the welfare reform act fueled substantial delinkage. Medicaid increasingly became a program for people with a more favorable social construction—working adults rather than welfare recipients. At least in this sense Medicaid distanced itself from the label "welfare medicine." The passage of welfare reform yielded other political benefits to Medicaid as well. An improved public image for those on welfare does not appear to have been a significant policy legacy of reform, even though many recipients now worked. But the new law negated welfare as a hot button issue with the public, and it became much less salient in subsequent election campaigns (Soss and Schram 2007). Medicaid supporters therefore had less reason to fear that antiwelfare sentiments would spill over to damage the program. The new law also improved Medicaid's standing among key Republicans in the forefront of welfare reform, such as Governor Tommy Thompson of Wisconsin. With this group, Medicaid transitioned from being seen as a cause of welfare dependency to being a vehicle for supporting women who did the "right thing" by leaving TANF to get jobs.

The Waxman Kids and CHIP

Important as the welfare reform act was, it represented only one front in the effort to divorce Medicaid eligibility from cash assistance. In key respects the concerted and persistent quest to insure more children surpassed welfare reform as a vehicle for delinkage. This quest had germinated before the arrival of the Clinton administration. During the 1980s Congress approved several measures that gave states the option of expanding Medicaid coverage. Legislation in 1987, for instance, permitted states to cover all pregnant women and infants with incomes up to 185 percent of the poverty line. Increasingly, however, Congress simply mandated that states act. From 1984 to 1990 Congress imposed nineteen directives on the states expanding Medicaid eligibility (Gilman 1998, 67). Of particular importance, a

1989 mandate required states to insure pregnant women and all children up to age six with incomes up to 133 percent of the poverty line. The next year Congress required states to phase in Medicaid coverage for all poor children from age six through eighteen by 2002. These federal initiatives did not spring from a broad bipartisan consensus. Presidents Ronald Reagan and George H. W. Bush, along with many of their fellow Republicans in Congress, opposed them. Nor did these initiatives reflect the triumph of representative federalism, with Congress responding to the wishes of governors or other state elected officials. To the contrary, governors from across the partisan spectrum disliked the mandates; forty-nine of fifty governors voted in 1989 for a resolution from the National Governors Association requesting a moratorium on them. The following year the National Conference of State Legislatures followed suit in a letter to Congress.

Rather, congressional action largely reflected the tenacious and skilled advocacy of Representative Henry Waxman (D-CA). Waxman bridled that some states, especially in the South, excluded many poor children from Medicaid coverage. In seeking to remedy this problem through mandates, Waxman benefited from the fact that the Democrats enjoyed substantial majorities in the House of Representatives throughout the 1980s and in the Senate from 1987 through 1990. In addition, he chaired a subcommittee of the House Energy and Commerce Committee that had jurisdiction over Medicaid. His success also stemmed from his qualities as a policy entrepreneur. He was an expert on health policy with broad political networks, keen negotiating skills, and an understanding of how to take advantage of budgetary rules. Among other things, he used his subcommittee chairmanship and his role on House–Senate conference committees to negotiate placement of the Medicaid mandates in massive budget reconciliation bills. The use of these omnibus measures made it much more difficult for the president to veto Waxman's Medicaid initiatives. Budget procedures in effect during the 1980s also allowed Waxman to mask the long-term costs of the mandates.[3]

The Waxman initiatives further established Medicaid as an insurer of poor children independent of whether their parents qualified for welfare. But they hardly constituted a great leap forward in shrinking the ranks of uninsured children. Between 1990 and 1996 the proportion of children without insurance drifted upward, from 13 to 15 percent.[4] The persistence of the problem combined with other forces to place children's health insurance squarely on the congressional agenda.

To Entitle or Not to Entitle?

By 1997 Republican leaders increasingly sensed that the bruising battle of 1995 and 1996 to convert Medicaid into a block grant and to cut Medicare had portrayed them as hardhearted. Public opinion had turned against them as they went toe to toe with President Clinton. Moreover, Clinton had soundly defeated the Republican candidate, Senator Robert Dole, in the 1996 presidential election. Faced with these defeats and an improved federal budget picture, some Republicans became interested in recasting the party's image on health care. As Republican senator Orrin Hatch of Utah put it when he endorsed CHIP, his party needed to demonstrate that it "does not hate children." He also noted with apparent satisfaction that *The National Review*, a conservative magazine, had referred to him as a "latter-day liberal" for his support of the measure (Pear 1997b).

Congress also grasped that it could count on bipartisan support from the governors in pursuing new initiatives to cover children. Testifying before Congress in early 1997, the NGA chair, Governor Bob Miller (D-NV), noted with pride that thirty-nine states had extended Medicaid eligibility for children beyond federally mandated levels and that some were implementing major expansions. Miller expressed support for new federal initiatives to cover more children, so long as the federal government did not impose additional eligibility mandates on the states, jeopardize current state activities to insure children, or "create an opportunity for shifting private-sector insurance costs to the public sector" (US Senate, Committee on Finance 1997a, 7–8). At a subsequent congressional hearing, top health officials from California, Florida, Iowa, New York, and Rhode Island extolled their states' initiatives to cover more children (US Senate Committee on Finance 1997b).

As proposals to insure more children surfaced in Congress in early 1997, a key question revolved around the role that Medicaid should play. Should lawmakers turn to Medicaid to boost coverage? Or should Congress craft a separate grant initiative? Members of Congress differed sharply in their responses to these questions. Some conservatives shunned both Medicaid and a new grant. Senator Phil Gramm (R-TX) took the lead in this regard, proposing to help children from families with incomes up to 200 percent of the poverty line by adding $3.5 billion to the Maternal and Child Health Block Grant. All fifty states had a long history of providing primary and some specialized care to the uninsured through this program. The Gramm initiative struck many in Congress as minimal, and it gained little traction (Smith 2002, 214–15).

A second proposal, cosponsored by senators John Chafee (R-RI) and Jay Rockefeller (D-WV), fully embraced Medicaid. It gave states the option to extend the Medicaid entitlement to children in families with incomes up to 150 percent of the poverty line at an enhanced federal match rate. The proposal called for a federal commitment of $15 billion over a period of five years (Smith 2002, 216–17). This initiative to extend Medicaid garnered substantial support, including that of President Clinton. Ultimately, however, it encountered stiff opposition from the NGA, which opposed expansion of the Medicaid service entitlement. The NGA also wanted a bill that gave states more discretion to shape program details.

Ultimately, Congress punted the issue of Medicaid expansion to the states. Melding a proposal by senators Ted Kennedy and Orrin Hatch with a bill from the

House of Representatives, Congress approved and the president signed the Children's Health Insurance Program as part of the Balanced Budget Act of 1997. The new law appropriated $40 billion over a period of ten years for states to expand coverage to uninsured children in families with incomes up to 200 percent of the poverty line, or 50 percentage points above a state's Medicaid eligibility standards in effect on March 31, 1997 (GAO 2007b, 4).[5] It authorized a federal match rate for CHIP some 15 percentage points higher than that of Medicaid. The CHIP allocation formula also differed from that of Medicaid. Rather than emphasize a state's per capita income, as Medicaid did, CHIP provided higher allotments to states that (1) had more children from low-income families *and* (2) more uninsured low-income children. This latter factor stood to benefit states that had historically done less to cover children through Medicaid.

In drawing down CHIP funds, states had three options: They could extend the Medicaid entitlement up the income ladder, create a separate program, or adopt a hybrid covering some CHIP children via Medicaid and others through a stand-alone initiative. Whichever option a state pursued, CHIP was a capped grant. Each state would receive an allocation from the federal government. States that chose a Medicaid expansion would receive an enhanced federal match via CHIP until they spent their allotment. Then they had to cover the newly eligible children at the federal government's lower, regular Medicaid match. In contrast, states that treated CHIP as a separate program would avoid this obligation. Once they spent their CHIP funds, they could suspend enrollment and establish waiting lists. States with a stand-alone program also gained more discretion to shape the service package offered to CHIP enrollees.[6]

States Reach for the Middle Class while Slighting Medicaid

CHIP rapidly became a popular program, with all fifty states participating. As CHIP evolved from the late 1990s to its reauthorization in 2009, two important policy patterns unfolded. First, the states steadily moved to expand eligibility for CHIP up the income ladder toward the middle class. By January 2009 forty-three states had used earnings disregards and other means to cover children living above 200 percent of the poverty line. Nine had set eligibility at 300 percent of the poverty line or higher; New Jersey led the way, at 350 percent. Policymakers in several other states had announced their intention to expand coverage further, with Massachusetts and New York setting their sights on a 400 percent eligibility threshold (Ross and Marks 2009, 6, 22, 25).

Second, in reaching for the middle class, states distanced themselves from the Medicaid entitlement. By the end of the Bush administration, the number of states covering all CHIP enrollees through a Medicaid expansion had shrunk to six, down from eighteen in the early 2000s.[7] In contrast, eighteen states—including such highly populous ones as New York, Pennsylvania, and Texas—insured all their CHIP beneficiaries in stand-alone programs. The remaining twenty-six states pursued hybrids, covering lower-income CHIP children under a Medicaid extension but assigning those from better-off families to a separate initiative. All told, thirty-three states insured more children through stand-alone CHIP initiatives. Separate CHIP programs enrolled more than twice as many children as Medicaid extensions. Several factors fueled this pattern. For instance, some policymakers thought that creating a distinct CHIP initiative would reduce any problems of stigma associated with Medicaid, thereby enhancing take-up rates. For others, the appeal of a distinct CHIP offering stemmed from the greater flexibility it gave them to shape program specifics. Above all, a stand-alone program allowed states to hedge fiscal uncertainty. Policymakers could take political credit for bold steps to enhance eligibility while reserving the right to suspend enrollments and establish waiting lists if demand surged beyond the state's willingness to meet it. A Medicaid expansion, in contrast, entitled people to services and was less controllable.

The Implementation Challenge

The Waxman amendments and the birth of CHIP ostensibly reflected a burst of policy liberalism. But from the outset issues persisted as to whether there would be a substantial gap between policy promise and program performance. Would the children who qualified for Medicaid and CHIP participate in the programs? The answer would depend heavily on the commitments, capacities, and coordination of federal, state, and local governments enmeshed in an enrollment labyrinth. Administrators had to find ways to recruit qualified children to the program and retain them when they came up for renewal.

Three implementation challenges threatened to function as termites in the foundation of take-up efforts. First, officials faced a *marketing challenge*. This partly involved making the target population aware of the programs and the fact that they could meet the eligibility criteria. Studies show that many uninsured people lack pertinent information in this regard (e.g., Kenney, Cook, and Dubay 2009).[8] The marketing challenge also entailed persuading parents to apply. Several factors might inhibit informed parents from enrolling their children. Immigrants insecure about their legal status often refrain from contacting public agencies, even though their children qualify for benefits. Stigma might also enter the picture. Although most low-income people greatly valued Medicaid, its image as "welfare medicine" persisted with some potential beneficiaries.[9] Still other families declined to apply because they believed the insurance added little value to their lives. Many low-income parents fathom that their uninsured children have a right to be treated in hospital emergency rooms; they often have access to neighborhood clinics. Failing to pay the transaction costs of enrolling them in Medicaid or CHIP would not, therefore, block access to all medical services.

Public agencies responsible for Medicaid enrollment have historically neglected to market the program. Their cultures and performance measurement systems typically placed little or no emphasis on maximizing take-up. Nor did most of these agencies have the financial or other capacities to undertake sophisticated and extensive marketing. The CHIP legislation provided some funding for outreach, but it remained an open question whether states would use these monies effectively.

Second, the *integrity challenge* threatened to erode participation in Medicaid and CHIP. This challenge revolves around a balancing act between two kinds of eligibility errors. Officials grasp that they can foster higher take-up if they reduce the transaction costs of application and renewal. They can, for instance, require less documentation of income, simplify enrollment forms, and permit applications by mail. Through these and other steps, officials can cut the level of false negative errors—that is, the denial of benefits to children who in fact meet the income and related criteria for enrollment. This also encourages people to apply because they find the process easier. All else being equal, however, the reduction of false negatives will tend to increase the incidence of false positive enrollment errors, that is, providing coverage to children who do not meet Medicaid or CHIP eligibility criteria (Mendeloff 1977). Hence, administrators must juggle any quest to streamline intake and retention processes to foster take-up against threats to "program integrity" in the form of these false positives. Policymakers and administrators have often assigned a special importance to fighting these errors of generosity. This partly stems from their symbolic overlay—the tendency of false positives to trigger concerns, deeply rooted in American culture, that social programs will throw open the gates to abuse by undeserving freeloaders. Officials sense that, when publicized, false positives can undercut public support for their programs.[10] Concern about these miscues also flows from the historic bias of federal "quality control systems" that penalized states for these errors while downplaying false negatives. To the degree that those who staff the enrollment gates stress the importance of avoiding false positives, take-up problems mount (Brodkin 1986; Fossett and Thompson 2006).

Third, the *fragmentation challenge* complicates take-up efforts. In dealing with outreach and enrollment for Medicaid, the federal government does not (as in the case of Social Security or Medicare) turn to a unitary bureaucracy with clear lines of hierarchical authority. Instead, take-up depends on the actions of countless loosely coupled networks of gatekeepers that vary greatly in their capacities and commitments. The issue here is not just that the federal government relies on the fifty states to manage enrollment practices. Within states, fragmentation and attenuated accountability lines rear their heads. Many state governments—including large Medicaid programs in California, New Jersey, New York, and Ohio—rely primarily on county governments to manage Medicaid enrollment.[11] As county employees, eligibility workers are formally accountable to the executives and legislators in these jurisdictions. These local officials may not share the enrollment priorities of state or federal Medicaid principals. County policymakers also possess great discretion to shape administrative capacity related to take-up—staffing levels, physical space, information technology and more. Some counties, for instance, have larger staffs per potential enrollee than others (Dutton et al. 2009, 46–47). Some do more than others to fight the chronic problem of turnover among frontline eligibility workers by offering better pay.

State Medicaid officials rely on many tools to assure that county eligibility workers reflect their policies and priorities (Dutton et al. 2009; Edwards et al. 2008). They issue directives, provide administrative subsidies, periodically audit local case files, fund training, sponsor information technology, and establish performance measurement systems. Some states pay private enrollment brokers (often community-based organizations) to identify and do the preliminary processing of Medicaid applicants (under the law, public officials must make the final decision). But these measures do not guarantee that counties will promote robust take-up rates for children. When state officials find county performance wanting, they must typically rely on negotiation and bargaining with local offices. When these efforts at persuasion falter, the ability of state administrators to realize their preferences at times depends on the capacity and willingness of local advocacy groups to sue county officials in court (Dutton et al. 2009, 15; Thompson 2001, 56). The large county role has prompted some historians to characterize Medicaid enrollment systems as featuring "fractured governance, diffuse authority, and a disjointed operational infrastructure" (Dutton et al. 2009, ii).[12]

State Medicaid officials who do not depend on counties for enrollment (e.g., those in Florida, Louisiana, and Massachusetts) still face a fragmentation challenge. Medicaid agencies frequently rely on other state departments to process applicants. In Florida, for example, the Agency for Health Care Administration has chief responsibility for Medicaid but depends on the State Department of Children and Families to operate enrollment processes. The latter also processes applications and renewals for welfare, food stamps, and other social programs (Edwards et al. 2008, 10). Under this circumstance, a state Medicaid director committed to enhancing take-up must persuade administrators in another department to prioritize this objective.

Fragmentation also flows from the decision of most states to establish separate CHIP initiatives with their own sets of gatekeepers. In California, for example, fifty-eight counties manage the bulk of all Medicaid enrollments under the supervision of the state Medicaid agency, the Department of Health Care Services. A separate state department, the Managed Risk Medical Insurance Board, contracts with a private vendor to provide a single point of entry for all CHIP applicants. So, too, New York relies on a centralized computer system and contracts with managed care plans to enroll children in CHIP while depending on county governments to process Medicaid applicants (Edwards et al. 2008). The establishment of a separate CHIP silo heightens challenges of administrative coordination. It raises the question of whether children eligible for Medicaid but not for CHIP will be smoothly referred by CHIP administrators to Medicaid, and vice versa. Failure to achieve a seamless administrative relationship causes children to fall between the cracks of the two programs and thus end up uninsured. Because the incomes of families fluctuate over time, the coordination challenge presents itself not only at the time of the initial application but also at renewal. So, too, as children become older they must often transition from Medicaid to CHIP.[13] States with separate CHIP initiatives vary considerably in the degree to which they have achieved a seamless relationship with Medicaid (e.g., Thompson 2003). Some studies suggest that creating a stand-alone CHIP initiative rather than a Medicaid expansion depresses take-up rates.[14]

The Clinton Administration Tries to Lead

The possibility that implementation challenges would derail promises to insure more children soon came to the attention of the Clinton administration. As the number of people on welfare declined, concern mounted that states had failed to delink their Medicaid enrollment processes from cash assistance. Contrary to expectations, many states reported declines in Medicaid enrollment of children. Concerned about this situation and wishing to achieve some kind of health care legacy, President Clinton in late 1997 voiced his dismay to the bureaucracy. The administrator of the Health Care Financing Administration (HCFA) told the media that “the President has talked to me personally about this and has made clear that he wants to see results” (Pear 1997a).

From that point until it left office, the Clinton administration attempted to reshape the enrollment labyrinth in order to foster the take-up of children. Its actions fell into three general categories. First, the president sought to rally an array of federal agencies to help with the problem. In early 1998 the president directed eight federal departments to report back within ninety days on their plans to foster take-up. By June 1998 this Interagency Task Force on Children’s Health Insurance Outreach had responded with a sixty-four-page report that listed 150 action steps. Each federal department promised to participate in the effort. The Internal Revenue Service, for instance, pledged to post information promoting CHIP enrollment in its 400 walk-in centers (Thompson 2001, 54–55).

Second, HCFA unleashed a stream of missives to state health and welfare bureaucracies. In January 1998, for instance, HCFA sent an official letter to state agencies reminding them to coordinate enrollment processes for cash assistance and Medicaid in a way that would not lead to inappropriate denials of Medicaid. Eight months later HCFA followed up with a more extensive letter recommending sixteen steps that states should take to increase Medicaid and CHIP enrollments. These recommendations included the adoption of a brief two-page application form for both programs, the elimination of asset tests, the extension of hours for eligibility workers, and the implementation of a follow-up process for families that started but failed to complete their applications. In a similar vein HCFA joined with another federal agency to issue a twenty-eight-page *Guide to Expanding Health Coverage in the Post–Welfare Reform World* in the spring of 1999 (Thompson 2001, 55–56). In addition to exhorting states to do more to foster take-up, HCFA increased its oversight and occasionally raised the specter of sanctions. Because President Clinton was concerned that some jurisdictions had established barriers to enrollment that violated federal requirements, in August 1999 he announced that HCFA would "conduct comprehensive on-site reviews" of Medicaid enrollment processes in all the states. The Clinton administration also employed the intergovernmental lobby as a conduit for encouraging states and localities to promote take-up. In this regard HCFA reached out to the NGA, the National Education Association, and the American Public Human Service Association, at times offering contracts to foster "best practice" (Thompson 2001, 55–57).

Third, the Clinton administration made public appeals and sought to rally the private sector to support take-up. In February 1998, for instance, President Clinton and the first lady visited the Children's National Medical Center in Washington to publicize efforts to enroll uninsured children in Medicaid and CHIP. A parent whose child had recently signed up for Medicaid as a result of a local outreach initiative was featured at the event. Federal officials also solicited support from businesses. For instance, ABC and NBC promised to run public service ads touting CHIP with a toll-free number (877-KIDS-NOW) that people could call for information. K-Mart pledged to put this number on shopping bags and diaper boxes in its stores (Thompson 2001, 54–55). Foundations also agreed to help. Of particular note, the Robert Wood Johnson Foundation committed $43 million to its Covering Kids initiative from 1997 to 2001. This initiative offered technical assistance to the states to simplify enrollment and sought to engage schools, businesses, churches, and other community leaders in efforts to market Medicaid and CHIP to eligible families (Wielawski 2009, 65–66).

The Bush Years: Take-Up Barriers Resurface

Advocates persisted in calling for streamlined enrollment during the Bush years. The Robert Wood Johnson Foundation, for example, poured an additional $70 million into grants aimed at increasing coverage for children and their families

(Wielawski 2009, 65). For its part the Kaiser Commission on Medicaid and the Uninsured tracked and routinely published reports on the states' progress in reducing enrollment obstacles. Although the Bush administration did not place as much priority on fostering take-up as the Clinton White House, it did not explicitly impede these efforts. By early 2006, however, two policy developments had occurred that threatened to enervate take-up efforts—one targeted at the perennial issue of "waste, fraud, and abuse," and the other at illegal immigrants.

War on Waste: The Improper Payments Information Act

Calls for different and often contradictory kinds of administrative reform persistently buffet the federal bureaucracy and compete for attention. One of the most persistent emphasizes the need to wage war on waste—to ferret out unnecessary spending and identify fraud (Light 1997). Strong temptations exist for policymakers to layer on additional control systems to further this fight. In addition to saving "taxpayer dollars" and penalizing lawbreakers, these initiatives play to cultural stereotypes about the lassitude of government bureaucracies. Policymakers often adopt new control systems with little assessment of their added administrative costs, implications for efficiency, or ramifications for other program objectives. The passage of the Improper Payments Information Act of 2002 reflected this pattern. This new law, which was part of President Bush's "management agenda" for reforming the operations of the federal government, won nearly unanimous support in Congress. The statute required the heads of all federal agencies to submit estimates of improper payments each year to the Office of Management and Budget and Congress. It targeted eligibility errors as one of several potential sources of inappropriate expenditures.[15]

For Medicaid, the new law threatened to exacerbate the integrity challenge by elevating the importance of curtailing false positive eligibility errors. For decades the federal government had required states to operate Medicaid Eligibility Quality Control programs. Under this system, states monitored eligibility determinations and claims processing in an effort to keep their erroneous outlays under 3 percent of total benefits paid. If states exceeded these levels, the federal government reserved the right to recoup the misspent funds. Increasingly, however, federal administrators had backed away from vigorous enforcement of this system. Among other things, they devolved substantial authority to the states to customize their quality control efforts. As of 2000 thirty-one states had obtained federal approval to operate pilot programs. This had the effect of allowing states to place a lower priority on minimizing eligibility errors. It meant that they could respond to entreaties to enhance take-up for Medicaid and CHIP with less concern that the federal government would penalize them if their efforts led to more false positives.

The movement of states to deal with quality control through pilot programs complicated federal efforts to obtain uniform information. The multiple methods states used made it difficult for federal administrators to compare error rates from one state to the next; officials could not compute a national payment error rate for Medicaid, which the Improper Payments Information Act required (Wachino and Ross 2008, 9, 22). To remedy this situation the Centers for Medicare and Medicaid Services layered a new approach called Payment Error Rate Measurement (PERM) on its old quality control system. PERM standardized the method that all states would use to estimate excess payments emanating from eligibility errors and other sources. Federal administrators pledged to review error levels in one-third of the states annually. The first PERM review of seventeen state Medicaid programs that included eligibility errors occurred in 2007. When the Department of Health and Human Services provided its first estimate of Medicaid's improper payments in 2008, the news for Medicaid was not good. Medicaid exceeded all other federal programs in waste, with more than 10 percent of its expenditures deemed "improper" (GAO 2009c, 12).

Eligibility errors were, of course, only one of several factors fueling improper disbursements. Nonetheless, many state Medicaid officials worried that the new measurement system would undermine efforts to maximize the take-up of children in Medicaid and CHIP. As one state official put it: "We've been focused on outreach and getting children enrolled and reducing the number of uninsured, but now it's not going to be about that. It will be all about the process. We'll have to be sure that everything in the file is darn right because the stakes are so high."[16] The introduction of PERM adds to the administrative costs of Medicaid and CHIP; it elevates the salience of avoiding false positive eligibility errors as a performance goal. But the impact of PERM depends largely on the degree to which the federal executive branch signals its concern to states about performance on this measure and threatens to penalize them. Presidential administrations focused on getting children insured could downplay PERM's significance. For policymakers who wish to retrench Medicaid, however, PERM and the annual reports on waste could become a valuable weapon in their political arsenals.

Barring the Medicaid Door to Illegal Immigrants

A second legislative initiative that threatened to sidetrack Medicaid and CHIP take-up sprang from the public resentment of illegal immigrants.[17] In the early 2000s this issue increasingly roiled American politics. One manifestation of this dyspepsia revolved around the perception that the "illegals" obtained government benefits at considerable cost to the taxpayer. In the case of Medicaid, the existing law declared that states could not offer benefits to people here illegally. To meet this requirement forty-six states simply required Medicaid applicants to attest that they were citizens. Four (Georgia, Montana, New Hampshire, and New York) mandated that applicants provide some supporting documentation. Federal administrators did not believe that the less demanding approach of most states resulted in significant numbers of illegal residents enrolling in Medicaid. But two Republican members of Congress from Georgia, representatives Nathan Deal and Charles Norwood, disagreed. Responding to concerns expressed by Governor Sonny Perdue of Georgia (R), they concluded that any approach short of extensive documentation represented state failure to enforce Medicaid law.[18] Acting on this view they inserted a provision in the Deficit Reduction Act of 2005 that required applicants and current Medicaid enrollees to document their citizenship.[19] The law established a short five-month time frame for compliance, insisting that states redesign their eligibility processes by July 1, 2006.

Because representatives Deal and Nathan were concerned that the US Centers for Medicare and Medicaid Services (CMS) might find a way to delay or water down the new requirement, they persistently communicated their preference for tough enforcement to the executive branch. In this regard and with an eye toward the upcoming congressional elections, the two representatives arranged for oversight hearings on illegal immigration and Medicaid to be held in Tennessee and Georgia in mid-August 2006. The hearings served two broad purposes. First, they provided a forum for nurturing a sense of grievance that illegal residents were "busting the bank" in the health care system and crowding out Medicaid benefits for deserving citizens.[20] As Representative Norwood put it, the nation faced "the outright theft of health care benefits for . . . low-income Americans by illegal aliens. . . . Fewer poor American citizens get Medicaid because illegal aliens get Medicaid." A state legislator from Georgia subsequently testified that some 12,700 people with disabilities remained on a Medicaid waiting list for community-based care because of the amount the state had to spend on the health care needs of the undocumented. Yet another witness claimed that the United States had become a "magnet" for chronically ill people who wanted to enter the country illegally to obtain services (US House Committee on Energy and Commerce 2006, 71, 78, 145).

Overall, the testimony had little to do with state Medicaid programs making errors by approving applications from illegal immigrants. Although Representative Dean justified the hearings with the claim that "document fraud" was "one of the biggest problems that we have in this country in every program," none of the testimony buttressed this claim (US House Committee on Energy and Commerce 2006, 45). Instead, the hearings focused on Medicaid costs for the undocumented that derived from providing occasional care to them in emergency rooms, or from the fact that some of the undocumented immigrants had children in the United States who, as citizens (because they were born here), qualified for Medicaid or CHIP.

In addition to nurturing a general sense of grievance against illegal immigrants, Deal and Nathan used the hearings to keep the heat on CMS to issue exacting regulations on documentation. The hearings represented the latest in a series of communications from House Republicans to the executive branch on the subject. For instance, key Republicans had protested when CMS indicated that it might permit states to accept signed affidavits from two blood relatives attesting to the applicant's claim of citizenship. CMS promptly retreated, and it began to allow such affidavits only in rare circumstances (*Inside CMS* 2006). At the hearings Representative Dean admonished the administrator of CMS to "stand firm" against pressures from advocacy groups to weaken the citizen documentation requirements (US House Committee on Energy and Commerce 2006, 3, 29).

Faced with a tight deadline established by Congress and continued pressure from House Republicans, CMS moved apace to develop an elaborate protocol for documentation. The agency published an interim rule in mid-2006 and a final regulation in 2007 (US Department of Health and Human Services 2007a). The new rule significantly increased the transaction costs for Medicaid applicants and enrollees seeking renewal. It insisted that they present a combination of original documents (no copies permitted), such as a passport, certificate of naturalization, or birth certificate. It also imposed new requirements on the children of illegal immigrants born after emergency room admissions. In the past, officials typically enrolled the newborns in Medicaid automatically. Now the parents would have to fill out a formal application and provide documents concerning citizenship and income for the child to be placed on Medicaid (Pear 2006). In these and other respects, the new federal requirements were far more exacting than those imposed by the four states that had long insisted upon citizen documentation (Boozang, Dutton, and Hudman 2006).

Most Medicaid administrators saw the new requirements as a costly administrative burden that would spill over to depress take-up rates for citizens. In a survey conducted in early 2007, twenty-two states reported declines in Medicaid enrollment due to the new rule (GAO 2007c, 4). For administrators in jurisdictions with high percentages of undocumented Hispanic citizens, the new requirements exacerbated the integrity challenge. Concerned not to experience a public relations nightmare if they extended benefits to the undocumented, many oriented their procedures toward avoiding false positive eligibility errors (Fossett and Thompson 2006).

Take-Up Rates as a Weapon against CHIP

The Improper Payments Information Act and congressional action against the undocumented immigrants presented new challenges for those committed to enhancing participation rates in Medicaid and CHIP. But neither represented signature initiatives of the Bush White House. As CHIP came up for reauthorization in 2007, however, presidential involvement increased dramatically. Take-up rates became an administrative weapon in the Bush administration's effort to reign in the middle-class creep of CHIP. State failure to do enough to foster Medicaid take-up became the justification for attacking CHIP.

As the time approached to reauthorize CHIP, it became apparent that the program had built supportive constituencies across the partisan divide. A significant push for expansion came from the governors. In late July 2007 the chair of the NGA, Tim Pawlenty (R-MN), indicated the "unanimous support" of that group "for a reasonable expansion of the program" (Pear 2007a, 2007b, 2007c). Arnold Schwarzenegger (R-CA) called for a $50 billion increase in CHIP over five years. Within Congress, Republican senator Orrin Hatch pledged to work again in bipartisan fashion with Senator Ted Kennedy (D-MA) and other Democrats to reauthorize and expand the program. The election of a Democratic majority to both houses of Congress in November 2006 further fueled momentum to expand CHIP.

But the Bush administration threw down the gauntlet. It supported a renewal of CHIP with an increase in funding so modest ($5 billion, one-tenth of what Schwarzenegger had proposed) that the Congressional Budget Office projected that enrollment in the program would decline (Pear 2007d). In addition to belated concerns about the mounting federal deficit, a kind of domino theory linked to conservative ideology drove presidential opposition. The White House sensed that a significant CHIP expansion that extended eligibility up the income ladder would fuel the program's progress in building a politically potent, middle-class constituency; it would thereby whet the public's appetite for government health insurance. Hence the White House worked to transform the debate over CHIP from a pragmatic give-and-take over how best to insure more children into a test of whether the country was on the road to "government-run health care" for all that would feature "a single-payer health care system with rationing and price controls" (Pear 2007a, 2007b, 2007d). During his last two years of office, President Bush vetoed congressional legislation to enlarge the program. Although significant numbers of Republicans joined them, the Democrats lacked the votes to override the vetoes.

The Bush administration's efforts to corral CHIP did not end with legislative vetoes. It also waged an offensive through the administrative process. The president had grown increasingly alarmed by the growing number of states seeking to extend coverage to children in families with incomes at 300 to 400 percent of the poverty line under the existing CHIP. To counter this middle-class drift in eligibility, the Bush administration decided to deny states' requests for amendments to their plans that would increase eligibility. In this vein CMS turned down proposals from such diverse states as Louisiana, New York, Ohio, and Oklahoma to expand coverage beyond 250 percent of the poverty line (Pear 2008). Beyond blocking states through the state plan amendment process, the Bush administration sought to employ a rarely used administrative device to roll back CHIP. In August 2007 CMS instructed states that they must achieve a take-up rate of 95 percent for children living below 200 percent of the poverty line in order to receive a federal match under CHIP to cover children beyond the 250 percent line. The states had one year to comply.

In taking this action the Bush administration skirted laws designed to foster deliberation and due process in the exercise of executive discretion. Because Congress was sensitive to the power that administrators might accrue, it had passed the Administrative Procedures Act in 1946. This policy structured a decision-making process for agencies when they officially interpreted a statute. Among other things, the act called upon these agencies to issue a notice of proposed rulemaking and offer opportunities for stakeholders and the public to comment. When issuing a final rule, agencies had to summarize these comments for the public record and provide a rationale for why they accepted certain suggestions and rejected others. The Bush administration found these procedures unappealing as a vehicle for curbing CHIP. Adherence to the Administrative Procedures Act would open the door to prolonged and extensive comments from opponents of the change. It might take more than a year to issue a final rule. Rather than endure this protracted process, CMS simply sent a letter to all Medicaid directors announcing the 95 percent take-up target for low-income children. CMS frequently uses official letters to provide guidance to the states on Medicaid. But up to this point it had not employed them to announce major administrative reinterpretations of the law.

The Bush directive had major implications for the states. When CMS issued the letter in the summer of 2007, fourteen states extended CHIP to children from families with incomes above 250 percent of the poverty line. Eleven more had passed legislation to cover this cohort but had yet to obtain federal approval for the expansion (Ryan and Mojerie 2008, 5). In theory states could insure these children if they achieved the 95 percent take-up rate for those below 200 percent of the poverty line. But state officials viewed this target as mission impossible. State-specific, calibrated data on take-up rates for children do not exist, but were generally understood to be well below 90 percent for low-income children (Confessore 2007). Medicaid administrators knew that they had no feasible way to reshape the enrollment labyrinth to achieve the take-up target that CMS had established. If the directive stood, it would for all practical purposes slam the door on federal subsidies for CHIP enrollees above 250 percent of the poverty line.

State officials fought back. A top Medicaid administrator in New Jersey, which had extended eligibility for CHIP to people living at 350 percent of the poverty line, said she "was horrified" by the Bush initiative and warned "it will cause havoc with our program and jeopardize coverage for thousands of children" (Pear 2007c). In early October 2007 Governor Eliot Spitzer (D-NY) announced that his state would join six others in filing a lawsuit to stop federal implementation of the directive (Kershaw 2007). Democratic members of Congress also denounced the Bush initiative and questioned its legality. In May 2008 the GAO (2008a) testified before Congress that the Bush administration had failed to comply with the requirements of the Administrative Procedures Act when it announced the take-up target.

Faced with these stiff political headwinds and the possibility of adverse court action, the Bush administration retreated. In early May 2008 CMS sent another letter to state Medicaid directors affirming that CHIP would continue to subsidize children from families with incomes above 250 percent of the poverty line so long as they remained continuously enrolled (Ryan and Mojerie 2008, 5). In August CMS announced that states unable to demonstrate a 95 percent take-up rate would not be penalized at this time. The Obama administration promptly killed the Bush initiative when it took office in January 2009.

State Responses to the Take-Up Challenge

The Clinton push to enhance take-up and the policy eddies set in motion during the Bush administration buffeted the states' efforts to enroll children in Medicaid and CHIP. In the face of these and other contending pressures, how much effort did the states exert to boost take-up? Three kinds of evidence cast light on the implementation vigor that the states achieved: (1) the degree to which the states managed to spend their CHIP grants rather than return money to the federal Treasury for reallocation; (2) the extent to which the states adopted best practices in managing enrollment processes; and (3) the degree to which data on take-up rates, enrollment, and insurance among children point to progress.

Did States Spend Their Grants?

In his seminal study of Italian governance, the political scientist Robert Putnam (1993) used the ability of regional governments to spend the money that the central authorities gave them for various purposes as one indicator of their performance. On the whole, regions in the south of the country did worse than their northern counterparts on this and other measures. A similar empirical test can be applied to states under CHIP. Unlike Medicaid, CHIP apportioned a specific capped amount to a state each year. A state had three years to spend this allocation. To accomplish this objective, a state had to find enough eligible enrollees and commit enough of its own revenues to draw down its entire CHIP grant (given its match rate). Failure to do so meant that the unspent federal monies would return to the federal government for redirection to states that had spent their CHIP grant and wanted more funding. Hence the question naturally presents itself: Did the states marshal the will and capacity to spend their grants?

Table 3.1 indicates how well jurisdictions did in this use-it-or-lose-it competition by examining the number of years a state had to return unspent CHIP funds to the federal government from 2001 through 2007.[21] The table divides the states into four categories based on this metric: pacesetters (zero to one year of returning CHIP monies), solid performers (two to three years), slow performers (four to five years), and stragglers (six to seven years). Two primary conclusions emerge from the table. First, most states did not get out of the starting blocks rapidly but over time learned how to spend their allocations. Overall, twenty-seven states failed to spend their CHIP allotment in four or more of the seven years. But states' performance on this measure improved over time. In the 2001–4 window, thirty-nine states returned money to the federal treasury at least twice. In the 2005–7 period, only twelve did. Second, states vary considerably on this measure of implementation vigor. The ten pacesetter states consistently managed to use up their grants and thereby garner transfers from less efficacious states. Six of the pacesetters are in the Northeast and Mid-Atlantic regions and had significant traditions of high Medicaid expenditures per poor person. At the opposite end of the continuum, twelve stragglers repeatedly struggled to spend their entire CHIP grants. Seven of them never managed to do so, from 2001 through 2007.

No parsimonious explanation for the states' variations on this measure of implementation vigor readily emerges. In some instances, the ability of states to manage the marketing, integrity, and fragmentation challenges of take-up probably mattered greatly. But explanatory factors other than administrative prowess in dealing with these challenges also played a role. In this regard, states could better position themselves to spend their grants if they simply made more people eligible. For instance, New Jersey as a pacesetter not only established the highest eligibility level for children living at 350 percent of the poverty line; it also obtained a federal waiver to cover adults under CHIP. Of the seven states with CHIP waivers to insure adults, three were pacesetters (Rhode Island and Wisconsin, in addition to New Jersey) and two (Arizona and Minnesota) were solid performers.[22] Whatever the precise explanatory forces at play, one cannot credibly claim that the failure of some states to spend their grants flowed from a lack of uninsured children. Virtually all states had significant numbers of low-income children who could qualify for Medicaid and CHIP. Two straggler states, New Mexico and Texas, had some of the highest rates of uninsured children in the country.

The Adoption of Best Practices

A second indicator of implementation vigor centers on a state's willingness to adopt widely endorsed best practices for Medicaid and CHIP enrollment. Notions about the virtues of these practices seldom emanate from the findings of rigorous social science research.[23] Instead, they spring from commonsense hypotheses

Table 3.1 Number of Years States Failed to Spend Their Entire CHIP Grant, 2001–7

State	*2001–4*	*2005–7*	*Total*
Pacesetters			
Alaska	0	0	0
Kentucky	0	0	0
Maine	0	0	0
Maryland	0	0	0
Massachusetts	0	0	0
New York	0	0	0
Rhode Island	0	0	0
New Jersey	1	0	1
North Carolina	1	0	1
Wisconsin	1	0	1
Solid performers			
Kansas	2	0	2
Minnesota	2	0	2
Mississippi	2	0	2
Missouri	2	0	2
South Carolina	1	1	2
West Virginia	2	0	2
Arizona	3	0	3
Florida	3	0	3
Georgia	3	0	3
Indiana	2	1	3
Nebraska	3	0	3
Pennsylvania	3	0	3
South Dakota	3	0	3
Slow performers			
Alabama	4	0	4
Illinois	4	0	4
Iowa	4	0	4
Louisiana	4	0	4
Michigan	4	0	4
Montana	4	0	4
Ohio	4	0	4
Arkansas	4	1	5
California	4	1	5
Colorado	4	1	5
Hawaii	4	1	5
North Dakota	4	1	5
Oklahoma	4	1	5
Virginia	4	1	5
Wyoming	4	1	5
Stragglers			
Idaho	4	2	6
New Hampshire	4	2	6
Oregon	4	2	6
Utah	4	2	6

Table 3.1 Number of Years States Failed to Spend Their Entire CHIP Grant, 2001–7

State	*2001–4*	*2005–7*	*Total*
Vermont	4	2	6
Connecticut	4	3	7
Delaware	4	3	7
Nevada	4	3	7
New Mexico	4	3	7
Tennessee	4	3	7
Texas	4	3	7
Washington	4	3	7

Note: A state has three years to spend an annual CHIP grant before the remaining funds are redirected to other states.

Sources: The 2001–6 data come from US Government Accountability Office (GAO 2007a, figure 9). Data for 2007 are from the Centers for Medicare and Medicaid Services, "Notice 72," *Federal Register* 102 (May 29, 2007): 29502–13, table 1, at 29511.

about factors that maximize outreach and reduce the transaction costs of application and renewal processes for those seeking benefits. No data set exists that comprehensively tracks the full range of preferred take-up practices. But the Kaiser Commission on Medicaid and the Uninsured routinely surveys states on a subset of them (e.g., Ross and Marks 2009). These surveys enable us to make some assessment of where states stand in adopting client-friendly enrollment practices.

Table 3.2 assays this subset as of 2009. The table's left-hand column lists twelve practices conducive to take-up. On balance, the table presents a mixed picture of states' progress in removing barriers to enrollment. To be sure, some steps have proven very popular. Nearly all states have abandoned asset tests and eliminated face-to-face interviews for both application and renewal. Most have adopted a joint application form for Medicaid and CHIP. Forty-one states refrain from premiums for the poor, and twenty-six do so for those people living below 151 percent of the poverty line. (Considerable evidence suggests that premiums discourage enrollment.)[24]

But the states have been more reluctant to adopt other client-friendly enrollment procedures. One way to trim transaction costs for beneficiaries is to reduce the frequency of eligibility reviews once they enroll. Historically, many states required Medicaid recipients to reapply every six months and admonished them to promptly report any changes in income that would make them ineligible for benefits. These practices fueled a churning of Medicaid enrollees where children and others lost coverage for certain periods. To reduce this churning, take-up advocates recommend that children be given continuous eligibility for twelve months regardless of any shifts in family income. Although thirty states have adopted this practice for CHIP, only eighteen have done so for Medicaid. In part out of a con-

Table 3.2 States Employing Client-Friendly Take-Up Practices for Medicaid and CHIP, 2009 (not including DC)

<table>
<tr><th></th><th colspan="2">No. of States</th></tr>
<tr><th>Practice</th><th>Medicaid</th><th>CHIP*</th></tr>
<tr><td>Initial enrollment</td><td></td><td></td></tr>
<tr><td>No face-to-face interview[a]</td><td>47</td><td>38</td></tr>
<tr><td>No asset test[a]</td><td>46</td><td>36</td></tr>
<tr><td>No income verification[b]</td><td>11</td><td>10</td></tr>
<tr><td>12-month continuous eligibility for children[c]</td><td>18</td><td>30</td></tr>
<tr><td>Presumptive eligibility for children[a]</td><td>14</td><td>9</td></tr>
<tr><td>Joint application for Medicaid and CHIP[a]</td><td colspan="2">35</td></tr>
<tr><td>No uninsured period required for enrollment[d]</td><td colspan="2">15</td></tr>
<tr><td>No premiums required below 101% of the federal poverty line[e]</td><td colspan="2">41</td></tr>
<tr><td>No premiums required below 151% of the federal poverty line[e]</td><td colspan="2">26</td></tr>
<tr><td>Renewal</td><td></td><td></td></tr>
<tr><td>No face-to-face interview[f]</td><td>48</td><td>38</td></tr>
<tr><td>No income verification[b]</td><td>12</td><td>11</td></tr>
<tr><td>Joint renewal form[c]</td><td colspan="2">21</td></tr>
</table>

Note: Where there are no separate Medicaid/CHIP boxes, we could not distinguish between them.

*A total of thirty-nine states had separate CHIP programs in the period during which these data were collected.

[a]*Source:* Ross and Marks (2009, table 5, 35–37).

[b]*Source:* Ross and Marks (2009, table 6, 38).

[c]*Source:* Ross and Marks (2009, table 7, 41).

[d]*Source:* Ross and Marks (2009, table 2, 27). States are allowed to have waiting periods in CHIP-funded Medicaid expansions with a waiver.

[e]*Source:* Ross and Marks (2009, table 10, 54).

[f]*Source:* Ross and Marks (2009, table B, 19–20; table 9, 49).

cern with avoiding false positive eligibility errors, the states have also been reluctant to rely exclusively on applicants' statements of income. Only one-fifth of the states do not require income verification in application and renewal processes for Medicaid and CHIP. Presumptive eligibility refers to the practice of provisionally enrolling children in Medicaid or CHIP while awaiting a final decision on applicant eligibility. Only a few states have adopted this practice.

Though not reported in table 3.2, the number of states adopting various client-friendly practices increased during the last decade (Ross and Marks 2009, 19). But backsliding occurred at times, especially in recessions. Grappling with the economic downturn of the early 2000s, for instance, Texas reduced its continuous enrollment coverage from twelve to six months. The state of Washington did the same. During the same period Wisconsin increased the documentation requirements for eligibility (Ross and Marks 2009, 4). Beyond application and renewal processes, states may also adjust marketing practices. When Florida found its enrollment growing faster than state officials preferred, they eliminated outreach funding. In these and other ways, some states have attempted to manage enrollment growth by tinkering with take-up practices (GAO 2007a, 34).

The Bottom Line

Data on take-up rates, program enrollments, and the insurance status of children provide a third lens through which to view Medicaid's durability. On balance, this evidence points to considerable progress in covering children. Estimates of participation rates by children in Medicaid and CHIP vary and are not routinely available on a state-by-state basis.[25] But various analyses point to progress. Medicaid take-up of qualified children rose from an estimated 72 percent in 1996 to more than 80 percent toward the end of the Bush administration. The participation rate for CHIP in turn grew from about 45 percent in 1998 (the year after Congress approved the program) to nearly 80 percent during the Bush years (Selden, Hudson, and Banthin 2004, 45; Kenney, Cook, and Dubay 2009, 3). Given Medicaid's enrollment labyrinth and the complexities of managing eligibility for a means-tested program, it remains unclear how much higher administrators can elevate the take-up rate.

Not surprisingly, rising take-up rates helped fuel growth in the number of children enrolled in Medicaid and CHIP. By 2008 Medicaid insured more than 29 million nondisabled children, an increase of more than 50 percent since 1992. Meanwhile, separate CHIP initiatives covered another 5 million.[26] The climbing enrollments of children in Medicaid and CHIP, along with the erosion of private health insurance, helped boost the share of the nation's children with public health insurance from 21 percent in 1997 to 34 percent in 2008.[27]

This growth in public coverage helped slim the ranks of uninsured children—from 13 percent in 1990, to 12 percent in 2000, to just under 10 percent in 2008. In contrast, the proportion of adults under sixty-five years of age without insurance grew from 17 percent in 1990 to more than 20 percent in 2008.[28] The insurance fortunes of children living at or below 200 percent of the poverty line (a group especially targeted by Medicaid and CHIP) also improved. The proportion of uninsured children below this income level dropped from 24 percent in 1999 to about 17 percent in 2008. Forty-five states witnessed declines in this measure, with eleven states having uninsurance rates for this cohort of less than 10 percent by 2008.[29] Some states made dramatic progress. The proportion of low-income children without insurance fell by more than 50 percent in six states, with Arkansas, Connecticut, and Indiana leading the way.

Although trend data on uninsured children point to progress, the limits to the states' capacity and commitment in dealing with the enrollment labyrinth also deserve to be noted. Of all children who remained uninsured in 2008, about two-thirds met the qualifications to be enrolled in Medicaid or CHIP (Kenney, Cook, and Dubay 2009, 3). Moreover, some states lag well behind others. As of 2008 the proportion of children living at or below 200 percent of the poverty line without insurance continued to exceed 20 percent in nine states; two of the country's five most populous states, Florida and Texas, had the worst rates, at 30 percent and 29 percent, respectively.

Breakthrough: CHIP Expansion

The 2008 election restored control of the presidency and both houses of Congress to the Democrats for the first time since 1993–94. Their victory broke the political logjam on CHIP and a year later led to passage of major health reform. Both events possessed significant implications for the ongoing quest to insure children.

The Democrats in Congress—no longer worried about a presidential veto, and seeking to establish momentum through some early wins—passed legislation reauthorizing CHIP by the end of January 2009. About a quarter of the Republicans in each house of Congress joined the Democrats in supporting the measure (Pear 2009). President Obama signed the bill into law on February 4, less than a month after taking office. The new legislation authorized $69 billion for CHIP for the 2009–13 period, more than double the funds that had previously been available to the states for the program (Kaiser Commission on Medicaid and the Uninsured 2009f). As in the past, the CHIP allotments to particular states would over time depend on a use-it-or-lose-it competition, with the more committed and capable states capturing funds from jurisdictions that failed to spend their grants. But unlike prior practice, laggard states would face a permanent decrease in their future CHIP allotments if they returned unspent money to the federal treasury.[30] Under the original program, the allocation formula did not penalize states in this way.

The CHIP reauthorization repudiated the view of the Bush administration that the program ought to focus on families with incomes less than 250 percent of the poverty line. Instead, the legislation permitted states to extend eligibility to 300 percent of the poverty line; moreover, it provided flexibility for states seeking to cover children above this income level to do so, albeit at a lower match rate.[31] The extension of CHIP benefits toward the middle class sparked strong objection from Republicans. Many of them feared that CHIP would become a Trojan horse for broader efforts to expand public health insurance. As Senator John McCain (R-AZ) put it, the bill should be seen as an effort "to eliminate, over time, private insurance in America" (Pear 2009).

The new law promised more enrollment growth for CHIP than for Medicaid because most states preferred to operate separate, capped programs. But it did not ignore Medicaid. To the contrary, it took aim at the take-up defects that had kept many qualified low-income children from Medicaid enrollment. In a sense the bill paid homage to the concerns of the Bush administration that many states had been more eager to expand eligibility to the middle class than surmount participation barriers for poor children. The new legislation proposed three initiatives to enhance participation rates. First, it authorized $100 million in funding for outreach. The Department of Health and Human Services would use 10 percent of these funds to wage a national enrollment campaign. The rest of the monies would go to state and local governments as well as other organizations (e.g., community-based groups) that submitted successful grant proposals to conduct outreach.

Second, the bill established a performance bonus system to encourage take-up for Medicaid.[32] To qualify for the bonus, a state had to adopt at least five of the eight user-friendly enrollment practices designed to reduce the transaction costs for applicants. These included measures discussed above, such as continuous eligibility for twelve months, the elimination of asset tests and interviews, and joint application forms for Medicaid and CHIP. The bill also touted new initiatives, such as Express Lane eligibility, whereby a state could use enrollment in other means-tested public programs (e.g., school lunches, food stamps, and Head Start) to determine that a child met one or more of the eligibility criteria for Medicaid or CHIP.[33] Success in obtaining a bonus also required a state to show Medicaid enrollment gains for children.[34] In this vein a state had to *exceed* an annual enrollment target of 4 percent growth for children in Medicaid. Over time, this target declined to 2 percent (Kaiser Commission on Medicaid and the Uninsured 2009b, 2009c, 2009d).

Third, Congress attempted to reduce some of the take-up burdens on states posed by initiatives to screen out illegal immigrants and implement PERM. In reauthorizing CHIP Congress responded to strong public sentiment against benefits for illegal immigrants by imposing citizen documentation requirements on CHIP applicants for the first time. To soften the impact, however, the law made it easier for applicants to prove their citizenship. Above all, it allowed Medicaid and CHIP to establish a data exchange with the federal government. Under this system, states submit the Social Security numbers of applicants to the Social Security Administration, which then informs state officials whether its records show that the applicant is a citizen. This initiative promised to pare the paperwork applicants had to provide to eligibility workers. The CHIP reauthorization also sought to tamp down prospects that concerns about eligibility errors and program waste would enervate the states' take-up efforts. It required CMS to issue new regulations on the PERM system to assure that the methods used to calculate error rates did not interfere with certain states' efforts to foster take-up (Horner et al. 2009, 12, 20).

Federal policymakers hoped that these steps, along with new funding for outreach and the performance bonus system, would boost participation rates for children. But before they could fully implement the provisions, the passage of comprehensive health reform in March 2010 altered the playing field. In November 2009 the House of Representatives passed legislation that would have repealed CHIP. Children eligible for CHIP in families with incomes above 150 percent of the poverty line would instead obtain subsidized coverage from the newly created health insurance exchanges. The remaining CHIP enrollees would move to Medicaid. The Senate, however, preferred to sustain CHIP, and it ultimately prevailed. Chapter 6 describes the role that CHIP continues to play under the ACA.

Implications for the Program's Durability

The policy developments assessed in this chapter have significant implications for Medicaid's durability. Four observations seem particularly pertinent. First, the distancing of Medicaid from stigmatization as welfare medicine strengthened the program. The passage of welfare reform in 1996, the approval of CHIP a year later, and the steady implementation of the Waxman mandates meant that growing proportions of nondisabled Medicaid enrollees under the age of sixty-five years were from working families. Eligibility for Medicaid became increasingly delinked from being on welfare. For its part CHIP helped legitimize Medicaid as the platform for its efforts to reach toward the middle class by offering coverage to children in families with incomes two, three, and even four times the poverty line. Moreover, CHIP's popularity enhanced take-up rates for Medicaid because states had to screen children for Medicaid eligibility before enrolling them in CHIP.

Second, much of the period featured growing, often bipartisan, support for expanding public insurance for children from the NGA and other elements of the intergovernmental lobby. This represented a marked change from the years before President Clinton. Throughout the 1980s the states had faced a steady barrage of unfunded, if incremental, Medicaid mandates. Forty-nine governors (including the then–governor of Arkansas, Bill Clinton) worked through the NGA to protest this development. Their resentment prompted many governors to join in Speaker Gingrich's failed attempt to convert Medicaid into a block grant in the mid-1990s. If Congress had persisted with unfunded mandates, Medicaid would have risked losing the support of this valuable constituency. But the 1990s and early 2000s featured much greater deference to the views of the states' policymakers. The Clinton administration's waiver initiatives and the Republican capture of Congress did much to propel devolution within the federal system. The passage of CHIP vividly illustrates this point. The governors fended off the efforts of some in Congress to cover more children by expanding Medicaid. Instead, they effectively pressed the case that the states should determine the vehicle for greater coverage. This could be a Medicaid expansion under CHIP or a new, separate program. CHIP became increasingly popular among the governors. When it came up for reauthorization in 2007, it elicited their bipartisan support. Gubernatorial commitment to the program helped prompt a significant minority of Republicans in Congress to support the bill.

Opposition from many governors also helped thwart the Bush administration's effort to curb CHIP expansions to higher-income families. When the federal government ordered the states to achieve an unattainable 95 percent take-up rate for lower-income children so as to extend CHIP to children living above 250 percent of poverty, many governors complained. Some joined in a suit against federal officials. Their opposition, along with that of others, prompted the White House and CMS to abandon attempts to roll back CHIP eligibility.

To be sure, catering to gubernatorial preferences for CHIP came at some cost to Medicaid. If Congress had covered more children through a Medicaid expansion rather than CHIP, it would have avoided creating yet another administrative silo to compound the complexities of the enrollment labyrinth. It would have shunned waiting lists and reinforced the right of children to health insurance. The actions of governors and other state-level policymakers with respect to CHIP reinforces the point that they are generally much more supportive of Medicaid as a fiscal entitlement for the states than as a service entitlement for enrollees. Thus, the political support that governors often provide Medicaid involves trade-offs related to the program's durability.

Third, the quest to insure more children highlights the particular problem of lagging large states in the quest to achieve national goals via intergovernmental grants. The states varied greatly in their commitment and capacity with respect to Medicaid and CHIP. Some were much more inclined than others to extend eligibility beyond the minimum floor set by the federal government. The states also differed greatly in their implementation vigor. Some wound up looking the federal gift horse in the mouth. They could not get their CHIP monies spent and returned dollars to the federal bureaucracy to be reallocated to competing states. Some states moved much more aggressively than others to adopt best take-up practices and master the enrollment labyrinth. Given the differences among the states in their political cultures, institutions, proclivities, and capabilities, one would expect state take-up rates for CHIP and Medicaid to vary appreciably. Nor should one be surprised that the rates of uninsured children living below 200 percent of the poverty line varied from the single digits in some states to 30 percent in others. The problem of lagging large states arises when the most populous jurisdictions demonstrate less commitment, capacity, or both in implementing a federal program. The actions of these states disproportionately affect whether a grant program has a significant impact on some national problem. Chapter 6 probes this issue in the context of two such states—Florida and Texas.

Finally, Medicaid's experience illustrates that the implementation of a means-tested health policy in the context of American federalism presents a persistent challenge to program durability. It makes the program more susceptible to subterranean erosion. Basing benefits on income and assets means that both administrators and potential beneficiaries face a moving target. Whether people qualify to be enrolled fluctuates over time with their financial well-being. This leads to the construction of complicated administrative systems to process and monitor the eligibility of individuals. The demands on these systems would be less if the public and policymakers had a high tolerance for false positive eligibility errors. That way, administrators could in more single-minded fashion dedicate themselves to establishing and maintaining user-friendly take-up practices. But concerns about fighting fraud, waste, and abuse make enrollment management a balancing act—a struggle to minimize the trade-off between reducing false positives and false negatives. To further complicate matters, policymakers at times send sharp signals that they want eligibility workers to assign importance to criteria unrelated to income—in the case of Medicaid, to the documentation of citizenship.

The enormous administrative fragmentation fueled by American federalism magnifies the take-up challenge. Turning the system around becomes more difficult. It means that even top-level officials can seldom rely on hierarchical authority to spur change; instead, hortatory, negotiating, and other skills related to network design and management become pivotal. The transaction costs of change increase.

Although means-testing heightens the risk of erosion, this chapter shows that the concerted efforts of policymakers, administrators, and other stakeholders can galvanize improvement. Over time, most states learned how to spend their CHIP monies, and there was a considerable diffusion of best enrollment practices. Take-up rates went up, and the number of children without insurance went down. The guidance, stipulations, and incentive systems embedded in the law reauthorizing CHIP promise to enhance take-up still further. The health reform act of 2010 takes additional steps to streamline enrollment processes. But these actions will not solve the take-up challenge once and for all. More improvement will require key stakeholders to evince persistent commitment, vigilance, and acumen. They will need to care about something that policymakers chronically tend to slight: how to build the capacity for effective public administration.

Notes

1. The program has also at times carried the label of the State Children's Health Insurance Program, or SCHIP. To simplify matters, I use the acronym CHIP throughout.

2. Conservatives cited a study by two Harvard University professors estimating that at *any point in time* 65 percent of those on welfare would eventually be on the rolls for that long (Haskins 2006, 6). If, however, one considers all those who had been on AFDC for a given period (including many briefly receiving benefits who then left the rolls), this percentage would be smaller.

3. Specifically, Waxman took advantage of budget rules established by the Gramm-Rudman-Hollings deficit control act of 1985. In 1990 Congress replaced this law with the Budget Enforcement Act, which made it much harder to obscure the long-term costs of Medicaid mandates. For the details, see Gilman (1998, 130–33).

4. Data are from the *Current Population Survey* of the US Census Bureau; see www.census.gov/hhes/www/hlthins/historic/index_old.htmf.

5. Maintenance-of-effort provisions required states to preserve or expand their existing eligibility criteria for Medicaid.

6. CHIP also enlarged state discretion to impose premiums, deductibles, and copayments.

7. According to CMS, the Medicaid expansion states as of 2008 were Alaska, Hawaii, Maryland, Nebraska, New Mexico, and Ohio. All the data in this paragraph come from CMS.

8. Kenney, Haley, and Pelletier (2009, 12) found that more than 20 percent of uninsured low-income parents had not heard of Medicaid. Only 24 percent of the uninsured thought their children would be eligible for the program.

9. Estimating the effects of stigma is difficult. Stuber and Kronebusch (2004), for instance, found that certain perceptions of stigma reduced the propensity of low-income people to enroll in Medicaid. More recent surveys suggest that stigma may not significantly depress take-up. In this vein, Kenney, Haley, and Pelletier (2009, 8, 12) report that more than 80 percent of the uninsured and Medicaid enrollees see the program as very or somewhat good. More than 80 percent of the uninsured say they would try to enroll in Medicaid if someone told them they were eligible. The survey points to factors other than stigma that could undercut take-up. For instance, nearly half of the uninsured believe that "there is a place nearby that offers affordable medical care for people without health insurance." This perception could lead them to be less aggressive in seeking Medicaid coverage.

10. Social science research suggests they are right to be concerned. Cook and Barrett (1992, 121) found that public support for social programs declines when people believe they feature high levels of waste, fraud, and abuse or other manifestations of ineffectiveness.

11. In 2010 New York policymakers moved to reduce greatly the role of counties in Medicaid eligibility processes.

12. Although a large county role increases the complexity of managing enrollment, I know of no studies that systematically compare take-up rates in state-centered and county-centered implementation structures.

13. Hudson (2009, w698) notes that this often occurs because of a "stair step" profile whereby at certain family income levels younger children are eligible for Medicaid and the older ones for CHIP.

14. Studies by Kronebusch and Ebel (2004) as well as Hudson (2009) support this view; Wolfe and Scrivner (2005) in contrast conclude that separate CHIP programs reduced the probability of targeted children being uninsured. Kronebusch and Ebel as well as Wolfe and Scrivner use data from the *Current Population Survey* from the early 2000s. Hudson relies on data from the *Medical Expenditure Survey* from 1995 to 2005.

15. The law also targets reimbursement for ineligible services, duplicate payments, expenses for services not received, and payments that did not take into account applicable discounts.

16. This quotation comes from Wachino and Ross (2008, 19).

17. Efforts to restrict the access of the undocumented to Medicaid intersect with the broader issue of "membership" and equity in distributional policy. See Stone (2002, 42–43).

18. Perdue's strong support for the provision discouraged the NGA from taking a position on the issue. See Ku and Pervez (2010, 7, 12).

19. In 2006 Congress exempted certain Medicaid enrollees from these requirements including those on Medicare, certain Supplemental Security Income recipients, and children in foster care (Ku and Pervez 2010).

20. Representative Charles Norwood used the phrase "busting the bank" (US House Committee on Energy and Commerce 2006, 97).

21. It would also be useful to know the amount of funds a state returned. However, these data were not readily available.

22. These data come from CMS as of January 20, 2009. I considered only states that had at least 20,000 adult enrollees under a CHIP waiver as of fiscal 2007.

23. For research that more rigorously assesses the implications of different take-up practices, see, e.g., Kronebusch and Ebel (2004), Stuber and Kronebusch (2004), and Wolfe and Scrivner (2005).

24. See Kenney and Yee (2007) and Martin (2007). States may partly refrain from this practice because of the administrative burdens of collecting premiums.

25. The participation rate, or take-up rate, equals the number enrolled in a program who meet the eligibility criteria divided by the total number of individuals in an area who could meet the criteria for enrollment.

26. The data on Medicaid come from Kaiser State Health Facts, www.statehealthfacts.org/comparemaptable.jsp?ind=200&cat=4. According to CMS, CHIP covered an additional 2 million children through Medicaid extensions. These 2 million are included in Medicaid's enrollment data. Overall, CHIP enrollments approximated 7 million.

27. These data are from the National Health Interview Survey, table 1.2a, p. 5, www.cdc.gov/nchs/data/nhis/earlyrelease/200909_01.pdf. Though CHIP and Medicaid make up the lion's share of those covered, "public health insurance" also includes Medicare (for certain children with disabilities), other state-sponsored initiatives, and military plans.

28. These data come from the current population survey of the US Census Bureau, www.census.gov/www/hlthins/historic/index.html and www.census.gov/hehs/www/hlthins/historic/index_old.html.

29. To reduce errors due to limited sample size in smaller states, the Census Bureau relies on three-year averages. These data as well as those in the following paragraph are from www.census.gov/hhes/www/hlthins/liuc99.html and www.census.gov/hhes/www/hlthins/liuc08.xls.

30. A state could choose to receive 110 percent of what it had spent on CHIP in fiscal 2008, what it projected it would spend in 2009, or the allotment it had received (but not necessarily spent) in 2008. The law guaranteed that states would receive whatever allotment they chose in 2010 adjusted upward by health care inflation and child population growth within its borders. This meant that states receiving supplemental CHIP funds due to the failure of other states to spend their allotments could claim it as part of their baseline allocation. Under the new law states had two years to spend their allotments before having their base reduced for failure to spend the monies.

31. States receive the Medicaid rather than the more generous CHIP match rate for new expansions to children living above 300 percent of the poverty line (Horner et al. 2009, 3).

32. Congressional willingness to fund the bonuses remains an open question. Congress approved a $3.5 billion cut in CHIP performance bonuses for fiscal 2011 (Baker 2011).

33. See Kaiser Commission on Medicaid and the Uninsured (2009d). A state could also earn credit for three other practices. It could employ presumptive eligibility whereby a full eligibility decision occurs after enrollment. It could do administrative renewals such as drawing on income data available from other public records to renew automatically those who continued to be eligible. Finally, a state could launch a premium assistance program whereby it committed Medicaid or CHIP funds to certain group health and employer-sponsored coverage.

34. The initial baseline for establishing enrollment gains was July 2008. States that expand Medicaid eligibility for children after July 1, 2008, could count newly qualified children for bonus purposes the third year of implementation (Kaiser Commission on Medicaid and the Uninsured 2009c).

CHAPTER FOUR

Government by Waiver

The Quest to Transform Long-Term Care

In late April 2005 a House of Representatives subcommittee on health opened a hearing on the need to reform long-term care under Medicaid to contain its "spiraling costs."[1] In his opening remarks at the session, Representative Charles Norwood (R-GA) observed that "Medicaid . . . is quickly becoming a welfare program for middle-income families. With clever estate planning and asset protection schemes, individuals can qualify for Medicaid and receive long-term care at taxpayer's expense" (US House Committee on Energy and Commerce 2005, 5). Norwood's statement recognizes a point made in the first chapter: that long-term care has done much to create a middle-class constituency for Medicaid. In recognizing the contribution of long-term care to the program's durability, the needs of the elderly for nursing home care have appropriately drawn attention (e.g., Grogan and Patashnik 2003).

But it is important to reach beyond this focus in at least two ways. First, Medicaid also provides long-term care to people under sixty-five years of age with disabilities, many of whom come from middle-class backgrounds. This constituency includes the parents of children with intellectual or other developmental disabilities who see Medicaid as a lifeline when they cannot meet the needs of their offspring.[2] It encompasses those who have suffered severe accidents or related events leaving them paralyzed, cognitively damaged, or otherwise impaired. Some observers suggest that these and other congeries of people with disabilities provide Medicaid with political leverage that surpasses that generated by the elderly (Vladeck 2003).

Second, and of central concern to this chapter, Medicaid's durability stands to benefit from efforts to overcome the program's historic bias toward providing long-term care in nursing homes and other large institutions. This quest to rebalance Medicaid long-term care in the direction of HCBS occupied center stage from 1993 through 2010 and intersects with issues of Medicaid's durability in several ways. It has the potential to reinforce Medicaid's appeal to key constituencies. Many Americans have come to value the access that the program provides to nursing homes and other institutions. But HCBS tends to be more appealing to great numbers of them—especially people with disabilities. Many also see rebalancing toward HCBS as a step toward enhancing the appropriateness and the quality of long-term care services—a key bottom-line dimension for assessments of Medicaid's vitality. Rebalancing also affords an opportunity to plumb the implications of Medicaid waivers. While fueling the spread of HCBS, waivers have also eroded Medicaid as a formal legal entitlement. How can these competing developments be reconciled from the perspective of Medicaid's durability?

This chapter opens by assessing the particular challenges that Medicaid faces in serving the elderly and people with disabilities. The origins and nature of Medicaid's institutional bias with respect to each group receive attention. The chapter then traces the efforts of the Bill Clinton and George W. Bush administrations to encourage states to offer a greater share of long-term care services via HCBS, primarily through the unprecedented use of program waivers. It documents the appeal of this policy tool to federal and state officials. The chapter then assesses the way in which these program waivers facilitated vertical policy diffusion, as manifested by passage of the Deficit Reduction Act of 2005. This law reinforced the devolutionary thrust unleashed by the waivers. It ratified many practices that the states had adopted through them. The chapter then explicates the ways in which both the waivers and the Deficit Reduction Act have curbed the Medicaid entitlement. While expanding access to HCBS, federal and state policymakers have worked to limit the potential for an unmanageable surge in demand. The chapter concludes by examining the implications of these developments for an understanding of American federalism and Medicaid's durability. The increasing importance of executive branch action at both the federal and state levels comes under the microscope. So, too, does the paradoxical possibility that weakening the Medicaid entitlement enhances the program's growth.

Medicaid's Institutional Bias

As noted above, the elderly and people with disabilities absorb about two-thirds of Medicaid spending. Many of these enrollees have serious medical conditions, and Medicaid covers their expenses either directly or by paying Medicare's premiums, deductibles, and copayments (in the case of the dual eligibles). Much of the benefit that the elderly and people with disabilities receive from Medicaid, however, resides less in its coverage of conventional medical services than in its subsidy for long-term care. Such care gives them basic assistance with the activities of daily living. About one-third of all Medicaid dollars go to long-term care, with the bulk of these monies flowing to nursing homes and other institutions. States range from spending 15 percent of their Medicaid budgets on long-term care (New Mexico) to 64 percent (North Dakota).[3] Although the elderly and people with disabilities share an interest in Medicaid long-term care, they also differ in their specific perspectives and needs; ultimately, they compete with each other for Medicaid resources. These differences have occasionally surfaced even as the two cohorts have joined hands to fight Medicaid's institutional bias. Before probing the politics of HCBS, therefore, certain distinctive features of each group of beneficiaries and the institutions that serve them warrant attention.

The Elderly and the Nursing Home Complex

The vast majority of older Medicaid enrollees are dual eligibles, with Medicare subsidizing most of their acute care needs. Medicare, however, provides very limited long-term care, instead passing the ball to the states to provide these services. About half of all Medicaid dollars for enrollees from sixty-five to seventy-five years of age support long-term care; this expenditure share rises to nearly three-quarters for those recipients age seventy-five years and older (Holahan, Miller, and Rousseau 2009, 13). The chronic afflictions of older people range from severe, as with Alzheimer's disease and certain forms of dementia, to relatively minor, as with modest difficulties in walking. The reigning framework for assessing an individual's need for long-term care stresses the inability to perform certain "activities of daily living" (ADL) and other "instrumental activities of daily living" (IADL). ADLs consist of such basic functions as bathing, toileting, grooming, eating, and dressing. IADLs focus on whether an individual can use the telephone, do laundry, keep house, administer his or her own medications, and handle financial matters. The more ADL limitations a person has, the greater the likelihood that he or she will wind up in a nursing home. Sixty-five percent of those in nursing homes have three or more ADL limitations; another 17 percent have one to two (Miller and Mor 2006, 15).

Eligibility for Medicaid long-term care depends, of course, not only on ADLs and IADLs but also on income level. In this regard, there are multiple pathways to enrollment. If older people have few assets and low incomes (i.e., below 75 percent of the poverty line), they can qualify for the Supplemental Security Income program (SSI) (Holahan, Miller, and Rousseau 2009, 4). This status brings them the full package of Medicaid benefits. Most elderly people, however, have too much income to qualify for SSI because they receive Social Security. Moreover, Congress moved in 1996 to close the SSI gates to the parents of immigrants who had followed their children to the United States and received neither Social Security nor Medicare (Kaushal 2010). In part as a result of these factors, the elderly constitute less than 20 percent of the approximately 7.5 million SSI enrollees (US Social Security Administration 2009, 30). The states, however, possess considerable discretion to extend Medicaid coverage to low-income people other than via SSI. In the case of long-term care, many of them authorize eligibility for older people with ADL limitations who have incomes up to 300 percent of the requirement for SSI eligibility (a little above 200 percent of the poverty line). Elderly people may also qualify for Medicaid when they "spend down" to eligibility by paying for health care costs that Medicare does not cover. Many older Americans go on Medicaid after they enter a nursing home and deplete their savings. Most of the elderly do not have sufficient assets to pay for one year in a nursing home out of their own pockets (Miller and Mor 2006, 21).[4]

Medicaid's founding legislation mandated that states participating in the program cover nursing home care. This development spawned a rapid expansion of nursing home beds and the growth of for-profit nursing home chains in the late 1960s and early 1970s (Smith and Feng 2010, 32). As of the 2000s more than 15,800 nursing homes with some 1.7 million beds provided care; nearly all participated in Medicaid and Medicare (National Center for Health Statistics 2009, 407). Close to 70 percent of nursing home residents are on Medicaid, and the program accounts for more than 40 percent of all spending for care in these facilities (Kaiser Commission on Medicaid and the Uninsured 2011, 11). Hence, nursing home operators have a huge stake in federal and state policy concerning certification for participation in Medicaid, payment rates, and quality assurance. Although older people make up the great majority of Medicaid enrollees in nursing homes, these institutions also provide care to younger recipients with a range of disabilities.

Concerns about the quality of nursing home services have dogged Medicaid from the start. Many complained that these facilities basically functioned as debilitating warehouses for the elderly. Scandals have sporadically erupted involving gross abuse and neglect of nursing home residents along with fraud. In the period before 1987, the quality standards applied to these facilities tended to be minimal and inconsistent from one state to the next. In the widely read 1980 book *Unloving Care: The Nursing Home Tragedy*, Bruce Vladeck (who went on to head the Health Care Financing Administration under President Clinton) summed up concerns about these institutions. Though acknowledging the most egregious nursing home abuses, he concluded that these "may be less distressing in the aggregate . . . than the quality of life in the thousands that meet the minimal public standards of adequacy. In these, residents live out the last of their days in an enclosed society without privacy, dignity, or pleasure, subsisting on minimally palatable diets, multiple sedatives, and large doses of television—eventually dying, one suspects, at least partially of boredom" (p. 4).

Concerns about quality eventually prompted Congress to forge an elaborate system of regulation and report cards for nursing homes in 1987. As a result, facilities participating in Medicaid and Medicare must meet basic standards of adequacy, as measured for 188 items clustered into 17 domains (e.g., dietary services, rehabilitation). States regularly conduct inspections to assure compliance, and the federal government posts nursing home deficiency ratings on a website. This regulatory system has in all probability improved the quality of care. But it has not vanquished concerns. A significant minority of facilities (about 5 percent by official federal estimates) continue to score poorly. Some states—such as Arkansas, Indiana, and Oklahoma—harbor higher proportions of low-quality facilities than others (GAO 2009b, 13, 15). Furthermore, nursing homes where Medicaid enrollees make up a higher percentage of residents tend to have more deficiencies (Amirkhanyan, Kim, and Lambright 2008). These lingering problems, along with the desire of the elderly to remain in their own homes or in assisted living, have kept up the pressure to expand HCBS.

Advocates for the elderly possess considerable political muscle with which to pursue their Medicaid objectives. For starters, they tend to benefit from a positive social construction. To be sure, the 1980s witnessed the ascendance of the "greedy geezer" image, with claims that older people siphoned off the lion's share of government budgets at the expense of the young. But even in its heyday complaints about intergenerational inequity more readily targeted the affluent, healthy elderly than those with low incomes in need of nursing care. By the 1990s this negative construction of the elderly became less common in public discourse. As noted in chapter 2, President Clinton and other Democrats fended off the Gingrich initiative to convert Medicaid into a block grant in part by framing the program as a vital lifeline for deserving older people. It was no accident that the president used a nursing home in Colorado as the setting for one forum to denounce the Gingrich proposal. The positive construction of the elderly persists. As one witness framed it at a congressional hearing in 2005, it is wrong to enact Medicaid changes that would "harm (the) countless number of older Americans who have worked all their lives, paid taxes, and have never been on public assistance" (US Senate Special Committee on Aging 2005, 34). This positive social construction also extends to the spouses of those in nursing homes. Medicaid law does not insist that they impoverish themselves and sell their homes to enable their husbands or wives to meet Medicaid eligibility criteria for long-term care.

Various interest groups promote the interests of Medicaid's elderly. AARP (formerly the American Association of Retired Persons) has, for instance, focused attention on long-term care for the elderly and backed the expansion of HCBS. On balance, however, AARP and other advocates for older people tend to be less vigorous in state policy processes than those speaking for people with disabilities.[5] A stakeholder in Minnesota noted, for instance, that AARP's support for HCBS had morphed into one targeted on expanding assisted living.[6] Another noted that many of the elderly in that state (especially those in rural areas) took a dim view of HCBS because they did not want a "stranger" coming into their homes.[7] On occasion, particular proposals prompt AARP to mobilize. In Minnesota, for instance, AARP fought a legislative proposal that threatened Medicaid payment rates to nursing homes for fear that it would trigger a decline in the quality of services. In this instance, AARP rallied local chapters to contact legislators and took out radio ads.[8] But at the state level, these kinds of AARP initiatives appear to be rare. To a substantial degree, lobbyists for nursing homes carry the ball for the elderly in state policy processes. They tend to be muted about HCBS, though some have branched out into providing such care. But they persistently stress the importance of Medicaid as one important avenue to long-term care for older people; they have championed increases in Medicaid payment rates to nursing homes.

People with Disabilities and the "Institutional Gulag"

The disabilities recognized by Medicaid assume countless forms, but five general clusters deserve note: (1) individuals with intellectual and such developmental disabilities as epilepsy, cerebral palsy, and autism; (2) people who suffer traumatic brain injuries or otherwise become incapacitated because of accidents or related events; (3) the mentally ill; (4) those with acute impairment of vision or hearing; and (5) people with AIDS (Crowley and O'Malley 2006).

This categorization does not mean that crisp medical definitions of disability exist. To the contrary, attempts at definition often expose sharp and heated philosophical differences. Historically, determinations of disability for adults have primarily rested not just on clinical judgments of an individual's infirmities but also on his or her ability to work.[9] Not surprisingly, therefore, applications for and enrollments in social programs for the disabled frequently increase in hard economic times when unemployment rises.[10] More recently, however, the disability rights movement has espoused a more basic and encompassing conceptualization of disability under the banner of individual empowerment. This view incorporates but goes far beyond the ability to work. It focuses on the fit between impairments and the broader "social, attitudinal, architectural, medical, economic, and political" fabric of society (Zola 1989, 401). For the disability rights movement, prejudicial attitudes, exclusionary practices, and the failure to invest adequate resources to reshape the physical environment (e.g., for transportation and architecture) do more to define "disability" within society than the physical or mental impairments of individuals per se (Skotch 1989, 380). For instance, "neurodiversity" advocates argue that efforts to remedy certain repetitive behaviors among children with autism at times miss the mark and should be redirected toward broadening societal definitions of "normal" behavior. Although the laws governing disability determinations for Medicaid rest on a much narrower, conventional notion, the more all-encompassing perspective of the disability rights movement has reinforced pressures for "independent living" and Medicaid-provided HCBS.

Uncertainties about disability do not end with its conceptualization. Even when laws go out of their way to crystallize standards and criteria for disability, eligibility determinations typically require complex, subjective judgments (Mashaw

1983). Most of the approximately 6.3 million people with disabilities who qualify for Medicaid do so by becoming eligible for the SSI program. The Social Security Administration has faced considerable oversight and constant second-guessing in its management of SSI enrollment (US Social Security Administration 2009, 30). The GAO has issued numerous reports exhorting SSI administrators to hone enrollment processes to reduce eligibility errors (e.g., GAO 1998, 1999). Political principals vacillate between actions designed to keep "cheats" off the rolls and concern that the agency has gone overboard in trimming them—efforts that often spark intense resistance from their constituents and fuel bad publicity (e.g., Derthick 1990). Though subject to much less oversight, state Medicaid officials face similar uncertainties when they make eligibility determinations for applicants with incomes too high for SSI. States vary greatly in the eligibility criteria they use to determine disability for purposes of Medicaid coverage (Kasper, Lyons, and O'Malley 2007, 2). Efforts to develop and enforce more objective criteria for disability status typically come up short. Ultimately, disability tends to become a "catchall bucket" into which officials can classify all sorts of people "who have real needs for which it is difficult or too uncomfortable to hold them personally accountable" (Vladeck 2003, 93). The indeterminacy and flexibility of the disability category make it vulnerable to external forces for expansion. It is no surprise, for instance, that with each edition of *The Diagnostic and Statistical Manual of Mental Disorders*, the official guidebook for mental health professionals, the list of potentially disabling conditions grows (Carey 2010).

A strong institutional bias in responding to people with disabilities had existed long before Medicaid. State institutions to house the mentally ill and those with intellectual disabilities date back to the nineteenth century. These large public facilities persisted into the twentieth century and sporadically underwent significant growth spurts. In the midst of the baby boom that followed World War II, for instance, many professionals counseled parents that they should place a retarded child in an institution in order to preserve the well-being of their families. Some physicians expressed frustration that inadequate space in state facilities for the intellectually disabled was contributing to family breakdowns. In response, states such as New York began to lift their earlier prohibitions on admitting infants and toddlers to these institutions (Trent 1994, 241–42). By the 1960s, however, housing the disabled in these large state complexes had fallen out of favor. Exposés of the neglect and abuse of residents at many state facilities, such as Willowbrook in New York, encouraged this trend. But the growing distaste for these large facilities did not lead federal policymakers to use Medicaid as a vehicle for deinstitutionalization. Instead, Congress responded in 1971 by giving states a Medicaid option to serve the developmentally disabled in another kind of large public institution: intermediate care facilities for the mentally retarded (ICF/MRs). States choosing this option would have the opportunity to obtain the federal Medicaid match for services they had previously funded out of their own resources. In exchange, they would need to submit to more federal oversight. Among other things, the new ICF/MRs would need to meet certain minimum federal standards for a safe environment, the employment of qualified professionals, and the active treatment of their residents.

Most states responded favorably to the federal invitation to create a new class of public institutions. By the time President Clinton took office, forty-two states housed some 62,000 developmentally disabled individuals in 434 large public institutions certified as ICF/MRs (GAO 1996). Many of these facilities were upgrades of the older institutions that had fallen out of favor. New Jersey, for example, served more than 400 people with intellectual and other disabilities at a 257-acre facility in Vineland. The state had established this institution in 1888, and one of its early superintendents had been a national leader in the movement to sterilize the mentally retarded and segregate them from the general population (Trent 1994, 175). The ICF/MRs have generally escaped high-profile scandals and the litigation that affected their predecessors. But concerns persist about the quality of services they provide. As of the mid-1990s annual surveys found that more than 5 percent of the ICF/MRs had been out of compliance with at least one of eight conditions for participation in the Medicaid program (e.g., active treatment programs, adequate staffing). Moreover, federal officials had evidence that the required annual surveys at times failed to unearth serious deficiencies. Some expressed concern that conflicts of interest afflicted the survey process because state governments simultaneously operated the ICF/MRs and monitored their compliance with federal standards. Under this circumstance, state inspection personnel might be tempted to pull their punches in citing quality deficiencies to avoid embarrassing the governor or other top officials (GAO 1996). It deserves emphasis that the ICF/MR complex serves many but not all Medicaid's institutionalized enrollees with disabilities. Nursing homes, state psychiatric hospitals, and other facilities also play a role. But this ICF/MR component looms large in defining Medicaid's "institutional bias."

In striving to shape who gets what from Medicaid, disability advocates possess significant political capital—arguably more than any other cohort of Medicaid enrollees. Thanks in part to the disability rights movement, which took off in the 1970s, this cluster of enrollees generally benefits from an increasingly positive social image. To be sure, variation persists. Those with a mental illness have made the least progress in escaping stigma. Those with physical disabilities who do not suffer from intellectual impairment may well have advanced furthest. But other people with disabilities have also gained ground. For instance, advocates for those with intellectual disabilities have made enormous strides in fighting stigma. In the early 1900s many leading experts viewed mental retardation as a predictor of moral degeneracy and criminality. They advocated harsh measures to keep this group out of the community to preserve social order (Trent 1994). By the early 2000s, in contrast, great segments of the public had come to see people with intellectual disabilities much more favorably. Leading advocacy groups had worked to eliminate use of the term "mental retardation," which they found degrading. They readily extracted apologies from public officials who made offhand pejorative references to the "retarded."[11] State agencies that had used "mental retardation" in their titles increasingly abandoned the term (Gottlieb 2010). The passage of the Americans with Disabilities Act in 1990 further testifies to the improved social and political standing of people with disabilities. This legislation drew the support not only of a Democratic Congress but also of a Republican president, George H. W. Bush. It represented an important symbolic expression of the need to respect the rights, dignity, and capacities of people with disabilities.

The political strength of people with disabilities also flows from their vigorous networks of advocates. Medicaid serves as the principal safety net for middle-class families facing catastrophic events, whether the birth of a child with acute disabilities, a daughter left severely impaired as the result of an accident, or a son facing the onset of mental illness. These parents tend to be vigilant, tenacious, impassioned supporters of Medicaid services for people with disabilities. They have helped create and energize a spectrum of advocacy groups. For instance, the Association of Retarded Citizens (later known as Arc) built an extensive grassroots organization to advance its concerns at the local, state, and national levels. At times, it sued state agencies to promote its agenda. It also worked to reshape the administrative organization of state governments so that the interests of people with intellectual disabilities did not get lost in the broader Medicaid bureaucracy. In New York State, for example, Arc teamed with other advocates to persuade policymakers to create the Office of Mental Retardation and Developmental Disabilities in 1979. Advocacy groups dominated by parents and providers have nurtured close working relationships with top administrators in this agency. By the 2000s Arc had established a formal collaboration with another group, United Cerebral Palsy, to become the American Association on Intellectual and Developmental Disabilities. Through this collaboration they combined forces to lobby in Washington while retaining separate organizations at the state and local levels.

Those with physical but not cognitive impairments have also emerged as vigorous advocates for people with disabilities. In the tradition of the civil rights movement, they have at times adopted more confrontational strategies, such as sit-ins, protests, and marches. Of particular relevance to Medicaid, since the 1970s they have demanded that resources be provided to promote "independent living" for people with disabilities (Skotch 1989, 393). When testifying before Congress and state legislatures, they have minced no words in denouncing nursing homes and other institutions. Many have presented lists of the abuses they have endured in "the institutional gulag." Advocates hold out little hope that institutions for people with disabilities can ever be satisfactory. As one of them told Congress, "Even in the 'good institutions' our people were not happy. If you do not have the basic freedoms, you don't enjoy living in one of the 'good' nursing homes, the 'clean' development center or the 'friendly' group home. We have seen many people, deprived of choice, become passive drones, drained of their humanity." Advocates contend that if people with disabilities are freed from institutions and provided with personal attendants, they can become "alive again" and contribute to their communities (US Senate Committee on Finance, 2004, 154, 288).

These advocates assign a high value to the personal privacy, dignity, and empowerment that independent living provides. As a woman with disabilities told a committee of state senators in South Carolina, "I want the legal right to say who comes in my bedroom and sees me naked—same as you do, Senator" (US Senate Committee on Finance 2004, 354). This quest for independent living has prompted these advocates to be front and center among those arguing for a rebalancing of Medicaid toward HCBS. They have decried the "tyrannical monopoly" of the nursing home industry, and they chafe at the fact that Medicaid requires states to provide nursing home care but makes personal assistance a state option.

Site visits to Florida, Minnesota, and Texas reaffirmed the importance of advocates for people with disabilities in state policy processes. This manifests itself in grassroots political activity. Advocates make their presence felt at election time by inviting candidates for the state legislature to meet with them. They are also active during legislative sessions, when they systematically visit the offices of legislators to make their views know. On certain days they stage rallies at the state capitol with members coming from across the state. Advocacy groups arrange meetings between those in attendance and the legislators who represent them. They hold special awards events to honor "champions" in the legislature who have supported the cause of people with disabilities.[12] Advocates also establish close relationships with state administrators who oversee Medicaid-provided HCBS. One of their legislative goals is inserting provisions in statutes requiring Medicaid administrators to confer with them on disability decisions made within the executive branch. To be sure, tensions exist among disability advocates. A tendency exits for persons with each type of disability (e.g., those with a traumatic brain injury, intellectual impairment, or autism) to pursue a particular agenda. In the view of some advocates, this fragmentation weakens the disability community in state policy processes. In Texas, for instance, one stakeholder bemoaned the lack of coordination between advocates for the developmentally disabled and people who have suffered traumatic injury as adults. He observed: "If we do (advocacy) in silos, it will be hard to get it done."[13] But on balance, advocates for those with disabilities emerge as persistent, politically potent supporters of HCBS.

Rebalancing by Waiver

The pressures to overcome Medicaid's institutional bias steadily picked up steam in the late 1960s and 1970s. Sensing the growing popularity of HCBS, federal and state policymakers looked for opportunities to promote it. Given the constellation of political forces, it is hardly surprising that Medicaid-provided HCBS made considerable headway starting in the 1980s. Far less predictable, however, was the vehicle for progress. Rather than formulate significant new policies requiring or inducing states to focus more on HCBS, Congress enacted a Medicaid two-step approach that elevated the power of the president and the bureaucracy to make decisions concerning these services. This approach featured the preservation of the existing Medicaid law while enlarging the authority of the executive branch to grant waivers from it.

In addition to mandating access to nursing homes, the Medicaid law (i.e., Title XIX of the Social Security Act) had long required participating states to provide a home health benefit. In this vein states would pay for intermittent home visits by a health professional to provide physical therapy, remediation for speech pathology, and other medical services. Although mandated, states varied considerably in the nature and amount of home health benefits they provided. In contrast, Medicaid law does not require states to provide personal assistance—that is, help with the basic activities of daily living. Instead, it gave states the option to do so. Throughout the late 1960s and 1970s, many states declined to implement this option. As of 2006 nineteen states still refrained from offering personal care through their regular Medicaid plans (Ng, Harrington, and Watts 2009).

In 1981 Congress, with the support of the Reagan administration, moved to coax states into expanding HCBS. The Omnibus Budget Reconciliation Act of that year implanted Section 1915c into the Medicaid law, which gave states the option of applying for a waiver to pursue HCBS. When approved by the federal executive branch, these waivers would allow states to circumvent key requirements of the Medicaid law. With federal approval, they could limit HCBS to specific geographic areas rather than face the customary Medicaid obligation to provide them statewide. They could precisely target services to particular categories of beneficiaries (e.g., certain of the developmentally disabled) in ways that would otherwise be impossible. The waivers also permitted states to cap the number of participants and establish waiting lists for HCBS. Congress insisted that the 1915c waivers be "cost neutral." This generally meant that the average per capita costs of the 1915c waiver had to be less than or equal to the projected expenditures for a comparable population treated in institutions (Shirk 2006, 10).

Now that the states had been granted the opportunity to customize HCBS to their particular circumstances, they moved apace to apply for waivers. Within limits, the presidential administrations of Ronald Reagan and George H. W. Bush accommodated them (Wiener and Tilly 2003). From 1981 to 1992 the number of HCBS waivers in operation grew from 6 to 155, while waiver expenditures jumped from about $4 million to $2.2 billion; 236,000 Medicaid enrollees received HCBS via waivers by the time President Clinton took office (Kitchener et al. 2005, 209; Miller 1992, 163–64). Although substantial, the HCBS waiver activity up to 1992 paled beside that under Bill Clinton and George W. Bush. This was largely because the Office of Management and Budget (OMB) became worried that the states might use their Section 1915c proposals in ways that were far from cost neutral. To defuse this prospect, it imposed the "cold bed" rule in the mid-1980s. This rule required a state to demonstrate that for each HCBS waiver participant, it had emptied a bed in a nursing home or other institution. This stricture inhibited states from submitting more ambitious waiver proposals and proved particularly galling to states that had moved earlier to restrict the supply of nursing home beds (Shirk 2006, 5; Wiener and Tilly 2003, 267). During the 1980s states often found negotiations with the federal bureaucracy over waiver approval to be arduous and protracted. For instance, it took Minnesota officials four years to obtain a federal sign-off on an HCBS waiver proposal, and it took Texas administrators three years. Delays frequently sprang from differences between national and state administrators over how to estimate the costs of the waiver (GAO 1989).

The Clinton Years: Proliferation and the Supreme Court's Intervention

The arrival of the Clinton administration in 1993 ushered in a more hospitable climate for Medicaid waivers. Having chafed under federal Medicaid restrictions when he was governor of Arkansas, the new president sought to empower the states to experiment with alternative approaches to the program. In 1994 officials took a major step to encourage HCBS waivers by eliminating the cold bed rule. This made it much easier for states to claim that their waiver proposals met the test of budget neutrality. States had only to show that the average cost for enrollees receiving HCBS was less than that of some institutional provider, such as a nursing home or ICF/MR facility. Unshackled from the cold bed rule and stringent federal interpretations of cost-neutrality, states rapidly moved to expand Section 1915c services (Wiener and Tilly 2003, 267–68). During the Clinton years the number of HCBS waivers increased by nearly 50 percent, to 231; the number of Medicaid enrollees covered by waivers grew by 225 percent, to 768,000; and Medicaid expenditures under the waivers ballooned by more than 470 percent, to $12.6 billion in 2000 (Kitchener et al. 2005, 209).

In 1999 the Supreme Court stoked the momentum for HCBS through its interpretation of the Americans with Disabilities Act.[14] As noted above, this law symbolically reinforced the legitimacy and status of people with disabilities as citizens with full rights. But the disability act also had more instrumental benefits.

Although advocates for the disabled complained that federal policymakers did not provide the resources and enforcement mechanisms to assure the law's effective implementation, it did open the gates wider for advocates to pursue their aims in the federal courts.

By the mid-1990s these advocates had trained their sights on Medicaid and HCBS. The case originated in Georgia, where officials had committed two women—one diagnosed with schizophrenia and the other with a personality disorder—to a psychiatric unit at the Georgia Regional Hospital in Atlanta. Over time, those treating each of the women concluded that their needs could be met in a community-based program, and the two enrollees concurred. State Medicaid officials did not, however, find a way to accommodate the request. The lawyers for the two women then sued Tommy Olmstead, in his capacity as commissioner of the Georgia Department of Human Resources, along with certain other officials. The plaintiffs argued that Georgia's failure to provide the two women with a community-based alternative violated their civil rights under the Americans with Disabilities Act. In June 1999 they scored a major though not complete breakthrough when the Supreme Court sided with them in its *Olmstead* decision. In general terms, the court noted that "institutional placement of persons who can handle and benefit from community settings perpetuates unwarranted assumptions that persons so isolated are incapable or unworthy of participation in community life"; it diminishes important "everyday life activities." More specifically, the Court agreed that enrollees were entitled to HCBS subject to three provisos: (1) that treatment professionals believed that community placement was appropriate, (2) that the affected enrollees wanted it, and (3) that "the placement can be accommodated, taking into account the resources available to the State and the needs of others with mental disabilities" (US Supreme Court 1999, 1, 15–16). Although in itself a significant triumph for disability rights activists, this third proviso also meant that state Medicaid programs could buy time or even stall in moving toward HCBS by pointing to budget and other resource constraints.

Although the *Olmstead* decision did not require state Medicaid programs to move immediately to fund HCBS for those with disabilities, it sparked a flurry of activity toward that end. Federal administrators sent a series of letters to state Medicaid directors providing guidance on how to comply with the Court's decision; they distributed seed grants to the states to develop comprehensive plans for shifting more enrollees to HCBS. By September 2001 forty states had task forces or commissions to address *Olmstead* issues (GAO 2001). For its part, Congress in 2000 approved the Real Choice Systems Change Grants, which authorized $240 million to assist states in building the infrastructure needed for individuals with disabilities to live in the community. By the mid-2000s the federal government had awarded about 240 of these grants to the states (US House Committee on Energy and Commerce 2005, 24, 26).

The Bush Administration Supports HCBS

The administration of George W. Bush also proved receptive to HCBS. Soon after entering office in 2001, top officials announced the New Freedom Initiative, which called for CMS to work with other federal agencies to identify the remaining barriers to HCBS and to recommend steps for surmounting them. This assessment led to adjustments in waiver practices. For instance, CMS clarified that the Section 1915c waivers could cover one-time costs, such as a security deposit on an apartment or fees to hook up utilities for people transitioning from institutions to the community (Shirk 2006). In 2002 the Bush administration launched the Independence Plus Initiative, which allowed waivers to be used for a cash-and-counseling model. This model empowered Medicaid recipients or their designated representatives with grants to pay caregivers of their choice. Rather than being required to receive services from a home health agency certified by Medicaid, they could employ a friend or relative to assist them (Crowley 2006).

These and other forces pushed HCBS waivers all the more to center stage during the Bush years. The number of Section 1915c waivers grew to about 280 in 2008, a greater than 20 percent increase from the final year of the Clinton administration.[15] All but two states were providing some portion of HCBS through these waivers. (Arizona and Vermont had no 1915c initiatives because they relied on comprehensive demonstration waivers to support HCBS.) The Bush years also witnessed growth in enrollments and expenditures via HCBS waivers. From 2000 to 2008 spending through these waivers more than doubled, rising to $30 billion. As of 2008 more than 1.2 million enrollees received HCBS under the banner of 1915c waivers, up more than 40 percent from the last year of the Clinton administration (Howard, Ng, and Harrington 2011).

Table 4.1 casts further light on the mounting importance of waivers relative to ordinary Medicaid channels as a vehicle for HCBS. Forty-one percent of Medicaid enrollees receiving HCBS did so via waivers. More dramatically, waivers accounted for nearly two-thirds of all Medicaid spending on HCBS. These aggregate figures mask the overwhelming significance of waivers in many states. Twenty-one states spent more than 90 percent of their HCBS Medicaid dollars through waivers; thirty-four committed more than 70 percent in this way.[16] (This variation among states receives more attention below.) In general, states used the waivers to target more expensive enrollees. As of 2006 Medicaid spent an annual average of more than $24,000 on each HCBS waiver participant, nearly triple the spending per HCBS enrollee provided through regular Medicaid channels (Howard, Ng, and Harrington 2011). Among waiver participants, people with disabilities overshadowed the elderly. The intellectually and developmentally disabled alone made up 40 percent of these participants and garnered more than 70 percent of waiver

Table 4.1 Role of HCBS Waivers Compared with Regular Medicaid Channels, 2008

	Enrollees		*Expenditures on HCBS*	
Waiver or Channel	*No.*	*%*	*Amount (billions of dollars)*	*%*
HCBS waiver	1,241,411	41	29.8	66
Regular home health	922,396	30	5.1	11
Regular personal care	902,943	29	10.1	23
Total	3,066,750		45.0	

Source: Howard, Ng, and Harrington (2011, 4–5).

dollars. Annual expenditures per enrollee in this cohort stood at nearly $42,000, substantially more than the comparable waiver figure for the elderly or other categories of the disabled (Ng, Harrington, and Howard 2011, 17–27, 32–33).

The Bush administration not only stoked the continued use of waivers; it also supported congressional initiatives to learn from state experiences with them and modify the Medicaid law. This effort bore fruit in the passage of the Deficit Reduction Act of 2005. Although certain provisions of this law sought to reduce the number of Medicaid enrollees receiving long-term care, others gave states new options to provide HCBS.[17] This episode casts light not only on issues of Medicaid durability but also on the dynamics of vertical policy diffusion in the American system of federalism.

Program Waivers and Bottom-Up Diffusion

Proponents of federalism have touted the virtues of the fifty states as the laboratories of democracy. They note that certain states innovate and test policies, which thereby enables other governments to make knowledgeable decisions about whether to adopt them. Diffusion occurs when officials gain information about policies or practices adopted by other governments and then act. They meld this information with insights into the circumstances that apply in their own jurisdiction to customize and enact a comparable policy. Most research has targeted horizontal policy diffusion, whereby policymakers in one state respond to developments in others.[18] Less studied but also important is vertical policy diffusion, whereby governments at different levels of the political system enact initiatives based on the policies or practices of another tier. Vertical policy diffusion can be bottom-up, top-down, or some mixture of the two. Top-down diffusion occurs when the federal government adopts policies or practices that then shape state initiatives. For instance, the legislation approving the Section 1915c waivers in

1981 signaled to the states that the federal government would be receptive to their rebalancing proposals.

Bottom-up diffusion underscores the potential for the federal government to learn from the practices of the states. This type of diffusion can assume several guises. One form involves the federal government learning from the states to forge new programs of its own. During the Great Depression of the 1930s, for instance, top federal officials distilled lessons from the experience of Wisconsin and other states in designing Social Security and a national program for unemployment compensation. Within the context of federal grant programs like Medicaid, vertical policy diffusion tends to stress either mandates or devolution. Mandate diffusion entails national officials observing that some states have engaged in beneficial practices and then requiring all states to emulate them. The Medicaid mandates of 1990 insisting that states phase in Medicaid coverage for all poor children fits this model. This initiative basically required lagging states to follow a practice that had already been adopted by most of their peers. Devolutionary diffusion entails national policymakers observing the initiatives of certain states and then acting to give other states more discretion or incentives to adopt these approaches. As will become evident in the following paragraphs, the Deficit Reduction Act fits this profile.

The existing literature suggests using a two-part test to determine whether two-part test bottom-up diffusion has occurred (e.g.,Weissert and Scheller 2008). First, the federal policy initiative should in some sense reflect state experiences. It should entail the federal government encouraging, adopting, or requiring policies and practices that the states have implemented. Second, there should be evidence that national policymakers have observed and thought about the states' experiences. Policy changes enacted with little or no awareness of what the states have done do not qualify as diffusion. Instead, policy congruence may have occurred for other reasons (Karch 2007, 30, 105). The degree to which those officials who are familiar with state HCBS practices have testified at congressional hearings provides one marker of the extent to which federal officials have considered state practices.

Some research indicates that federal policymakers tend to learn little from the states in the health care arena (e.g., Weissert and Scheller 2008). But in the case of the Deficit Reduction Act of 2005, its long-term care provisions meet the two criteria for vertical diffusion. Congress had devoted considerable attention to long-term care in the early years of the Bush administration. In the period 2001–5, Congress conducted at least thirteen hearings that dealt at least partly with the subject (e.g., US Senate Committee on Finance 2004). Those testifying at the hearings included governors (at least five), the executive director of the NGA, state cabinet-level officials responsible for long-term care, disability rights activists working in particular states, experts from think tanks that monitor Medicaid, and leaders of state advocacy groups for the elderly.[19] Nearly all the witnesses touted the virtues of expanding Medicaid HCBS. They differed, however, in their more precise policy preferences.

Disability rights advocates favored a Medicaid mandate for HCBS. They strongly supported the Medicaid Community-Based Attendant Services and Support Act, also known as MiCASSA. Championed by Senator Tom Harkin (D-IA), this legislation would have converted personal assistance from a Medicaid option for states to a requirement. A large share of Medicaid's elderly and disabled enrollees would thereby have gained the right to a personal attendant to assist them in their homes and communities. Having supported the measure since the late 1990s, disability advocates intensified their pressures on Congress to approve it in 2003. In early September of that year 160 people in wheelchairs from twenty states, many of whom had at one point been in nursing homes, staged a fourteen-day march from Philadelphia's Liberty Bell to the Capitol in Washington to support MiCASSA.[20] In April 2004 advocates testified at a hearing of the US Senate's Committee on Finance (2004, 5, 32) on behalf of the bill, as Senator Harkin stressed the need to get Medicaid out of the "Dark Ages" on HCBS. More than 90 national and 560 regional and local organizations concerned with disability rights petitioned Congress to support the legislation.

However, the proponents of MiCASSA ultimately came up dry. Republican leaders, whose party controlled both houses of Congress, opposed the measure, as did the Bush administration. Moreover, the forces of representational federalism stood in opposition. State governors, for instance, did not want a new mandate that would put more pressure on their state budgets. Although HCBS remained on the congressional agenda, the policy changes that eventually emerged had a devolutionary thrust.[21]

The Deficit Reduction Act of 2005 devolved new authority to the states to implement HCBS through the standard Medicaid program. It legitimated approaches that up to that point states had enacted through waivers. Specifically, the law enlarged the states' discretion in four main ways.[22] First, it permitted states to provide HCBS to seniors and people with disabilities with incomes up to 150 percent of the poverty line; and unlike waivers, states that took this option would not face a requirement that the action be budget neutral. Second, the law freed states from having to show that those receiving HCBS had functional impairments that would qualify them for admission to a nursing home or related institution. This step greatly expanded the potential pool of enrollees. Third, in a significant departure from Medicaid's status as an entitlement, the new law permitted states to cap enrollment, maintain waiting lists, and limit services to certain geographic areas rather than offer them statewide. As with waivers, states could keep the lid on program expansion. And fourth, the new law endorsed an approach to HCBS that the waivers helped incubate and encourage: cash and counseling. Under this model,

Medicaid provides monies directly to enrollees or their proxies. Subject to certain accounting controls, recipients use the funds to employ whom they want (e.g., family members, friends) to assist them, rather than rely on home health agencies that Medicaid had certified. The cash-and-counseling approach also permits "self-direction" in other spheres. States could, for instance, permit a Medicaid enrollee to use the funds to purchase a microwave, to install an accessibility ramp in his or her residence, or to take other steps to foster independent living.

Passage of the Deficit Reduction Act was a substantial triumph for state officials. It meant that they would no longer need to seek waivers from the federal bureaucracy to pursue certain HCBS initiatives. Instead, they could modify their state Medicaid plans with the full support of federal law. The new act buffered states from the possibility that subsequent presidential administrations could thwart HCBS by turning off the waiver spigot.

On the surface, passage of the act might also seem to support a theory of waivers as temporary learning devices for federal policymakers. Under this model, the waivers provide opportunities for vertical policy diffusion that could lead to changes in federal law; these changes would then obviate the need for their continued use. This progression might mollify the concerns of some advocates that waivers are a subterranean, opaque tool that can hinder their participation in policy processes. It might also assuage concerns about excessive departures from the rule of law via broad grants of discretionary authority to the executive branch (e.g., Lowi 1969).

The Deficit Reduction Act, however, did little to tamp down the states' interest in HCBS waivers. The new law did not repeal Section 1915c of the Medicaid law. Although the statute further empowered the states, it stopped short of giving them all the discretion that they enjoyed under the waivers. For instance, about 80 percent of the states used 1915c initiatives to cover enrollees with incomes above 150 percent of the poverty line (Kitchener et al. 2007, 28). The Deficit Reduction Act also continued Medicaid's "comparability requirement," which mandates that available services be equal in amount, duration, and scope for all enrollees in certain eligibility cohorts (Shirk 2006, 20). HCBS waivers gave states more of an opportunity to target specific groups for particular benefits (e.g., providing temporary personal assistance for children with disability "A" but not with disability "B"). These factors, plus the inertia of many HCBS initiatives, undercut the motivation of states to pare their use of 1915c waivers so long as federal administrators continued to approve them. Although some states turned to regular Medicaid channels to promote HCBS after 2005, waiver activity continued apace. From the time of the Deficit Reduction Act's passage until 2010, the George W. Bush and Obama administrations signed off on thirty-four new HCBS waivers submitted by twenty-three states. [23]

Although it was primarily focused on expanding health insurance for the non-disabled poor, the ACA of 2010 also took some steps to promote HCBS. It permitted the states to expand Medicaid HCSB to certain categories of individuals with incomes above 200 percent of the poverty line.[24] It also limited the states' discretion to cap enrollment, establish waiting lists, and confine services geographically for enrollees receiving HCSB through a state plan. The ACA's provisions to bolster the Medicaid service entitlement did not, however, extend to the great numbers of individuals receiving HCBS through Section 1915c waivers. If anything, the new statutory amendments made waivers more attractive to the states.[25] The health reform law also provided additional federal subsidies to expand HCBS. It allocated more money for demonstrations designed to move people out of institutions and into their homes and communities, and it promised states an enhanced federal match for five years if they did more to proffer HCBS to enrollees who would otherwise require care in an institution.[26]

Curbing the Medicaid Entitlement

The vast expansion of HCBS waivers and the passage of the Deficit Reduction Act have had significant implications for Medicaid's status as an entitlement. To be sure, they have not vitiated the federal government's open-ended obligation to match state Medicaid expenditures at a certain rate. But they have chipped away at Medicaid's initial statutory commitment to provide "equal" benefits to all who meet the eligibility criteria within a state's borders. Instead, states possess vast discretion to limit HCBS geographically, cap enrollments, and establish waiting lists. Of course, multiple factors have long weakened Medicaid as an entitlement in this sense. For instance, complex enrollment procedures, low payment rates to providers, and the geographic distribution of health care facilities have prevented Medicaid enrollees from receiving the "mainstream" services to which the law formally entitles them. Geographic variation in access within states has been present since the program's birth. What distinguishes the waivers and the Deficit Reduction Act is their endorsement of rationing as a policy principle rather than as an undeclared subterranean outcome of the implementation process. These developments mean that geographic inequalities in access to Medicaid benefits within many states will probably increase.

What factors have galvanized political support for curbing the Medicaid entitlement in this way? Three loom particularly large. First, the approach appeals to the fundamental preferences of governors and other state policymakers. Since 1995 most of them have resisted efforts to vitiate Medicaid as a blank-check fiscal obligation to the states, but they have been much less inclined to defend the program as a service entitlement. Many value the flexibility, state budget control, and greater freedom from court scrutiny that waivers and the Deficit Reduction Act provide. In this sense, these developments reflect the triumph of representative federalism. Second, the approach appeals to conservative forces at the national level, which have long been interested in reining in entitlements. Having been defeated in their efforts to convert Medicaid into a block grant in 1995 and again in 2003, they have gained some political solace from undercutting the program as a service entitlement.

Third, a widely shared perception of a possible "woodwork effect" has fueled concern about the cost implications of HCBS, even among those policymakers who are ideologically inclined to support entitlements for the elderly and people with disabilities. This cost concern does not primarily flow from the prospect of moving existing Medicaid enrollees from institutions to the community. In many cases, it would be cheaper to serve these enrollees in the community. Furthermore, the overall numbers transitioning out of institutions seem unlikely to be large. Although some advocates have argued that more than 60 percent of institutionalized Medicaid beneficiaries could be shifted to the community, others put the figure at 20 percent (US Senate Committee on Finance 2004, 31, 77; see also Mor et al. 2007). Many of the elderly, even among the less afflicted, find the prospect of leaving their nursing homes daunting. They generally have given up their homes and apartments; many have lost touch with neighbors and others who in the past informally assisted them. Still others develop "nursing home head," whereby in the absence of the need to keep up their basic skills, such as shopping and cooking, they lose confidence in their ability to perform these tasks (Reinhard 2010, 46). On balance, then, many policymakers see the costs of moving people from institutions to the community as manageable over a reasonable period. Their anxieties about the potential for an HCBS cost explosion spring from a concern that a spate of people not currently in institutions or receiving services from Medicaid will "come out of the woodwork" to apply for personal assistance.

Several factors raise concerns about the woodwork effect. Policymakers are aware of evidence suggesting that there is a great *pent-up demand* for HCBS. They understand that legions of spouses, parents, relatives, friends, and others freely provide vast amounts of personal assistance and home health care to the elderly and people with disabilities. One study notes that 80 percent of adults getting long-term care at home receive it from unpaid caregivers, and 14 percent have both paid and unpaid help. Another study estimates the value of this free care to be more than $257 billion annually (Miller and Mor 2006, 34–36); yet another analysis "conservatively" calculates the amount to be $350 billion (Gibson and Houser 2007). This means that easing eligibility requirements for Medicaid-provided HCBS could yield a gusher of demand. In addition to the potential pressures on government budgets, an issue related to the proper balance between government and civil society lingers in the background. Informal caregiving often imposes great stress and cost on those providing it. But survey data also suggest that it has rewards. One study found that nearly half these caregivers considered themselves to be more religious and spiritual as a result. Ninety percent felt that the person they cared for appreciated what they did; more than 70 percent said that their relationship with the individual improved as a result of their HCBS experience (Donelan et al. 2002, 229). Would greater Medicaid investment in HCBS undermine the intangible rewards of caregiving, thereby crowding out services that informal networks currently provide? Would it undermine the widely held norm that family members should bear the primary burden of assisting each other?[27] The available studies provide no definitive answer. It may be that properly calibrated Medicaid support for HCBS would enhance the informal care network and not trigger a surge in demand (Stone 1999). But policymakers cannot be sure.

Those on official waiting lists for Medicaid-provided HCBS also testify to the presence of pent-up demand. As of 2008 more than 393,000 Medicaid applicants were biding their time on these lists, about double the number in 2002; the waiting lists increased every year except one in the period 2002–8 (Ng, Harrington, and Watts 2009, 3).[28] Policymakers also sense that the inexorable aging of the members of the baby boom generation will lead to greater demand in the years ahead. Although they are likely to be healthier and less incapacitated than previous generations of older people, their sheer numbers seem sure to fuel applications. Although many elderly people detest the notion of moving to a nursing home, they are open to the prospect of receiving Medicaid-provided HCBS.

The *plasticity of the concept of disability* noted above also engenders concern about the woodwork effect. The indeterminacy and flexibility of the disability category make it vulnerable to expansion. Officials in most states constantly deal with strong pressures from providers, middle-class parents, and advocacy groups to extend the disability label to new impairments. They typically share a conviction that a growing array of borderline disabilities (e.g., certain forms of autism, epilepsy, attention deficit, and other psychological disorders) can and should be recognized by the Medicaid gatekeepers who determine eligibility for HCBS. Once enrolled, people with disabilities cannot be easily removed from the rolls. They and their families become accustomed to the support. They are more likely than nondisabled women and children to pursue every avenue of appeal if Medicaid officials reappraise and strive to strip them of their eligibility.

Although less salient to state officials, the *weakening of a supply side constraint* also bolsters concern about the woodwork effect. In an effort to constrain long-term care costs, policymakers in some states have worked to decrease nursing home beds. In a similar vein, a shortage of trained, certified home health workers and personal assistants in the labor market might conceivably function as a supply-side brake on HCBS demand (Miller and Mor 2006; Kaye et al. 2006). But the Section 1915c waivers and Deficit Reduction Act have endorsed the deprofessionalization of these services through the cash-and-counseling model—which, as noted above, empowers Medicaid enrollees to pick whom they like to assist them with activities of daily living, including friends, relatives, and acquaintances. Many individuals prefer these providers over "strangers" from home health agencies. By 2008 thirty-five states allowed or required some form of "consumer direction" for HCBS.[29]

In sum, concerns about the potential cost implications of the woodwork effect have stiffened the resolve of policymakers in their dealings with two of Medicaid's more politically potent constituencies: the elderly and people with disabilities. These cohorts have made progress in their quest for HCBS. But by weakening the service entitlement in Medicaid, policymakers have hedged fiscal uncertainty and reserved the right to shut the HCBS gates. It deserves note that the available studies suggest that the concerns of state officials about the costs of HCBS are far from groundless. Although these analyses are not definitive, they typically suggest that expanding HCBS boosts Medicaid costs for long-term care, at least over the short term.[30]

HCBS: A Glass Half Empty or Half Full?

Federal and state actions in the 1990s and 2000s spurred significant movement toward surmounting Medicaid's institutional bias. The amount and share of Medicaid funds going to HCBS steadily increased. By 2009 HCBS consumed 43 percent of the program's long-term care dollars. Although this is a significant step toward rebalancing, it does not mean that policymakers have "cured" Medicaid's institutional bias. The lengthy waiting lists for HCBS signal that there could still be additional rebalancing. Data from European countries also suggest that an appreciably higher proportion of long-term care could be delivered in a home or community setting (Gibson et al. 2003). Variation among state Medicaid programs yields a similar conclusion. Some states have gone much further than others in rebalancing. As of 2009 the proportion of Medicaid long-term care dollars spent on HCBS ranged from 14 percent in Mississippi to 82 percent in New Mexico.[31]

States vary appreciably in their commitment and capacity with respect to HCBS. Table 4.2 casts some light on this variation by sorting states into four clusters based on two indicators: HCBS expenditures per poor person, and the share of Medicaid long-term care dollars spent on HCBS. In the table, pacesetting states consist of those above the national mean on both indicators. Lagging states, in contrast, fall below the mean on the two metrics. The remaining states make up two categories of hybrids. More generous but less balanced states are above average in the Medicaid monies they spend on HCBS per poor person, but they are below the mean in the degree to which they have rebalanced. Less generous but more balanced states are below the national mean in their Medicaid outlays for HCBS per poor person, but they are above average in rebalancing.[32]

Table 4.2 identifies fifteen pacesetting states. Five of them (Alaska, Connecticut, Minnesota, New York, and Vermont) spent more than $3,000 a year on Med-

Table 4.2 States' Commitments to HCBS and Rebalancing, 2009

State	*HCBS Expenditures in Dollars per Person Living in Poverty*	*HCBS as Percentage of Long-Term Care Dollars*
US average	1,212.80	43.30
Pacesetting		
Alaska	3,132.27	64.87
California	1,321.31	54.17
Connecticut	5,192.27	45.49
Kansas	1,534.09	55.61
Maine	2,742.40	52.29
Massachusetts	2,263.41	44.34
Minnesota	3,438.16	64.67
Montana	1,228.80	46.28
New Hampshire	2,427.15	43.67
New York	3,227.32	45.73
Oregon	1,856.48	73.02
Rhode Island	1,983.82	46.10
Vermont	4,699.42	69.53
Washington	1,836.77	65.18
Wyoming	2,490.19	50.82
Generous but less balanced		
Iowa	1,664.90	39.67
Maryland	1,488.05	38.15
Nebraska	1,558.38	39.02
New Jersey	1,421.46	28.90
North Dakota	1,506.20	28.53
Pennsylvania	1,639.55	34.09
West Virginia	1,384.59	40.80
Wisconsin	1,463.56	43.27
Balanced but less generous		
Colorado	1,202.44	56.05
Hawaii	889.74	60.08
Idaho	933.06	46.20
Missouri	933.79	45.53
New Mexico	1,073.56	82.17
North Carolina	947.64	43.69
Texas	599.50	44.85
Utah	807.96	48.98
Lagging		
Alabama	571.06	29.78
Arizona	583.47	43.30
Arkansas	676.58	29.75
Delaware	1,101.05	35.83
Florida	588.38	36.45
Georgia	401.08	37.21
Illinois	647.93	31.48
Indiana	710.37	33.21

(Continued)

Table 4.2 States' Commitments to HCBS and Rebalancing, 2009

State	*HCBS Expenditures in Dollars per Person Living in Poverty*	*HCBS as Percentage of Long-Term Care Dollars*
Kentucky	633.86	32.02
Louisiana	1,199.23	38.26
Michigan	604.70	34.57
Mississippi	271.49	14.35
Nevada	457.38	41.55
Ohio	1,177.58	31.94
Oklahoma	1,150.28	41.60
South Carolina	762.15	39.01
South Dakota	1,023.81	40.59
Tennessee	632.71	34.34
Virginia	1,049.64	42.39

Note: HCBS includes standard home health services, personal care, targeted case management, hospice, and home and community-based care for the functionally disabled elderly, and services provided under home and community-based services waivers; the fiscal year (FY) runs from October 1 through September 30. All spending includes state and federal expenditures. Long-term care expenditures shown for Arizona include approximately $1.9 billion in payments to managed care organizations that we estimated to be used for long-term care services. These expenditures were allocated among the services shown based on nationwide patterns of spending for long-term care services.

Sources: Medicaid data are from the Urban Institute and Kaiser Commission on Medicaid and the Uninsured estimates, based on data from Centers for Medicare and Medicaid Services-64 reports, 2011, www.statehealthfacts.org/comparetable.jsp?typ=4&ind=180&cat=4&sub=47; Census Bureau Historical Poverty tables 2 and 21, www.census.gov/hhes/www/poverty/data/historical/people.html.

icaid-provided HCBS per poor person, and five (again Alaska, Minnesota, and Vermont, along with Oregon and Washington) devote more than 60 percent of their long-term care outlays to HCBS. The states in this category come from all regions of the country except the Southeast. At the other end of the continuum, nineteen states are lagging in HCBS effort. Six states in this group (Alabama, Arkansas, Illinois, Kentucky, Mississippi, and Ohio) apportion less than one-third of their Medicaid long-term care monies to HCBS. States in the Southeast make up about half this cluster.

Eight states qualify as relatively generous but less balanced. These include states such as New Jersey and Pennsylvania, which spend considerable sums on Medicaid-provided HCBS but have not been able to overcome their historical legacy of heavy investment in nursing homes and other institutions. They have been less committed or strategically adept than comparable states in closing or otherwise trimming placement in these facilities. By contrast, New York also had a formidable institutional legacy but engaged in what one observer has termed "by far, the largest, most rapid, and successful closure of state-operated institutions in the United States".[33] A final cluster of eight states falls into the category of being more balanced but less generous. These states hover just above the national average in the proportion of long-term care dollars devoted to HCBS but trail in expenditures on these services per poor person. Texas serves as an interesting case in this regard. Though the state has one of the most penurious Medicaid programs in the country (see chapter 2) and spends only $600 per poor person on HCBS, its key policymakers have been relatively committed to rebalancing. In 2001 advocates persuaded the Texas legislature to support an initiative called Money Follows the Person, which allowed Medicaid enrollees in nursing homes to use the money the state was spending to institutionalize them to pay for HCBS (Reinhard 2010, 45). Impressed with this initiative, Congress endorsed the approach in the Deficit Reduction Act of 2005.

Given the importance of waivers in facilitating HCBS, the question naturally rises: Are pacesetting states more disposed to channel funds through waivers than the other clusters? The answer appears to be "no." Both pacesetting and lagging states, on average, spent about 80 percent of their Medicaid HCBS dollars through waivers. In general, all clusters of states find waivers appealing. Certain pacesetters, such as Minnesota and Oregon, have depended heavily on Section 1915c initiatives to push the envelope in their efforts to be HCBS leaders. Oregon spends 99 percent of all its HCBS Medicaid dollars through waivers, and Minnesota spends 87 percent. More conservative, lagging states have also gravitated toward waivers. Georgia and Mississippi, for instance, spend more than 90 percent of their HCBS Medicaid outlays this way. The allure of waivers in more conservative states springs from the high levels of targeting and expenditure control they permit. Lagging states often see waivers as a relatively inexpensive way to provide a particular form of HCBS to a narrowly defined group of recipients.

Although the great majority of states across the four clusters have found HCBS waivers alluring, there are some significant exceptions. California qualifies as a pacesetter, but it allocates only 29 percent of its Medicaid HCBS outlays through waivers. Another pacesetter, New York, allots about half its HCBS dollars in this way. Both these states have historically been more willing to provide personal assistance to all Medicaid enrollees with limitations on activities of daily living. California's commitment to this option dates back to 1973, during the administration of Governor Ronald Reagan and before the availability of Section 1915c waivers. Certain lagging states, such as Louisiana and Nevada, have also been relatively reluctant to spend through waivers. The former spent 49 percent of all HCBS dollars through waivers, and the latter spent 47 percent. The exact reasons for their lack of aggressiveness on this metric remain unclear. Given the new HCBS discretion provided to states under the Deficit Reduction Act, these states may remain content to rely on regular Medicaid channels rather than waivers to provide HCBS.

Medicaid's Durability and the Fabric of Federalism

HCBS developments not only illuminate the evolution of Medicaid; they also point to shifts in American federalism with implications for Medicaid's durability. As noted above, the story of HCBS is largely about devolving greater authority to the states to shape the nature and amount of services. It is about the rise of "executive federalism" as an intergovernmental force, in which waivers rather than new legislation play a dominant catalytic role (Gais and Fossett 2005).

The power relationships and processes between the national and state governments in the case of the HCBS waivers depart considerably from a standard model applied to intergovernmental implementation by policy scholars. This model spotlights the pervasive bargaining and negotiation that transpire between federal and state administrators as they resolve differences in preferences and priorities (e.g., Agranoff and McGuire 2004). As the next chapter shows, this model has frequently described intergovernmental relations in the case of the comprehensive demonstration waivers authorized under Section 1115 of the Social Security Act. To some degree, it also applied to HCBS waivers in the 1980s. Federal administrators in that decade frequently cast a skeptical eye on the cost projections of state waiver proposals and pressed for modifications. Protracted bargaining and negotiation often ensued. But with the advent of the Clinton administration and continuing under Bush and Obama, federal administrators assigned cost containment a lower priority. Instead, waivers increasingly came to embody a model of intergovernmental "licensing" (Weissert and Weissert 2008b). Although some negotiations between national and state officials occur under this model, much interaction is routine. State administrators present the requested information on a boilerplate application form. Federal officials check to make sure the application is complete and conforms to program requirements. They seldom attempt to impose their particular policy and administrative preferences on the waiver. Within broad program parameters, the waivers represent a triumph for devolution; they are bottom-up and state-driven. And once the waivers have been approved, federal officials conduct little oversight and almost automatically renew them.[34]

The low level of intergovernmental friction over the Section 1915c waivers in part reflects the substantial bipartisan consensus on the merits of HCBS. Despite their deep ideological differences on many issues of health policy, Democratic and Republican leaders generally concur that it is better to serve people in their homes and communities than in large institutions. So long as the states paid at least modest attention to the principle that HCBS waivers needed to be cost neutral, neither the Clinton nor George W. Bush administration had an incentive to oppose them. The Supreme Court's *Olmstead* decision further fueled the expeditious processing of waivers. To be sure, lower courts have interpreted this ruling cautiously and have been reluctant to issue sweeping mandates requiring states to expand community services (Rosenbaum and Teitelbaum 2004). Still, federal and state officials must live with the possibility of more aggressive court intervention if they make little or no progress in reducing waiting lists for HCBS or otherwise appear indifferent to *Olmstead.*

In addition to departing from a model of intergovernmental bargaining and negotiation, the experience with Section 1915c waivers suggests the need to reconsider the long-standing metaphor of "picket fence federalism" that scholars have applied to the states' implementation of federal grants. As articulated by former North Carolina governor Terry Sanford (1967, 80) and the political scientist Deil Wright (1978, 61–63), this metaphor focuses on the alliance between federal and state administrators in implementing grant programs. It notes that these program professionals tend to have similar educational backgrounds and outlooks. And it underscores the frustrations of both governors and top political appointees in assuring the responsiveness of this alliance of specialists to broader policy priorities. In this metaphor's depiction of policy implementation, it assigns a major role to "vertical functional autocracies," "balkanized bureaucracies," and "bureaucratic baronies" (Wright 1978, 63). Picket fence federalism also highlights the barriers to administrative coordination and integrated service delivery born of the proliferation of narrow grant programs (i.e., the "pickets"). Each grant program involves its own set of bureaucratic players and standard operating procedures.

Although the concept of picket fence federalism continues to illuminate some aspects of Medicaid implementation, it also has limits. Above all, it undervalues the degree to which waivers have frequently become tools of presidential and gubernatorial leadership. As a rule, waivers do not reflect the triumph of program specialists in the bureaucracy over top political executives—a core implication of the picket fence metaphor. In the nation's capital, Medicaid waivers became central to the presidencies of Clinton and George W. Bush. Both administrations viewed the Section 1915c waivers as critical to their policy goal of fostering HCBS. They supported moving the waivers from a bargaining to a licensing model. HCBS waivers have seldom become the signature initiatives of governors in the way that some Medicaid demonstration waivers have (this is discussed in chapter 5). At times, significant tensions have surfaced between governors and the administrative agencies responsible for Medicaid.[35] But it would be wide of the mark to portray most governors as frustrated, passive observers of a runaway professional bureaucratic complex in the case of HCBS. Governors have tended to sympathize with the 1915c waivers and the concept of deinstitutionalization. The NGA has supported HCBS and promulgated best practice models. Moreover, governors typically fathom that HCBS waivers can be part of a broader agenda to shift costs for certain services from the state's own purse to the federal government. They also appreciate the way in which waivers have weakened the service entitlement provisions of Medicaid and thereby have mitigated the risk of uncontrollable spending.

With general support from political executives, the specialized program professionals central to picket fence federalism do much to shape the specifics of HCBS. Some of the highly specific Section 1915c waivers target such limited numbers of people in such constrained geographic areas that they do resemble pickets.[36] But on balance Medicaid administrators are working in a program so broad in scope, so accommodating in the discretion it gives them, and so massive in terms of the funding it provides that the term "picket" is not really apt. In the context of American federalism, Medicaid is better seen as a pillar surrounded by pickets.

In developing Section 1915c waivers, state officials typically sustain close relationships with key stakeholders. Advocates for the elderly and those with disabilities press their case. So, too, do the providers of long-term care, whether in institutions or local communities (e.g., Castellani 2005, 174–76). In some instances, advocates evolve into providers. In New York State, for example, the Association for Retarded Citizens in the 1960s and 1970s became a formidable statewide advocacy group for those with intellectual disabilities. It was the lead plaintiff in a lawsuit brought against the state to foster deinstitutionalization. By the 1990s, however, it had also morphed into the largest network of private providers receiving Medicaid dollars to deliver HCBS to the intellectually disabled.[37] The top executives of the state's Office of Mental Retardation and Developmental Disabilities met frequently with this association and other service providers to discuss payment rates, new program initiatives, and other Medicaid matters (Castellani 2005, 174–76, 203, 215). The exact relationship between different interest groups and Medicaid agencies in forging HCBS waivers varies from state to state. At times, entrepreneurial professionals in the Medicaid bureaucracy lead in persuading stakeholders outside government that certain waiver proposals have merit. In other cases, states feature a more client-driven pattern where advocates and providers for the elderly and people with disabilities markedly shape the waivers; professionals in the bureaucracy serve more as their representatives than their partners. This alliance of the bureaucracy and interest groups operates under the watchful eye of the state budget office and at times the governor and certain state legislators (e.g., Castellani 2005, 225).

The shifting patterns of federalism driven by the Section 1915c waivers fueled support for Medicaid among state officials. State Medicaid administrators worked with their federal counterparts in relatively frictionless fashion and gained greater leeway to shape HCBS. State elected officials also benefited. Legislators could engage in casework for applicants on HCSB waiting lists. They could on occasion accommodate advocates for the elderly and people with disabilities by importuning the bureaucracy to seek a waiver pertinent to their districts. The fact that HCBS was optional, rather than a federal mandate, allowed them to claim more political credit for promoting it. For governors, the new patterns of federalism generally sent the signal that Medicaid was not a program that handcuffed them. The emergence of HCBS waivers as "licenses" meant that they seldom had to intervene with federal administrators to win approval for state requests. The vertical policy diffusion leading to the Deficit Reduction Act cemented into place new HCBS options without imposing significant new mandates on the states. Nor did the *Olmstead* ruling demand immediate Medicaid spending on HCBS. Through the Medicaid waiver process, governors and the NGA could increasingly have their cake and eat it, too; they gained impressive new powers to shape Medicaid without needing to forgo the federal government's open-ended funding commitment. The deal that many governors had forged with Speaker Gingrich in 1995 (less money for more discretion via a block grant) grew less appealing.

HCBS and Medicaid's Durability

The implications of HCBS developments for Medicaid's durability go beyond their role in generating support from the intergovernmental lobby. They had an impact on other factors affecting the program's durability. Those who stress the importance of sustaining Medicaid as a legal entitlement have cause for concern. Clearly, the waivers and the vertical policy diffusion that occurred in their wake have chipped away at this entitlement through enrollment caps, waiting lists, and targeting by geographic area and beneficiary group. Advocates for the elderly and disabled who fought for an enforceable Medicaid right to personal assistance in the home and community met defeat.

From a broader perspective, however, one may well see an *entitlement paradox*. Curbing the Medicaid entitlement in this way probably spurred greater Medicaid spending on HCBS than would have otherwise occurred. State officials face great pent-up demand for HCBS. The waivers and Deficit Reduction Act stoked the states' confidence that they could incrementally expand HCBS coverage without being overwhelmed by a surge in demand. Curbing the entitlement permitted state officials to apply the brakes and drive at slower speeds—to avoid getting on a runaway budget train. A step-by-step expansion of HCBS benefits became less risky for them, both politically and fiscally. If pursuing the HCBS option required state officials to entitle large categories of enrollees to these services everywhere within their borders, they might well have been more reluctant to expand this benefit.

Without question, state Medicaid programs spent more on long-term care services in general and on HCBS in particular. In the 1999–2007 period, for example, Medicaid outlays for HCBS grew by 95 percent in inflation-adjusted dollars while institutional expenditures rose by 15 percent. The number of Medicaid enrollees in institutions held about constant during this time, while those receiving HCBS grew by some 50 percent (Ng, Harrington, and Kitchener 2010, 25). This pattern becomes all the more impressive when one recalls that much state spending on the elderly and people with disabilities is optional rather than mandated by the federal government. As of 2007 a total of 85 percent of Medicaid outlays on the elderly fell into the optional Medicaid category, as did 67 percent of the funds spent on people with disabilities. In contrast, optional spending on children accounted for 15 percent of the Medicaid funds directed at them, and at nondisabled adults, 63 percent.[38]

This higher level of optional spending reflects the substantial political muscle in state politics of service providers and certain other advocates for the elderly and people with disabilities. The nursing home and other institutional benefits that Medicaid had long proffered built support for the program among the middle class. With HCBS on the rise, advocates for people with disabilities and many of the elderly had even more reason to go to bat for the program. They viewed Medicaid-provided HCBS as a far more attractive benefit than institutional care. Although state policymakers buffered themselves from HCBS demand by curbing the Medicaid entitlement, pressures for further expansion of this benefit will persist.

The rise of HCBS has almost certainly strengthened Medicaid by enhancing the quality of its long-term care services. Placing enrollees in institutions who can as readily be served in their homes and communities frequently fuels dissatisfaction, discomfort, and even greater disability among them. Some research suggests that HCBS ushers in greater life satisfaction and social activity among enrollees (Grabowski 2006). The advantages of HCBS loom even larger in the face of evidence that nursing homes with greater proportions of Medicaid enrollees tend to have more quality deficiencies. To be sure, one must avoid viewing Medicaid-provided HCBS through rose-tinted glasses. The federal government and the states have done less to establish a quality assurance system for HCBS than for nursing home care. Throughout the 1990s and into the 2000s CMS provided little guidance to the states on how to assure HCBS quality. In their requests for Section 1915c waivers and their periodic progress reports, the states have typically paid scant attention to the issue. Although some states have relied on such practices as case management, beneficiary surveys, and complaint systems to guard against inferior service, reports of medical and physical neglect sporadically surface. One CMS audit of a state found that more than one-fourth of elderly HCBS waiver enrollees did not receive any of the personal care services that Medicaid had authorized, and another 49 percent received only half of them (GAO 2003a, 3, 20, 36). Nor do most states conduct mortality reviews for disabled enrollees who die while receiving HCBS. In some instances, these deaths reflect improper treatment. For instance, a sixty-three-year-old man with significant cognitive disabilities living in a community group home choked to death on a sandwich, even though he was supposed to be fed pureed food (GAO 2008b, 2). In yet other cases, those providing HCBS have physically abused enrollees (e.g., Hakim 2011).

Although quality concerns about HCBS persist, the fact remains that most Medicaid enrollees strongly prefer it to institutional care (Ng, Harrington, and

Kitchener 2010, 27). For many young people with disabilities, the value of independent living trumps quality concerns. As one advocate for the disabled communicated to the US Senate's Committee on Finance (2004, 289), "There will be risks. Some attendants may not be reliable. We may be stranded without needed help." But he went on to affirm that "no risk involved with attendant care can compare to the terror of even one day of so-called life in a nursing home. It is our life. It is our risk to take. Dignity entails risk. The government is not our mother or father and we are not children." Comments such as this should not gainsay the quality problems that many may encounter with Medicaid-provided HCBS or the desirability of improving quality assurance. Nor should it obscure the other quality issues that dual eligibles face in coordinating their medical and long-term care.[39] But on balance, the rise of HCBS has in all likelihood had a positive impact on the health of the elderly and people with disabilities as well as the quality of their lives.

Notes

1. Some of the information and themes of this chapter draw from Thompson and Burke (2009).

2. Until recently, "intellectually disabled" people were referred to as the "mentally retarded." The latter nomenclature still persists in many settings (e.g., the labeling of certain kinds of institutions, the organization charts of government).

3. These data are from the Kaiser Commission on Medicaid and the Uninsured, www.statehealthfacts.org/comparetable.isp?=178&cat=4.

4. Some policymakers believe that the adult children of people who need long-term care work with estate lawyers to divest their parents of assets so they can qualify for Medicaid. At times, this occurs. But the Medicaid expenses created by this practice appear to account for a very small percentage of the program's long-term care costs (see, e.g., O'Brien 2005),

5. My site visits to Florida, Minnesota, and Texas uniformly reinforced this view.

6. Interview 13, September 22, 2010.

7. Interview 11, September 24, 2010.

8. Interview 16, October 4, 2010.

9. In the case of children, disability decisions rest on assessments of whether they achieve "functional equivalence" relative to "normal" peers (GAO 1998, 3).

10. See Stone (1984). In this vein, the official report of the US Social Security Administration (2009, 4) predicted an increase in SSI claims due to the severe economic recession of 2008.

11. In early 2010 White House chief of staff Rahm Emanuel issued a formal apology after the *Wall Street Journal* reported that he had called certain political liberals "retarded." He met with officials from the Special Olympics to express his regrets over his use of the "R word" (Zeleny and Stolberg 2010).

12. They use the term "champions" in Minnesota; interview 13, September 22, 2010.

13. Interview 31, March 10, 2011.

14. For an overview of the events leading to passage of the Americans with Disabilities Act, see Switzer (2003).

15. This estimate derives from a baseline number provided by Kaiser State Health Facts for 2006 plus CMS reports of waiver actions in 2007 and 2008. See www.statehealthfacts.kff

.org/comparabletable.jsp?ind=240&cat=4&sub=62&yer=17&typ=1&so and www.cms.hhs.gov/MedicaidStWaivprogDemoPGI/MWDL/list.asp?listage=53.

16. These percentages were derived from data furnished by the Kaiser Commission on Medicaid and the Uninsured, www.statehealthfacts.org/comparetable.jsp?typ=4&ind=180&cat=4&sub=47.

17. The law sought to make it harder for people to qualify for Medicaid by divesting themselves of their assets, provided new incentives for individuals to purchase long-term care insurance, and (as discussed in chapter 3) imposed greater citizen documentation requirements for eligibility.

18. For an overview of this literature, see Karch (2007). I follow Karch in seeing diffusion as a broad category encompassing policy "learning, emulation, or imitation" (p. 140). Students of policy learning tend toward more restrictive definitions. For example, May (1992, 333) contends that "learning implies improved understanding, as reflected by an ability to draw lessons about policy problems, objectives or interventions. The lessons are not necessarily refined understandings of policy cause and effect that might emerge from formal evaluations or policy experiments." Rather, they often reflect a kind of "trial-and-error learning." Although I adopt the broad category of diffusion, I suspect that the Deficit Reduction Act would meet May's standards for learning.

19. I relied on the Congressional Information Service to compile a list of the hearings and those who testified.

20. See Center for an Accessible Society, "Advocates on 144-Mile 'Free Our People' March on Congress: Want to Live 'at Home, Not in Nursing Homes,'" www.accessiblesociety.org/topics/persasst/freeourpeoplemarch.html.

21. Disability rights advocates have continued to fight for more access to HCBS through legislation called the Community Choice Act. The proposal would allow any person deemed eligible for care in an institution to receive it in a home or community setting.

22. See Crowley (2006) for an overview. The Deficit Reduction Act also authorized Money Follows the Person demonstrations, whereby participating states would receive an enhanced federal match for a time to move enrollees from institutions to the community. It also allowed states to extend Medicaid "buy-in" coverage to children with disabilities in families with incomes up to 300 percent of the poverty line.

23. See CMS, "Waivers," www.cms.hhs.gov/MedicaidStWaivProgDemoPGI/MWDL/lis.asp.

24. The legal changes pertained to Section 1915i of the Social Security Act. The ACA established an eligibility threshold set at 300 percent of that required to qualify for SSI.

25. Stakeholders in the disability community doubted that states would take advantage of the opportunity to provide HCBS under the new terms of the ACA. They anticipated that state fiscal stress and the broad entitlement would be key deterrents (Coughlin 2010).

26. The law extended the Money Follows the Person Rebalancing Demonstration Program through September 2016 and allocated additional monies. And the Community First Choice Option promised an enhanced federal matching rate of six percentage points for reimbursable expenses for five years. Though not part of Medicaid, the ACA also established a national insurance program funded by voluntary payroll deductions to provide HCBS to individuals should they need it.

27. See Levitsky (2008, 564).

28. State Medicaid officials reported that most of those on waiting lists had already met the program's eligibility criteria (Ng, Harrington, and Watts 2009, 11).

29. Consumer direction does not always entail substantial discretion to hire and fire service providers. At times it refers to the shaping of service allocation budgets (Ng, Harrington, and Watts 2009, 11).

30. See Grabowski (2006) and Ng, Harrington, and Kitchener (2010, 27). Kaye, LaPlante, and Harrington (2009) suggest that under certain circumstances HCBS expansion may reduce Medicaid spending on long-term care.

31. These data are from www.statehealthfacts.org/comparetable.jsp?typ=4&ind_180&cat+4&sub=47.

32. In thirty-eight of fifty cases, a state's HCBS expenditure per poor person also predicts its placement relative to the mean on HCBS participants per poor person. Discrepancies between the two indicators in a handful of cases emanate from such factors as differences in provider payment rates and the HCBS case mix among the states. With respect to the case mix, for instance, a state might score above the mean on the expenditure measure but below it on the participation metric because it has disproportionately focused its HCBS efforts on more expensive enrollees, such as those with intellectual and developmental disabilities.

33. Among other things, New York guaranteed employees of state institutions protection against layoffs, assuaged local communities by finding alternative uses for the abandoned facilities (e.g., Willowbrook became a campus of the City University of New York), and worked effectively to establish an HCBS infrastructure at the local level (Castellani 2005, 238, 249–50).

34. See GAO (2003a). On some occasions, however, issues surface that lead to protracted negotiations between federal and state officials. A Minnesota Medicaid administrator described a "painful process" of negotiation over an ongoing Section 1915c waiver that took six months (interview 8, September 24, 2010).

35. In this vein an official at the NGA noted that some tensions exist between it and the National Association of State Medicaid Directors. The latter group tends to be more liberal than the governors. He said he knew of two Medicaid directors who lost their jobs because their activities via the National Association of State Medicaid Directors were out of sync with the preferences of their governors (interview 6, September 2, 2010).

36. To reduce administrative and related costs, federal and state officials have demonstrated increasing interest in consolidating multiple, narrow-gauge waivers into an overarching one.

37. In some states, such as Minnesota, Arc has refrained from becoming a provider out of a concern that it might compromise its advocacy role; interview 13, September 22, 2010.

38. These percentages refer to the Medicaid monies spent on optional enrollees and services; see Courtot and Artiga (2011, 10).

39. For example, Medicare payment practices encourage hospitals to discharge Medicaid patients back to nursing homes or to HCBS settings as quickly as possible. If they are discharged prematurely, many of the dual eligibles wind up being readmitted to hospitals (Ng, Harrington, and Kitchener 2010, 27). Special efforts to coordinate Medicaid long-term care with Medicare acute care have also made limited headway and face several barriers (Grabowski 2009).

CHAPTER FIVE

Demonstration Waivers and the Politics of Reinvention

Within a month after taking office in January 1993, President Bill Clinton appeared at the winter meeting of the National Governors Association, a group with which he had been affiliated for twelve years as governor of Arkansas.[1] The president spoke words the governors wanted to hear. Clinton deemed the process that the federal bureaucracy employed to evaluate Medicaid demonstration proposals as "byzantine and counterproductive." He asserted that "for years and years, governors had been screaming for relief from a cumbersome process by which the federal government had micromanaged the health care system affecting poor Americans." He vowed to bring relief by directing federal administrators to consult with the NGA and develop plans to streamline the waiver process within sixty days (Friedman 1993).

The Clinton initiative signaled the start of a significant transformation in Medicaid politics and American federalism. As described in chapter 4, Clinton had accelerated the approval of HCBS waivers by eliminating the cold bed rule and easing pressures on states to assure cost neutrality. But his speech before the NGA addressed a topic much broader in scope. Clinton and many other governors envisioned demonstration authority under the Social Security Act as a springboard for states that wanted comprehensive Medicaid reform. This development promised to take the devolution of Medicaid authority to heights far beyond the substantial discretion that states had acquired through the more targeted HCBS waivers.

Section 1115 of the Social Security Act, which Congress approved in 1962, provides the primary provenance for Medicaid demonstration waivers. It was endorsed by President John F. Kennedy, and it gives the federal executive branch authority to experiment with alternative state approaches to program delivery. Unlike the HCBS waivers, it explicitly envisions the 1115 initiatives as a tool for policy learning by requiring that state demonstrations be formally evaluated. Throughout Medicaid's first quarter century, presidential administrations approved relatively few demonstrations. This changed with the arrival of Clinton. The period from 1992 to 2010 featured an outpouring of demonstrations, with many states using them to reinvent their Medicaid programs.

This development possesses implications not only for the fabric of American federalism but also for Medicaid's durability. After tracing how the Clinton and George W. Bush administrations fueled the proliferation of waivers, this chapter zeroes in on their substance. The federal executive branch authorized waivers for myriad purposes—the adoption of managed care, eligibility expansions for adults, the introduction of market reforms, restructuring via mechanisms that resembled a block grant, emergency response, the leveraging of broader health system reform, and more. Did the substance of these waivers strengthen or weaken Medicaid? The chapter then examines whether the demonstrations helped states serve as laboratories of democracy fostering the diffusion of well-tested policy ideas. Did the waivers create a knowledge base and dissemination dynamics that augmented Medicaid's durability? I then examine concerns about waivers from the perspective of democratic process. Whatever their substantive benefits, do waivers represent the triumph of a kind of executive federalism that scotches the effective participation of legislative bodies and key stakeholders in the policy process? The answer to this question is not only important in its own right. It also has implications for the legitimacy of waivers as a policy tool for program enhancement and, more generally, for Medicaid's ability to generate political support. A concluding section plumbs the ways in which the waivers have created positive policy feedbacks through the administrative process that bode well for the program's durability.

The Rise of Demonstration Waivers

Before 1993 the federal bureaucracy used its Medicaid demonstration authority quite sparingly, approving just fifty waivers in nearly three decades (Vladeck 1995, 218). Waiver processes during this period tended to reflect a top-down approach, with the federal government typically driving the topical agenda. Federal officials generally stressed the research component and limited the demonstrations' durations. In 1982 and 1983, for instance, HCFA used Section 1115 and other types of waiver authority to test various hypotheses about the efficacy of managed care for Medicaid in six states (Freund et al. 1989). Only one of the 1115 waivers given during this period, Arizona's managed care program, typified the kind of comprehensive reforms that marked the Clinton years.

As the 1980s unfolded OMB employed the concept of "budget neutrality" to constrain waivers. OMB had grown concerned that federal administrators and the states might use demonstration waivers to launch innovations that would drain the federal Treasury at a time of growing budget deficits. Historically, HCFA had neither promulgated guidelines on waiver costs nor built the capacity to project and track these costs with any precision. No statutory provision required it to do so (unlike the HCBS waivers). In 1983, however, OMB insisted that federal administrators adhere to the principle of budget neutrality in their waiver reviews

(Anderson 1994, 227). In general terms this meant that the demonstration could cost the federal government no more over its duration than if the state had continued to operate its existing Medicaid program.[2] OMB's growing political muscle in the waiver process prompted a sharp decline in the number of Medicaid demonstrations approved in the late 1980s (Dobson, Moran, and Young 1992, 79). State policymakers increasingly chafed at the federal government's reluctance to accept and approve their proposals. One governor even editorialized in the *New York Times* that the administration of George H. W. Bush had "put its courage in the closet" concerning state experimentation.[3]

The Clinton Administration as Watershed

The Clinton administration wasted no time in signaling that a new day had dawned for Section 1115 waivers when it took office in January 1993. The president ordered federal administrators to work with the NGA to streamline the processes for dealing with state waiver requests. They moved promptly to comply. Of particular importance, HCFA (1994, 23, 960) published a notice in the *Federal Register* promising several steps to speed up 1115 reviews. The agency vowed to establish a well-defined schedule with target dates for reaching a decision on state waiver requests. It pledged to maintain, "to the extent feasible, a policy of one consolidated request for further information" when it responded to a state's proposal. Federal administrators also agreed to expand preapplication consultation and to provide more technical assistance to states that wanted waivers. To reduce delay, proposals would receive concurrent rather than sequential review from HCFA, OMB, and any other pertinent federal agencies. Moreover, federal officials promised to commit the staff and other resources needed for a "sound and expeditious" review (no small matter in the face of a likely increase in the volume of waiver applications and relatively constant staffing levels).

The 1994 notice also announced that the federal government would abandon the stringent approach to budget neutrality that had done so much to thwart waiver approvals. Federal administrators promised to examine the cost neutrality of a demonstration project over its entire life, not on an annual basis (the prior practice). They also pledged to be more open to state ideas on how to calculate future Medicaid expenditures under the waiver. This more flexible stance on "cost neutrality" soon sparked criticism from fiscal watchdogs. Appearing at a congressional hearing in 1995, for instance, the US comptroller general, Charles A. Bowsher, warned that "waivers could lead to a heavier financial burden on the federal government." He complained that HCFA had interpreted the budget neutrality requirement so loosely as to make it almost meaningless (Pear 1995b).

Reinforcement under Bush

Upon entering office in 2001, President George W. Bush successfully proposed to change the name of the Health Care Financing Administration to CMS. But this did not signal the rejection of the Clinton administration's posture on demonstrations. The new administration continued to interpret the budget neutrality of waiver proposals flexibly and soon came under criticism from the GAO (2004b) for its permissiveness. Federal officials also renewed most of the Section 1115 waivers that states had obtained during the Clinton years. In other respects, however, the Bush administration pursued new directions. For instance, it permitted states to use two additional pots of money to subsidize their waivers. One was Medicaid's Disproportionate Share Hospital program. The federal government had long permitted states to use certain Medicaid funds to aid hospitals and related institutions that provided relatively large amounts of care to the uninsured and Medicaid enrollees. Now the federal bureaucracy stressed that states could use demonstrations to reprogram this subsidy to fund insurance expansions for individuals. The Bush administration also ceded states more discretion over CHIP grants. The 1997 legislation creating this program had permitted states to apply for waivers to cover the parents of CHIP children. Federal officials now took the additional step of allowing states to apply for waivers under CHIP that would insure childless adults.

In August 2001 the Bush administration further articulated waiver themes that it would welcome by announcing the Health Insurance Flexibility and Accountability (HIFA) initiative. HIFA signaled to the states that federal administrators would be more flexible than ever in approving proposals that altered the Medicaid benefit package, modified eligibility rules, targeted benefits to certain geographic areas, and established enrollment caps. HIFA encouraged states to adopt private market approaches, such as enrollee cost sharing and premium assistance for individuals to purchase private insurance. In exchange for this flexibility, states were expected to propose ways to expand health insurance coverage, especially for those with incomes below 200 percent of the poverty line (Coughlin and Zuckerman 2008). In addition to HIFA the Bush administration announced a Pharmacy Plus demonstration initiative in January 2002 to enhance the opportunity for states to cover the drug costs of low-income seniors and people with disabilities who did not meet current eligibility criteria.

States responded to signs of a new federal flexibility by flocking to submit demonstration proposals. During the Clinton administration, thirty-nine states submitted 89 waiver requests, and thirty states won approval for 66 initiatives. By the end of the Bush administration nearly every state had submitted a Section 1115 waiver proposal at one time or another, and CMS had approved more than 150 of them (Thompson and Burke 2007, 978). Although states did not invariably implement or renew their waivers, many demonstrations endured over the years.

As of early 2010 thirty-two states plus the District of Columbia ran their Medicaid programs at least partially through 1115 waivers. States operated more than 50 waivers, with the numbers ranging from 1 in seventeen states to 4 in Arkansas.[4]

The Varied Substance of Waivers

The demonstration waivers launched under Clinton and George W. Bush varied greatly in their substance. Some of the more significant initiatives involved moving Medicaid enrollees to managed care, expanding coverage to adult populations, and embedding market-based features in the program. The Bush administration attempted to use them as a vehicle for promoting backdoor block grants. The waivers also loomed large in efforts to deal with emergencies, such as Hurricane Katrina, and in the attempts of some states to restructure their health care systems.

The Allure of Managed Care

As the 1990s dawned most states relied on a fee-for-service model to serve Medicaid beneficiaries. This model allowed enrollees to access nearly any provider willing to see them. These providers then forwarded their bills to Medicaid for payment. Officials in many states found much to criticize in this model. They believed that it undervalued preventive care and thwarted the effective coordination of services. They knew that access barriers persisted because many doctors refused to accept Medicaid payment rates or practiced in places that were geographically inaccessible to low-income people. Nor did critics believe that the model kept the lid on costs. Fee-for-service systems rewarded providers for delivering more care. This tempted providers to deliver services of dubious or no value to obtain more reimbursement. At the extreme, "Medicaid mills" provided so much excess care as to spark accusations of waste, fraud, and abuse. Critics also believed that the insufficient attention to preventive care meant that Medicaid enrollees wound up with more acute and costly ailments. They noted that inadequate access prompted many Medicaid beneficiaries to seek care from hospital emergency rooms, which billed the program at higher rates than providers in the community.

Given these and other concerns, state policymakers increasingly saw managed care as an attractive alternative. Under this model states would contract with managed care organizations to serve Medicaid enrollees. To obtain a contract these entities would need to demonstrate that they had a network of providers that would afford access to high-quality care. The managed care plans would assign enrollees to a primary physician, who would oversee their care and use of specialists. Appropriate payment methodologies, such as capitation (i.e., paying a flat amount per enrollee) would discourage the provision of excess services. To assure that managed care organizations did not scrimp in the provision of care, state administrators could monitor data on encounters and other indicators of access and quality. In sum, managed care increasingly emerged as a way for state Medicaid programs to have their cake and eat it, too. States could simultaneously pare Medicaid costs while enhancing access and quality.

Although attractive to many state officials as a model, managed care had been difficult to achieve through ordinary Medicaid channels. The receptivity of the Clinton administration to demonstration waivers now opened the door to states that wanted to pursue it. During the 1990s federal officials approved seventeen comprehensive waivers that moved large numbers of Medicaid enrollees into managed care (usually with eligibility expansions as well). States such as Minnesota, Maryland, Missouri, New York, Oregon, and Tennessee transformed their Medicaid programs in this way. Maryland, for instance, obtained federal approval for a HealthChoice demonstration that pledged to move 80 percent of its Medicaid enrollees into managed care within one year. Initially, the state awarded contracts to nine organizations, which received risk-adjusted capitation payments (i.e., more money for signing up Medicaid enrollees with more acute health problems). In six months starting in July 1997, the state transitioned 300,000 enrollees into these managed care organizations (Chang et al. 2003, 392–93). The Bush administration also supported waivers promoting this approach, and as of June 2008 more than 70 percent of Medicaid enrollees were in some form of managed care.[5] The proportion ranged from 100 percent in Tennessee to 0 in Alaska and Wyoming. All but three states had placed more than half their enrollees in managed care. To a much greater degree than with Medicare or employer insurance, managed care left its mark on Medicaid.[6]

The degree to which managed care under Medicaid has lived up to its early promise remains unclear. In terms of cost, the evidence from Wisconsin and certain other states points to some initial savings. But this approach did not yield the savings of 5 to 10 percent relative to fee-for-service programs that some of its proponents thought it would (Hurley and Zuckerman 2003, 234–35; Levinson and Ullman 1998; Sparer 2008, 47). Part of the issue here is that managed care under Medicaid did not follow the money. State Medicaid programs have tended to enroll relatively healthy adults and children in these arrangements rather than the elderly and people with disabilities. The latter groups consume a disproportionate share of program expenditures. In New York State, for instance, the 60 percent of Medicaid enrollees in managed care account for only 14 percent of the program's outlays (Sparer 2008, 47).

Considerable fog also shrouds managed care's implications for access to high-quality services. Some studies reach pessimistic conclusions. For instance, an analysis based on a national sample of white, non-Hispanic women reported that managed care yielded a drop of 2 percent in the number of prenatal visits for Medicaid enrollees and an increase of 3 to 5 percent in the incidence of inadequate prenatal care (Kaestner, Dubay, and Kenney 2005). Nor do studies focused on health outcomes consistently make the case for the superiority of Medicaid managed care over the traditional fee-for-service model (e.g., Kaestner, Dubay, and Kenney 2005; Levinson and Ullman 1998). Other studies, however, point to sanguine effects. For instance, research on Rhode Island in the early 1990s found significant increases in the adequacy of prenatal care utilization among Medicaid mothers seeing physicians in private offices after the state enrolled them in managed care via a waiver (Griffen et al. 1999). Evidence from Wisconsin points in a similar direction (Levinson and Ullman 1998, 367). Still other studies note reductions in the inappropriate use of emergency rooms in the wake of managed care under Medicaid (Hurley and Zuckerman 2003, 235).

Nonetheless, whatever the limits of the available evidence gauging its relative efficacy, managed care under Medicaid has met a political test of success. Having moved to adopt it, few state policymakers have returned to the fee-for-service approach that historically dominated Medicaid. And several states have pledged to use waivers or other means to move more of the elderly and people with disabilities into managed care.

Waivers Spark Coverage Expansions

Nearly half the states employed demonstrations to expand Medicaid coverage to new groups of low-income people (Coughlin and Zuckerman 2008, 214). During the Clinton years, several states linked eligibility expansions to their managed care initiatives. For instance, Minnesota during the administration of Governor Arne Carlson (R) won approval of a Section 1115 waiver in 1995 that allowed it to supplement its regular Medicaid program with MinnesotaCare. Through a series of incremental steps this initiative eventually extended coverage to pregnant women and children with incomes up to 275 percent of the poverty line along with certain uninsured, low-income adults. Other states also launched ambitious initiatives. In 2001, for example, the administration of Governor George Pataki (R) in New York forged a demonstration called Family Health Plus. This initiative extended Medicaid coverage to low-income uninsured adults with and without children. By the time Pataki left office in 2007, Family Health Plus covered about a half million people (Sparer 2008, 2). For its part, New Jersey under Governor Christine Whitman (R) initiated New Jersey FamilyCare in 2001. This waiver allowed uninsured children with incomes up to 350 percent of the poverty line to obtain CHIP or Medicaid coverage. Certain uninsured adults also became eligible (Holahan and Pohl 2003, 186). As of early 2010 this program enrolled 267,000 adults and 638,000 children.[7]

As significant as these and other demonstrations were in expanding Medicaid coverage, none loomed as large as the Massachusetts waiver of 2006. This waiver—

the product of intense negotiations between Republican governor Mitt Romney, a legislature controlled by the Democrats, and the Bush administration—became a catalyst for the state's success in achieving near-universal health care coverage. It also became the inspiration for federal policymakers when they passed major health care reform in 2010. The role of the waiver process in galvanizing path-breaking reform in Massachusetts and the nation comes under the spotlight in chapter 6.

As with the HCBS waivers, states pursuing eligibility expansions through demonstrations have the option to curb the Medicaid entitlement. Capping enrollments is one way to do this. Most states with waivers for coverage expansions, including Minnesota and New York, have shunned caps (Coughlin and Zuckerman 2008, 215–17). But others, such as New Jersey, have decided to hedge fiscal risk in this way. The imposition of caps typically leads to on-again, off-again enrollment as states encounter fiscal stress. New Jersey has sporadically suspended new enrollments in FamilyCare as budget difficulties have surfaced. States also possess considerable discretion to depart from the Medicaid entitlement by modifying service packages. In this vein, the administration of Governor Mike Leavitt (R) in Utah initiated a demonstration in the early 2000s that dramatically sliced benefits. This waiver extended coverage to parents and other uninsured adults with incomes up to 150 percent of the poverty line. It financed this Medicaid expansion by trimming the health benefit package and imposing certain types of cost sharing on current enrollees. The newly "insured" group of adults obtained insurance that covered primary care but not hospital services, except for emergency room use. Utah officials promised the new Medicaid beneficiaries that case managers in the Utah Department of Health would try to connect them with specialists willing to offer them free care if they became acutely ill. They also negotiated with the hospitals to provide these new beneficiaries with a limited amount of charity care. Utah, however, is the exception. Most states with demonstrations tended to preserve the Medicaid benefit package for newly eligible groups.

State initiatives to extend Medicaid coverage to new populations did not invariably succeed. Some states fell short of achieving their enrollment goals (Coughlin and Zuckerman 2008, 224). In certain states, especially Tennessee and Oregon, ambitious demonstrations did not prove politically durable. Led by Governor Ned McWherter (D), Tennessee won federal approval for a bold initiative called TennCare in 1993. Under the waiver the state not only moved all Medicaid enrollees into managed care but it also allowed those without insurance to enroll in Medicaid by paying a premium adjusted to their incomes. TennCare was launched in 1994 and soon added more than 400,000 previously uninsured people to the state's Medicaid rolls; the ranks of the uninsured in the state dropped sharply. Within a year, however, TennCare faced acute cost pressures and resistance from some providers. Policymakers moved to freeze enrollments for certain categories of beneficiaries. By the early 2000s Governor Phil Bredesen (D) persuaded federal administrators to approve a stripped-down version of TennCare. The modified waiver rolled back eligibility levels to below 200 percent of the poverty line (Holahan and Pohl 2003, 201).

A major waiver in Oregon also suffered setbacks. The state had initially won approval in 1993 for a demonstration (the "Oregon Health Plan") to cover all uninsured poor adults. In the 1990s this waiver boosted Medicaid enrollments and helped pare the state's uninsurance rate. A bipartisan coalition supported the proposal in budget battles, and voters approved increases in the state's cigarette tax to fund the demonstration. In 2002 Governor John Kitzhaber (D) led efforts to expand Medicaid coverage still further through a new waiver. This demonstration, which was approved in 2002, promised a 50 percent expansion in enrollments by extending coverage to single adults and couples with incomes up to 185 percent of the poverty line. To keep costs down, officials required the expansion group to contribute to cost sharing and reduced the benefit package to an estimated 78 percent of the value provided to lower-income Medicaid enrollees. The waiver also allowed officials to cap enrollments. Thanks in part to the cost-sharing requirements, applications for the program lagged expectations. Moreover, deteriorating economic and political circumstances prompted officials to cap enrollments as of 2006. The projected increase in beneficiaries did not occur, and the proportion of Oregonians without insurance grew (Oberlander 2007).

The limits to the durability of Medicaid coverage expansions in Oregon and Tennessee have attracted considerable attention (e.g., Hurley 2006; Oberlander 2007). But one should guard against excessively weighting the experiences of these two states in judging the efficacy of demonstrations in facilitating coverage expansions. Though suffering setbacks, neither Oregon nor Tennessee emerged as a poster child for Medicaid erosion. From 1992 to 2008 Oregon experienced a 33 percent increase in enrollees per poor person; Tennessee achieved 56 percent growth on this measure (see chapter 2).[8] Moreover, eligibility expansions via waivers in states such as Massachusetts, Minnesota, and New York have endured and grown. Some states have pursued waivers for coverage expansions since the passage of the ACA. In November 2010, for instance, federal administrators approved a demonstration sought by California called the Bridge to Reform. This waiver led to the enrollment in Medicaid of nearly 200,000 nonpregnant adults with incomes up to 200 percent of the poverty line by late 2011.[9]

Waivers and Market Reforms

Waivers, especially during the Bush years, also became vehicles for promoting privatized, market-friendly models within Medicaid. Federal officials encouraged states to pursue several variations on this theme. One was greater cost sharing.

States that wanted to charge premiums or impose other costs on Medicaid enrollees won greater freedom to do so. Supporters of this approach believed that consumer cost calculations ought to be more central to the health care system. In this view enrollees with a greater financial stake in their health care would use services more wisely. States displayed some interest in cost sharing. Out of thirty-three demonstration waivers approved or renewed during the Bush years, 70 percent featured some mix of premiums, deductibles, or copayments. Most states employing this approach did not impose cost sharing on their lower-income enrollees, instead applying it to expansion populations further above the poverty line. With the exception of the Oregon waiver discussed above, most states refrained from imposing major costs on enrollees (Coughlin and Zuckerman 2008, 215–17, 222).

Market-friendly ideas have also manifested themselves in demonstrations that foster greater reliance on private organizations to shape and administer Medicaid benefits. The rise of managed care in the 1990s was a significant step in this direction. The Bush administration encouraged other variations on this theme. One of its initiatives promoted demonstrations where Medicaid provided premium assistance to firms to enroll low-income workers in an employer-based plan. States such as Arkansas, Idaho, Illinois, and New Mexico pursued waivers of this kind in the early 2000s. On balance, however, these initiatives have played a small role in Medicaid coverage expansions (Coughlin and Zuckerman 2008, 227–28).

The Bush administration also welcomed waivers that stressed competition among private plans and consumer choice. A Florida demonstration approved in 2005 stands front and center in this regard. Spearheaded by Governor Jeb Bush (R), the Florida waiver sought to move Medicaid away from a "defined-benefit" program that entitled all enrollees to similar benefits to a "defined-contribution" program, whereby each Medicaid enrollee would choose among alternative plans offered by private insurance companies. The state launched the program in Broward and Duval counties, which encompassed nearly 10 percent of the state's Medicaid enrollees. Although Florida imposed certain requirements on the plans, the demonstration gave managed care organizations considerable freedom to depart from the standard Medicaid model in designing their benefit packages. The plans could vary appreciably in their provider networks, preferred drug lists, cost sharing, services covered, and requirements for prior authorization.[10] The state promised to pay a specific risk-adjusted premium to the health plans per Medicaid enrollee. In an effort to keep the established managed care organizations responsive, the demonstration also encouraged the creation of alternative provider service networks in the designated counties. This gave hospitals, whose administrators disliked the treatment they received from managed care organizations, an opportunity to create their own Medicaid plans to compete for enrollees.[11]

The demonstration emphasized consumer choice, with Medicaid beneficiaries informing themselves of the differences among the plans and picking the one best suited to their needs. Florida contracted with a private vendor to counsel enrollees on these choices. Medicaid enrollees could use a toll-free telephone number to reach a long-distance call center to obtain information (Coughlin et al. 2008). Florida officials hoped that this would spur the development of a "smart market," with informed consumers stimulating competition among the plans to offer more cost-effective services.

Evidence on the efficacy of the Florida waiver has yet to emerge fully. Clearly, however, officials have encountered significant implementation challenges. Initial reports indicated that about 30 percent of Medicaid enrollees were not aware of the alternative plans, let alone how they varied. Half the enrollees neglected to choose among the health plans and were therefore assigned to one by state Medicaid officials. The Florida experience reinforces the more general finding that understanding and acting on health plan information (achieving a form of health care literacy) poses substantial problems not only for the general population but also especially for Medicaid enrollees who have less education and often face a harried existence trying to make ends meet (Coughlin et al. 2008).

Waivers as Backdoor Block Grants?

The George W. Bush administration failed in its legislative effort to convert Medicaid into a block grant. But it strongly encouraged states to consider this possibility via a waiver. States that proved amenable to this approach would gain vast flexibility to reinvent their programs but would need to accept a five-year global cap on their Medicaid expenditures. A state that surpassed the cap would need to pay the excess out of its own resources. Most states resisted this approach. Officials in Minnesota, for instance, declined to pursue a waiver of this kind despite considerable pressure from the Bush administration.[12] However, two states, Vermont and Rhode Island, proved receptive. Their respective experiences illustrate the degree to which states prove savvy in negotiating their global caps.

The administration of Governor Jim Douglas (R) in Vermont pursued two major demonstrations in 2005—one for medical services and the other for long-term care. These waivers gave the state new flexibility to trim benefits, boost cost sharing, and limit enrollment. They also allowed the state to use federal funds to subsidize non-Medicaid health costs. In the case of long-term care, Vermont officials committed to increasing the proportion of services delivered in a home or community setting rather than a nursing home. By mid-2008 the state had expanded Medicaid eligibility to people with moderate disabilities in hopes of reducing their need to enter nursing homes at a later point (Crowley and O'Malley 2008). The Douglas administration proved skillful in negotiating a generous cap on Medicaid outlays. The cap substantially surpassed the amount that would ordinarily be derived from a historical analysis of Medicaid spending in the state. Expenditures from the first three years of the demonstrations indicate that Vermont faced little risk of exceeding its global budget target (Artiga 2009a, 6). Under the waivers, Vermont's Medicaid program has continued to rank among the most generous in the country in terms of Medicaid enrollees and expenditures per poor person (see chapter 2).

Rhode Island's officials at first appeared less savvy than their counterparts in Vermont in negotiating a munificent cap. Facing a budget shortfall, Governor Donald Carcieri (R) sought to save $358 million in Medicaid costs by submitting a demonstration proposal to the Centers for Medicare and Medicaid Services in 2008.[13] In exchange for enhanced flexibility, including the ability to establish waiting lists, the state proposed a five-year limit on Medicaid spending of slightly more than $12 billion. Medicaid stakeholders in Rhode Island promptly protested that the cap would be insufficient to meet the needs of low-income people, especially as the recession took hold in 2008. Think tanks in Washington provided analyses echoing these concerns.[14] In early January 2009 the state's congressional delegation in Washington—two senators and two members of the House, all Democrats—sent a letter to Carcieri questioning the wisdom of the waiver. The letter complained that the cap was set too low and "could pose serious risks to the Medicaid program." It urged the governor to defer the request until it became evident what monies Rhode Island might receive under a stimulus package the Obama administration planned to propose.[15] But Carcieri persisted and the Bush administration approved the waiver on January 16, 2009, five days before President Obama took office. Subsequently, however, passage of Obama's stimulus bill significantly increased the federal government's share of Rhode Island's Medicaid costs. Moreover, observers increasingly gravitated to the view that the global budget Governor Carcieri had negotiated was a generous "sweetheart deal" with the Bush administration. The global cap greatly exceeded what the state projected it would spend on Medicaid in the absence of the waiver (Cross-Call and Solomon 2011).

Conceivably, federal administrators could negotiate a global budget that significantly restrained Medicaid spending in a state. On balance, however, the limits of demonstrations as vehicles for backdoor block grants stand out. Most states resisted pressures to adopt them. Officials in Vermont and Rhode Island negotiated munificent global caps that allowed them to remain in the top quartile of states in Medicaid spending per poor person. Moreover, the waivers typically run for five years, after which officials can return to the standard fiscal entitlement.

Fire Alarm Waivers

In a vast departure from the original conception of demonstrations as carefully crafted research vehicles for policy learning, the federal government has employed them as an emergency response mechanism. At no time was this more evident than in the wake of Hurricane Katrina, which devastated New Orleans in 2005. To help ameliorate the health care dislocations that Katrina precipitated, the Bush administration encouraged states to apply for temporary Medicaid coverage for certain groups of evacuees. States that obtained waivers not only included those at or near the geographic center of the storm, such as Louisiana and Mississippi; it also incorporated more remote jurisdictions—such as Idaho, Montana, and Rhode Island—where some evacuees from New Orleans had settled. Eventually, thirty states obtained Katrina waivers and provided temporary Medicaid coverage to more than 100,000 people (Artiga 2009a, 7). Although the Clinton administration had not used waivers to meet natural disasters, it was not immune from using them for other forms of rescue. In the mid-1990s, for instance, top federal administrators rushed through approval of a demonstration to bail out the financially troubled Los Angeles County health system. Unlike the Katrina initiatives, this waiver proved to be far from temporary; it was extended well into the early 2000s after renewals.

Other Uses of Demonstrations

In addition to using Section 1115 waivers under Medicaid to foster managed care, coverage expansions, private market initiatives, backdoor block grants, and emergency responses, states have employed them for myriad other purposes. The federal government has, for instance, approved twenty demonstration waivers to expand family planning services (Thompson and Burke 2007, 980). In 2004, for instance, Minnesota initiated a waiver that extended Medicaid eligibility for these services to uninsured women and men between fifteen and fifty with incomes up to 200 percent of the poverty line.

Beyond targeted initiatives like family planning, the federal government has at times acceded to state requests to use waivers to promote broad, basic reforms in their health care systems that go well beyond the nitty-gritty of Medicaid eligibility, service packages, delivery mechanisms, and financing. New York State provides a particularly vivid example. In 2003 Governor George Pataki appointed a Health Care Reform Working Group to consider ways to streamline and improve the state's health care system. The deliberations of this group yielded a briefing paper in 2005, which New York officials shared with federal Medicaid administrators.[16] Above all, the paper contended that New York needed to move beyond "piecemeal reform" in reducing excess capacity in its hospital and nursing home sector.[17] Through "acute care rightsizing" and "long-term care reform and restructuring," officials sought to curtail New York's proclivity to treat individuals in institutions rather than less costly outpatient settings. The working group claimed that the excess capacity of the current health care system imposed a "significant financial burden" on Medicare, Medicaid, and other payers. Consistent with these themes, the state legislature agreed to create a Commission on Health Care Facilities in the Twenty-First Century to recommend facility closures and reconfigurations.

Policymakers understood, however, that this downsizing effort stood little chance of success without additional federal funds. The briefing paper thereby became the rationale for a Section 1115 waiver proposal. Claiming that the state's 1997 managed care demonstration had saved the federal Treasury $7 billion, the state requested additional Medicaid monies to subsidize the restructuring effort. After considerable negotiations, federal administrators signed off on the waiver in October 2006. Under the terms of the New York Federal–State Health Reform Partnership, the federal government pledged up to $300 million annually over a period of five years to promote reform. In exchange, New York State agreed to meet certain federal milestones, such as increasing the Medicaid monies recovered from fraud and abuse inquiries, decreasing hospital utilization, and implementing a single point-of-entry system for applicants seeking long-term care. The state would need to demonstrate savings of $1.5 billion to offset the commitment of additional federal funds and satisfy the requirement that the demonstration be budget neutral.

Policy Diffusion: States as Laboratories?

The outpouring of Section 1115 waivers represented a triumph for devolution as states gained new freedom to try alternative approaches to Medicaid. The question persists, however, as to whether the demonstrations lived up to their role in advancing states as laboratories for policy learning. Throughout Medicaid's first twenty-five years, federal administrators had generally taken the research and evaluation function of waivers seriously. They wanted state waiver experiences to be independently evaluated with the most rigorous social science methods that could feasibly be applied. Ideally, such research would provide a more robust knowledge base for policymakers concerning how to make Medicaid more cost-effective. It could galvanize enlightened policy diffusion. In fact, however, the proliferation of demonstrations as a tool for devolution marched hand in hand with the atrophy of systematic evaluation. This development by no means foreclosed the possibility that the waivers would fuel policy diffusion and contribute to Medicaid's durability. But it did mean that any such diffusion would draw limited succor from carefully crafted research.

The Atrophy of Formal Evaluation

The application of rigorous social science methods to state-level demonstration projects has never been easy. Random assignment to treatment and control groups, carefully crafted multistate comparisons, before-and-after testing, and other components of sophisticated evaluation have typically proved difficult to achieve.[18] The Clinton administration understood that imposing finely honed research designs would be all the more difficult as it deferred more to states' preferences. In this vein, federal administrators promulgated guidelines in 1994 signaling that they would be more flexible and less exacting in reviewing the research protocols that states submitted as part of their waiver proposals (Thompson and Burke 2007, 983).

While adopting a more permissive approach, however, federal officials still hoped for some knowledge gains. In 1993 HCFA's director of research and demonstrations, Joseph Antos (1993, 182), asserted that a more state-driven, streamlined waiver approval process featuring a more "laissez-faire approach" could still yield valuable research. So, too, the agency's top administrator, Bruce Vladeck (1995, 220), reaffirmed the role of the demonstrations in testing "good ideas" to determine their "real-world effects." He underscored that federal officials would rely on independent evaluators to assess states' efforts. The agency subsequently contracted with well-qualified organizations (at times collaborating with private foundations) to promote several rigorous studies. In the late 1990s, for instance, HCFA sponsored a cash-and-counseling demonstration in Arkansas, Florida, and New Jersey. As noted in chapter 4, this approach empowered those needing home and community-based services to hire assistants and manage the care they received rather than rely on a home care agency designated by Medicaid. With financial support and encouragement from the Robert Wood Johnson Foundation, federal administrators contracted with Mathematica Policy Research to design and implement a rigorous evaluation. The approach featured random assignment of Medicaid enrollees to the traditional agency model and to the experimental cash-and-counseling alternative. Ultimately, the evaluation studies pointed to the superiority of the new consumer-directed approach on several fronts (e.g., Carlson et al. 2005).

On balance, however, the Clinton administration's commitment to providing states with more flexibility, the surge in demonstrations, workload pressures at HCFA, and declining research budgets triggered a federal retreat from formal evaluation. The HCFA placed less pressure on states to present cogent evaluation plans in their waiver proposals. It backed away from contracting with an independent evaluator for each waiver and instead increasingly relied on state self-evaluations. Although some states took this obligation seriously, these self-assessments often failed to cast much light on the efficacy of the demonstrations (Thompson and Burke 2007, 984).

The George W. Bush administration downplayed the research component of Section 1115 waivers even more. Top administrators at the newly renamed Centers for Medicare and Medicaid Services further reduced funding for evaluation. They placed little pressure on the states to document their research plans in their waiver proposals. States varied greatly in the attention they paid to the subject. For instance, Illinois, South Carolina, and Wisconsin submitted Pharmacy Plus demonstration proposals that contained fairly detailed research protocols.[19] In contrast, Florida submitted a proposal of this kind that devoted only two paragraphs to evaluation methods. Federal administrators approved all of them (Thompson and Burke 2007, 984). In the case of fire alarm waivers, such as those for Katrina victims, states provided minimal descriptions of what they had done for those covered under the waivers. Bush administration officials also dragged their feet in releasing the findings of some studies that were undertaken.

Policy Diffusion Anyway?

The atrophy of formal evaluation in the waiver process undercut efforts to build a better knowledge base about variations in state Medicaid approaches and their cause–effect dynamics. It also reflected a substantial drift away from the original legislative thrust of Section 1115 and federal practices before the Clinton administration. But this development did not slam the door on prospects for policy diffusion based on the waivers. It did not rule out that any such diffusion might bolster Medicaid durability by encouraging more states to pursue cost-effective approaches.

For horizontal diffusion to occur, two conditions must hold. First, policy actors in Jurisdiction A must have significant information about one or several demonstrations in other states. Second, policymakers in Jurisdiction A must act on this information to adopt policies and practices based on those demonstrations. The adoption will seldom be an exact replica. Instead, customization occurs as Jurisdiction A adapts the approach to its particular circumstances (Karch 2007).

During the past two decades prospects for meeting the first precondition of policy diffusion have increased appreciably thanks to advances in information technology. Search engines such as Google make it much easier to track information. The Centers for Medicare and Medicaid Services and many state Medicaid agencies have developed Web pages that afford access to basic waiver documents. With e-mail, officials in different jurisdictions can more efficiently exchange information with each other. Moreover, a gaggle of think tanks and professional associations monitor Medicaid and disseminate information about demonstrations. These include such entities as AcademyHealth, the National Academy for State Health Policy, and the Kaiser Commission on Medicaid and the Uninsured. More general agents of representative federalism, such as the NGA (which houses a best practices center) and the National Association of State Medicaid Directors, also provide conduits for information. So, too, job mobility among top Medicaid officials as they move from one state to another can facilitate the flow of information. At times states hire major consulting firms, such as Health Management Associates, to assist them in designing initiatives. These firms employ former Medicaid administrators who can share knowledge born of their work experience in particular states and their current networking. These and other information sources contribute to a robust supply of "ordinary knowledge" about Medicaid demonstrations—insight rooted in casual empiricism, tacit understanding, common sense, and thoughtful speculation (Lindblom and Cohen 1979, 12).

The abundance of ordinary knowledge about the state demonstrations does not guarantee that policy diffusion will occur. A precise mapping of the degree to which the Medicaid demonstrations sparked horizontal policy diffusion is not feasible. Clearly, however, some diffusion of this kind occurred. For instance, one study suggests that states proved "highly discriminating" in drawing lessons from the managed care demonstrations of other jurisdictions in customizing their own versions. Policymakers learned, for instance, to shun approaches that ran sharply against the grain of local provider sentiment and practices (Hurley and Zuckerman 2003, 241). Horizontal diffusion also surfaced in the case of the cash-and-counseling waivers designed to empower people with disabilities to direct and manage their home and community-based services.

Bottom-Up Vertical Diffusion: Limits and the Big Bang

Vertical bottom-up policy diffusion resulting from the demonstrations is somewhat easier to appraise. Did national policymakers modify federal law or administrative rules to facilitate the adoption of the approaches embedded in the Medicaid demonstrations?[20] As was noted in chapter 4, this might occur through a federal mandate requiring states to follow the policies and practices that a waiver had illuminated. It can also occur in a devolutionary way, with Congress modifying the Medicaid law to give states the option of pursuing an approach that had previously been proscribed. Additionally, the federal government might provide states with greater financial incentives to adopt the approach spawned by the waiver. Whatever the exact federal action, a second prerequisite of diffusion must also be present: evidence that national policymakers relied on ample information about the demonstrations to guide their decisions.

With one major exception, the demonstrations during the 1990s and early 2000s featured very limited bottom-up diffusion. To be sure, some signs of diffusion present themselves. For instance, the carefully evaluated cash-and-counseling demonstrations testing the virtues of client direction in the case of HCBS helped fuel momentum to endorse the expansion of this approach in the Deficit Reduction Act of 2005. But this kind of episode tends to be the exception. One can certainly find instances where federal policymakers passed laws to encourage practices featured in the demonstrations. But it appears dubious that federal action emanated from a careful consideration of states' waiver experiences.

Consider, for instance, the mass migration of Medicaid enrollees to managed care in the 1990s. States led the way with their demonstrations, and Congress also stepped on the accelerator. The Balanced Budget Act of 1997 devolved new authority to the states to pursue managed care through ordinary Medicaid channels without obtaining a waiver.[21] But this development appears to have been less about federal policymakers learning from the states than being swept up in the political momentum that managed care enjoyed as a policy solution in the 1990s (Oliver 2001, 284). Most state managed care demonstrations had not been operating for long enough by 1997 for federal officials to have much information about their efficacy. A case does exist that federal policymakers sensed from the demonstrations that managed care could be implemented without scandal. Before the 1990s state managed care initiatives had a checkered past. Fraud and other forms of implementation failure had surfaced with a vengeance in California and elsewhere (Thompson 1981, 127–28). The absence of egregious episodes of failure in state approaches to managed care may have persuaded some members of Congress that states were up to the task. But beyond this, the managed care demonstrations hardly make a robust case for bottom-up diffusion.

The Bush administration evinced little interest in learning from the Section 1115 waivers. Instead, it attempted to foster top-down diffusion by encouraging the states to try approaches it favored on ideological grounds. In essence it acted more as a teacher of the states than a student of them. It held strong views on how to improve Medicaid through a private market approach. This approach touted enrollee choice and cost sharing, flexible benefit packages, premium support for employers, greater use of private contractors to implement Medicaid, and alternative financing approaches for the program. Shortly after taking office, it invited states to submit waivers featuring these themes under its Health Insurance Flexibility and Accountability initiative. This effort did not spring from a desire to test the efficacy of these approaches in the states. The Bush administration displayed little interest in evaluating the waivers and further cut the budget for research. Rather, the initiative reflected the hope that states could be persuaded to adopt the favored practices. "Try it, you'll like it" might well have been the motto. Ultimately, the Bush administration worked with Republican leaders in Congress to insert many of these market provisions into the Deficit Reduction Act of 2005. This law granted states new discretion to impose cost sharing on Medicaid enrollees, to alter Medicaid benefits, and to employ other market tools without a waiver. But this legislative victory reflected the triumph of Republican ideology rather than lessons that federal officials had soaked up from the state demonstrations that featured these elements. Even if national policymakers had been interested in assaying the pertinent state demonstrations, most of the waivers had not been operating long enough to yield many lessons.

Though touted as devices for policy learning, the demonstrations had up to 2005 played a small role in fostering bottom-up policy diffusion. Subsequently, however, a dramatic exception to this pattern occurred. The Bush administration approved a Medicaid demonstration waiver in Massachusetts that profoundly shaped major health care reform in 2010. This waiver established Medicaid as the platform for an ambitious attempt at near-universal coverage. In 2008 the three major Democratic candidates for president—Hillary Clinton, John Edwards, and Barack Obama—proposed health care plans that drew heavily on the Massachusetts model (Hacker 2010, 866). In forging the ACA of 2010, federal policymakers also turned to the experience in that state. The nature and dynamics of this big bang of bottom-up policy diffusion receive attention in chapter 6.

Waivers, Federalism, and Democratic Governance

The surge in demonstrations has ushered in major changes in state Medicaid programs. In doing so, waivers have also raised issues of democratic governance. Whatever their substantive benefits, do they threaten the rule of law by delegating too much discretion to the federal executive branch? Some observers believe the answer is "yes." In this vein, Jonathan Bolton (2003, 91,135) treats the rise of Section 1115 waivers as "the case of the disappearing statute." He argues that allowing the federal executive branch to replace Medicaid with "a patchwork of customized state programs" threatens to become "a statutory mouse hole hiding an elephant." In essence, "the Medicaid program enacted by Congress could cease to exist in any recognizable form." Bolton's concern looms all the larger in the face of complaints from some advocates that waiver processes fall short in meeting appropriate standards of administrative law, or "bureaucratic justice" (e.g., Edwards et al. 2007). Concerns here center on whether waiver processes are sufficiently transparent, respectful of due process, and consistent in providing opportunity for public input.

The political scientists Thomas Gais and James Fossett (2005) articulate a separate, albeit related, concern in arguing that the proliferation of waivers underpins a new model of governance, which they call "executive federalism." Under this model, major decision sites shaping policy increasingly shift to the executive branch at the federal and state levels. While noting the value of demonstrations in fostering policy innovation, Gais and Fossett register concern that the waivers may be eroding a core feature of the American political system: checks and balances. They also observe that waivers have become a vehicle for avoiding national policy debates, even while major program changes diffuse throughout the country (p. 487). In essence, the program drifts into a new configuration with little explicit consideration by policymakers. Gais and Fossett also portray congressional oversight of waivers as "weakened by the need for individual delegations to support requests from their own states" (p. 511).

Issues of waivers and democratic governance are important in their own right. They also have implications for program durability. If key Medicaid stakeholders come to see waiver processes as cutting democratic corners, they may move to complicate and constrain the use of this policy tool. In turn, this development could undercut the propensity for these waivers to enhance Medicaid in innovative and substantively important ways (as many of the demonstrations have done). It would further vitiate the potential for constructive horizontal and vertical policy diffusion. So, too, it could undercut Medicaid's support in the states as governors and others feel increasingly handcuffed in dealing with the program. They may resent the red tape and added transaction costs of the waiver process even if they can ultimately get their proposals approved. Hence, it is important to assay the criticisms of waivers from a governance perspective.

The question of how much discretion legislative bodies should delegate to the executive branch has long been a bone of contention among political scientists and jurists (e.g., Lowi 1969). In part the debate rests on different normative perspectives. Rather than exhaustively parsing Medicaid waiver processes through the lenses of these competing perspectives, I explore a more specific empirical question: What role have legislative bodies at the national and state levels played in the waiver process? To the degree that Congress and state legislatures keep a watchful eye on waiver decisions in the absence of precise laws, problems of democratic governance diminish. In essence, legislators could compensate for lack of a priori statutory control through post hoc monitoring, influencing waiver decisions made within the bureaucracy, and intervening with legislation when they find the executive branch insufficiently responsive.

Congressional Attentiveness

At the national level, there is considerable evidence of congressional attentiveness to and involvement with waiver processes.[22] In the period before 2000 much congressional activity aimed at promoting waivers. Signs of this pattern had occurred before the arrival of the Clinton administration. In the 1980s Congress occasionally took the initiative in writing a demonstration into a statute or preventing the bureaucracy from terminating an ongoing waiver (Dobson, Moran, and Young 1992, 80; Anderson 1994, 245–46). Congressional involvement intensified during the Clinton years. The outpouring of waivers under Clinton and the Republican takeover of Congress in 1995 fueled much greater oversight of the waiver process. Congressional committees repeatedly summoned administrative officials to testify. Congress conducted at least five sets of major hearings on Medicaid in 1995–96; one focused exclusively on the Section 1115 waivers and the others partly dealt with them (US House of Representatives, Committee on Commerce 1996a, 1996b, 1996c; US Senate, Committee on Finance 1995, 1997c). Congress also called on its analytical arm, the GAO (1995a, 1995b), to prepare reports on the waivers.

Some of this oversight reflected a genuine effort to learn more about the demonstrations, but most of the hearings developed the theme that the waiver approval process was still hopelessly bureaucratic and resistant to states' preferences. Committee chairs invited a gaggle of officials to testify about federal delays in approving waiver requests from such major states as Florida, Illinois, and New York. Appearing before Congress in June 1995, for instance, Illinois governor Jim Edgar (R) complained that the "HCFA has delayed and delayed and delayed" in responding to his state's waiver request. "The bureaucrats ask questions. We rush to respond. And then we wait and wait. The bureaucrats then ask more questions" (US House Committee on Commerce 1996a, 23–24). Edgar concluded that federal administrators would rather "fiddle and quibble" than act promptly. In chastising the Clinton administration at these hearings, members of Congress frequently resorted to such visual props as huge stacks of paper (three feet high in one case) representing a state's correspondence with HCFA over a waiver request. On one occasion, the committee chair had these stacks brought into the room in a wheelbarrow (Thompson and Burke 2007, 996). In these and other ways, the 1995–96 hearings supported the theme that waivers were a poor substitute for a block grant in devolving greater authority to the states.

President Clinton's veto of a Medicaid block grant and his reelection in 1996 brought these "show trial" hearings to a close. This did not, however, signal an end to congressional support for waivers. Members of Congress continued to do casework for state officials if they needed assistance in persuading federal administrators to approve waivers. Beyond this, Congress enacted pro-waiver statutory measures. A provision approved in 1997 mandated that states' renewal requests automatically be granted for three years if the federal bureaucracy failed to act with six months. Another measure in 2000 clarified that despite any changes in federal law, states could continue to operate their programs under waiver authority at least until they came up for renewal (Smith 2002, 302–3).

Although Congress has generally supported the enhancement of state discretion via the demonstrations, it has at times intervened to curb the waiver practices of the executive branch. Consider in this regard developments during the George W. Bush administration. Starting in 2003 the Republicans controlled both houses of Congress and the presidency. Under unified party government, legislative leaders usually lack the electoral incentive to embarrass or confront the executive branch and tend to trust it more (Huber and Shipan 2003). Moreover, the Republicans demonstrated considerable party discipline in furthering much of the president's agenda. Given these circumstances and Congress's favorable disposition toward waivers, one would predict minimal formal oversight and substantial deference to the executive branch on Section 1115 initiatives. This is not, however, the picture that emerges. To be sure, Congress did not stage highly visible hearings on the waivers. But the Senate Finance Committee was far from passive. It requested several reports from the GAO (2002, 2004b, 2004d) on the Bush administration's waiver initiatives, and in at least two cases it prevailed when the executive branch proved indifferent to its concerns.

The first episode involved the Bush administration's practice of approving waiver requests to redirect CHIP funds to insure childless adults. By the end of 2003 such states as Arizona, Illinois, New Mexico, and Oregon had won the blessings of the Centers for Medicare and Medicaid Services for such initiatives. The GAO (2002, 2004a) advised Congress that these waivers violated the CHIP statute. Concerned about this development, senators Charles Grassley (IA), the ranking Republican on the Senate Finance Committee, and Max Baucus (MT), the ranking Democrat, wrote the secretary of health and human services, Tommy Thompson, in 2002 asking him to stop these approvals. But Thompson declined. In the face of executive branch recalcitrance, Grassley and Baucus inserted provisions in the Deficit Reduction Act of 2005 that prohibited the Bush administration from approving any new demonstration that reallocated CHIP funds to childless adults.

This statute also provided Congress with another modest victory in its skirmishes with the executive branch. As indicated above, the Bush administration had used its demonstration authority to allow states to extend Medicaid coverage to survivors of Hurricane Katrina. In doing so, it resisted claims from senators Grassley and Baucus that the executive branch lacked the statutory authority to initiate these waivers. Despite resistance from the White House, Congress implanted provisions in the Deficit Reduction Act that explicitly authorized and reshaped the Katrina waivers (Park 2005). Among other things, the law required the federal government to pay the state's share of the Medicaid match for services to this target group.

Congress Targets the Administrative Process

When the Democrats regained control of Congress after the 2006 election, they also sought to constrain the executive branch's discretion in dealing with waivers. Unlike their Republican counterparts, however, they focused on the bureaucracy's processes for approving waivers. Their initiative responded to the complaints of some stakeholders that Medicaid waiver processes failed to meet standards of administrative due process. Historical perspective helps illuminate the dynamics that unfolded.

The Administrative Procedures Act of 1946 requires federal agencies under many circumstances to issue notices of proposed rulemaking in the *Federal Register* and to solicit public comment. The executive branch has, however, long possessed considerable latitude to decide which administrative decisions must conform to this law. Federal Medicaid administrators did not believe that this law applied to many of their program decisions, including those concerning waivers.

However, as the Clinton administration opened the door to state reinvention initiatives via demonstrations, it saw some formalization of approval processes as desirable. HCFA decided to use the *Federal Register* to pursue a double-barreled approach to transparency and public notice. One barrel targeted the federal government. Starting in 1994 federal administrators pledged to place periodic notices in the *Federal Register* announcing all new demonstration proposals and the status of those under review (i.e., approved, disapproved, withdrawn, pending). They also promised to develop a list of organizations that would be notified whenever a state submitted a waiver request and to allow at least thirty days for public comment.

Federal officials aimed the second barrel at state waiver processes. They required states seeking waivers to describe and obtain federal approval of the approach they used to solicit public comment. To help states clear this hurdle, HCFA specified five practices, the adoption of any one of which would incline it to sign off on a state's processes. States could (1) hold public hearings concerning the Section 1115 request, (2) form a commission that held such hearings, (3) obtain state legislative approval of the proposal, (4) provide formal notice and opportunity for comment via the state's administrative procedures act, or (5) publish a waiver notice in the newspapers.[23]

The Clinton administration remained committed to these formal processes throughout most of its two terms. By 1998, however, HCFA faced a significant reorganization, the turnover of key personnel including its top administrator, the need to foster the Y2K computer transition for the new millennium, and the implementation demands of health care initiatives embedded in the Balanced Budget Act of 1997 (Smith 2002). In the wake of these workload pressures, federal officials stopped implementing the formal procedures they had adopted in 1994. Notices of waiver action no longer appeared in the *Federal Register*. Administrative oversight of state waiver processes diminished. The Bush administration pushed devolution to the states still further. States would no longer need to describe their efforts to obtain public input in any detail. Instead, they could check a box on a form indicating that they had done so.

A review of waiver proposals in the wake of these developments suggests that most states still exerted effort to inform the public of major waiver proposals and to invite public comment. Still, the devolutionary shift sparked restiveness in some quarters of Congress and among advocacy groups. In 2002 a GAO report took federal administrators to task for permitting some states to obtain waivers with little public input. In response to this criticism, CMS sent a letter to state Medicaid directors in May 2002 reaffirming its commitment to enforcing the 1994 guidelines concerning public notice at the state level. The agency also worked to improve Web access to waiver documents.

But concern persisted. In 2006 sixty national organizations sent a letter to the Senate Finance Committee about the lack of opportunity for input on waiver proposals once the federal bureaucracy received them. In December of that year, a special Medicaid Commission established by the Bush administration also endorsed greater public notice and opportunity for comment at the federal level (GAO 2007d, 17–18). A few months later, AARP released a report called *Let the Sunshine In: Assuring Public Involvement in State Medicaid Policy Making* (Edwards et al. 2007). This report asserted that the "hallmarks of effective involvement of the public include transparency, meaningful opportunities for engagement, and availability of accurate, objective and timely information" (p. iv). It found variation among the states in the degree to which they lived up to these ideals and considerable dissatisfaction among many stakeholders with waiver processes. The study proffered thirteen recommendations that targeted both the federal government and the states. Among other things, it called upon Congress to establish minimum standards for public participation in state waiver processes and to require a public notice-and-comment procedure at the federal level (pp. 18–19).

The Democratic takeover of both houses of Congress in 2007 unleashed a gusher of oversight hearings and related inquiries concerning the Bush administration's practices. In this vein, three Democrats with substantial leverage over health policy—Henry Waxman (CA), John Dingell (MI), and Frank Pallone (NJ)—joined with Senator Sherrod Brown (D-OH) to request that the GAO (2007) again examine the waiver process. This time the office zeroed in on the decision making that surrounded the approval of major waiver proposals in Florida and Vermont. Both had sparked controversy among liberal advocacy groups. The office credited the two states with having done much to foster transparency and opportunities for public comment on their waiver proposals. It noted, however, that some advocacy groups remained dissatisfied with the process at the state level. More fundamentally, the office voiced concern that CMS had not afforded opportunity for stakeholder input after receiving the proposals. The agency did not post the proposals on its website before approving them. It signed off on the Florida waiver in an uncommonly swift sixteen days. Ultimately, the office recommended that Congress consider requiring the federal bureaucracy to beef up processes for public notification and comment, at a minimum enforcing the policies that HCFA had forged in 1994 (GAO 2007d, 20).

The intergovernmental lobby rejected this view. The NGA and National Conference of State Legislatures firmly believed that the states could be trusted to assure that waiver processes achieved transparency and opportunities for public comment. To superimpose another notice-and-comment opportunity at the national level would reward lobbies that had resources to obtain leverage in Washington but not in particular states; it would heighten transaction costs and foster delay. The Bush administration sided with the intergovernmental lobby. Responding to the GAO, the acting CMS administrator, Leslie Norwalk, averred that the "states are in the best position to decide which public input process will be most effective."

At the federal level "legislation requiring the Department to build a new public input process would create redundancy and slow the demonstration approval process, delaying states' creative approaches to expanding coverage" (GAO 2007d, 27).

The opposition of the Bush administration headed off efforts to impose new procedural requirements on waiver processes. The arrival of the Obama administration in 2009, however, opened the door to change. Ultimately, reformers used the ACA as a vehicle. The new law required the secretary of health and human services to design a "process for public notice and comment at the state level, including public hearings, sufficient to ensure a meaningful level of public input." The statute also mandated that federal administrators craft a procedure for obtaining such input once they received a waiver proposal from the states.[24] Congress also bolstered reporting requirements. The law obligated states to submit annual progress reports on their demonstrations and the secretary of health and human services to deliver an annual report on actions regarding waiver applications. All told, the new statutory provisions increased formal access points for advocates in the policy process and supplemented the information conduits available to Congress to monitor waiver developments. In this way, it stood to boost the legitimacy of demonstration waivers as a valuable policy tool among key Medicaid stakeholders. But the statutory changes meant that states eager to launch waivers would face more procedural hurdles and delay—factors that could fuel tension between the intergovernmental lobby and the federal government.

In sum, demonstration waivers at the national level have become a major tool of executive action. Different presidential administrations have strongly shaped their number and substance. But it would be going too far to portray Congress as a passive observer in the waiver arena. Its members work with officials from their home states to shape waiver decisions. Oversight occurs with the assistance of the GAO and communications from advocacy groups. When the executive branch strays too far from congressional preferences, the lawmakers have altered Medicaid policy to constrain administrative discretion.

Variation in State Legislative Practices

A thorough assessment of executive federalism must go beyond Congress to consider state legislatures. To what degree have demonstration waivers enlarged the power of the executive branch at their expense? The answer is far from clear. Unquestionably, many of the comprehensive demonstrations signal the importance of gubernatorial leadership as exemplified, for instance, by Jeb Bush (R) in Florida, John Kitzhaber (D) in Oregon, Ned McWherter (D) in Tennessee, George Pataki (R) in New York, Mitt Romney (R) in Massachusetts, and Christine Todd Whitman (R) in New Jersey.[25] These and other governors made Medicaid reinvention through waivers signature initiatives. Moreover, the absence of gubernatorial support for a demonstration almost certainly spells its demise. Although governors loom especially large in the story of Section 1115 waivers, however, state legislatures should not be portrayed as uniformly acquiescent to the executive branch. In this regard three observations seem particularly pertinent.

First, most legislatures have sufficient capacity to influence the waiver process. All else being equal, legislatures with higher salaries, larger staffs, longer legislative sessions, and no term limits have a better chance of holding their own vis-à-vis the executive branch (Kousser 2005; Huber and Shipan 2003). States vary considerably on these measures of professionalism. Experts suggest that ten legislatures (primarily though not exclusively in the most populous states) achieve high levels of professionalism and twelve rank low. The remaining twenty-eight fall into the moderate, or hybrid, category of professionalism.[26] Evidence suggests that state legislatures with at least a moderate level of professionalism have the potential to make a meaningful impact on waiver processes (Edwards et al. 2007).[27]

Second, significant numbers of legislatures not only have the capacity to shape waivers but also the inclination. In a few cases, such as Minnesota, their involvement has been dramatic. In the early 1990s a bipartisan group of legislators known as the "Gang of Seven" began working on a waiver proposal to obtain federal Medicaid funding for a coverage expansion. The "gang," which consisted of four Democrats and three Republicans from both legislative chambers, ultimately reached agreement. Among other things, their proposal pledged to extend Medicaid coverage to children and pregnant women in families living at up to 275 percent of the poverty line. Though he did not play a prominent role in legislative deliberations, Governor Arne Carlson (R) supported the proposal. Federal administrators approved the demonstration in 1995 and again when it came up for renewals. The waiver continues to provide a key template for the Minnesota Medicaid program.[28]

This episode is not an isolated example of legislative involvement in Minnesota. Led by Senator Linda Berglin (D) from Minneapolis, a member of the Gang of Seven, the Minnesota legislature has been front and center in shaping the evolution of Medicaid. Berglin has spent nearly four decades in the Minnesota legislature and won wide respect as a tenacious and knowledgeable policy entrepreneur. One stakeholder referred to her as a "czar" in the health policy arena and another as "dogged and brilliant."[29] State Medicaid administrators acknowledge her enormous expertise, albeit with some concern that she "micromanages" them.[30] Virtually all stakeholders acknowledge that a waiver or other initiative to modify Medicaid would stand little chance of success without Berglin's support. Surveys rank the Minnesota legislature as medium in terms of its professionalism. Of critical importance, however, its members do not face term limits. This has allowed Senator Berglin to build expertise over a period of nearly forty years. She has also benefited from the fact that the Democrats controlled the Minnesota Senate for decades.[31] The vast majority of state legislators, whether in Minnesota or elsewhere, know little or nothing about Medicaid waivers. Senator Berglin and the Gang of Seven illuminate the influence a legislature can achieve based on the knowledge and engagement of a few members.

Few, if any, states replicate the activism of the Minnesota legislature in the Medicaid policy arena. Still, legislative engagement with waivers often occurs. Often, the demonstrations require approval by the legislature either before or after submission to the federal government. Although governors and state Medicaid bureaucracies tend to have the upper hand in shaping them, legislators frequently extract concessions. When Governor Jeb Bush of Florida proposed the market-based demonstration described above, for instance, his party controlled both houses of the Florida legislature. The state House of Representatives worked to accommodate his views. But leaders of the state Senate greeted the Bush proposal with skepticism and dragged their feet. They created a select committee on Medicaid reform to hold hearings on the initiative around the state. Thanks to Senate resistance, the legislation authorizing the demonstration contained many departures from the version the governor preferred.[32] The level of legislative involvement in state demonstration processes in all fifty states is unclear.[33] But a study of eight states found substantial legislative engagement in waiver processes in three states (California, Florida, and Texas), occasional involvement in three (Connecticut, Illinois, and Indiana), and limited engagement in two (Michigan and Nevada) (Edwards et al. 2007, 12, 21).

Third, governors run risks if they attempt to be too unilateral in their waiver actions—if they seek to exercise power without persuasion. Consider the case of Governor Pataki in New York State.[34] Less than a hundred days after taking office in 1995, his administration submitted a major demonstration proposal to federal officials. This waiver proposal required the vast bulk of Medicaid beneficiaries to enroll in managed care plans, including those with "special needs," such as substance abusers, the mentally ill, and those afflicted with AIDS. In submitting the waiver proposal, the Pataki administration introduced a sharp-elbows variant of executive federalism. The Medicaid politics surrounding managed care in the early 1990s in New York had featured broad participation by the executive branch, the legislature, local officials, and key interest groups. In contrast, Pataki and his newly appointed health commissioner, Barbara de Buono, acted more unilaterally with minimal consultation of these stakeholders. Medicaid politics in New York thereby morphed from a more incremental, consensual, slow-but-steady model to a more contentious, executive driven, big-bang mode (Sparer and Brown 2002).

The Pataki administration soon learned, however, that this approach to waivers typically shifts politics from the state to the national arena. Between 1995 and 1997 an array of New York stakeholders pressed their case with the federal bureaucracy, the White House, and members of the state's congressional delegation in an effort to modify the waiver. Among other things, advocates stressed that managed care organizations lacked the experience and capacity to serve special needs populations effectively. The Pataki administration countered this effort by rallying its Washington allies, such as Senator Alfonse D'Amato (R-NY), to pressure federal administrators to approve the partnership plan. Intense and protracted negotiation between state and federal officials occurred. Ultimately the Pataki administration retreated from its position that special needs enrollees ought to be rapidly moved to managed care. With these and related changes, the waiver won federal approval in July 1997, about two years after its submission.

Waivers and Democratic Governance in Perspective

The Section 1115 waiver process does not meet pristine standards of democracy with legislative bodies front and center in debating and crafting major policy changes. Instead, the executive branch at the federal and state levels assumes center stage. The vast discretion delegated to chief executives and administrators in the waiver process does not, however, invariably enhance their power or shunt legislative bodies to the sidelines. At the national level, the White House and CMS exert considerable influence over the contents of waivers. But the processes leading to the more transformative demonstrations are, as one career administrator at CMS put it, "very, very political."[35] Members of Congress, governors, and other stakeholders monitor the waiver process and voice their views to officials in the executive branch in order to shape its outcomes. In general Congress emerges as a watchful, mostly consenting, but at times contentious player in dealing with demonstration waivers. For their part, state legislatures vary considerably in the degree to which they shape Section 1115 waivers. These legislatures tend to be less professionalized and less capable of oversight than Congress. But in some states, such as Florida, they play a more important formal role in the waiver process than Congress does at the federal level. This is because in certain states the governor's office must obtain a vote of approval from the legislature before it can implement the waiver. This approval authority and other political assets often allow state legislatures to leave their mark on waivers and on rare occasions to originate them. Overall, the processes leading to major demonstration waivers appear more open, fluid, and in a sense "democratic" than those associated with the conventional model of "picket fence federalism" discussed in chapter 4. That model focuses on relatively autonomous bureaucracies at the national and state levels working with key legislators and interest groups out of the public view. In contrast, demonstration waivers have tended to be highly visible initiatives with governors and presidents significantly involved.

In evaluating waiver processes, one should not view steps to strengthen the role of legislative bodies through rose-tinted lenses. Whether in Washington or the states, legislative processes frequently fall short as vehicles for representative democracy and sound policy. The increasing propensity of Congress to roll major program changes into massive omnibus budget acts often leaves key stakeholders and the public in the dark during policy formation (Quirk and Binder 2005). Meanwhile, the policy processes in state capitols typically receive minimal media coverage—all the more so in the face of fiscal pressures on newspapers to cut staff. Nor can one gainsay the corrosive impact of intense partisan polarization at the national level and in some states. These forces have given compromise a bad name and undermined the ability of legislative bodies to aggregate interests into coherent statutes. Some research suggests that legislative bodies riven by partisan polarization tend to be less productive in the amount and quality of laws they enact (McCarty 2007). At the national level polarization has helped fuel the growing use of the filibuster in the Senate, which diminishes prospects for legislative action. *Against this backdrop, waivers emerge as a salutary mechanism to galvanize policy adaptation and innovation in the face of legislative dysfunction.*

The administrative procedures that govern waivers also need to be placed in comparative context. At times, waiver processes have lacked transparency and failed to offer the public and key stakeholders opportunity to comment. On balance, however, these processes meet higher standards of public notice and due process than states typically achieve through regular Medicaid channels when they submit amendments to their state plans (Edwards et al. 2007, 5). The ACA takes additional steps to assure that waiver processes at the federal and state levels meet suitable standards of bureaucratic justice.

Implications for Program Durability

Having assayed issues of substance and process concerning the demonstrations, the core question remains: Have waiver developments vitiated or bolstered Medicaid's durability? Certain patterns suggest pessimism. The atrophy of waivers as vehicles for more rigorous social scientific assessment reduced their potential to contribute to a well-grounded knowledge base about the efficacy of different Medicaid approaches. Pessimists can also point to the role of demonstrations in weakening Medicaid as a legal entitlement. The waivers made it easier for the states to dodge Medicaid's statutory provisions that benefits must be offered statewide, that enrollees must be protected from cost sharing, and that beneficiaries must be able to choose among providers. They opened the door for states to thin benefit packages under the banner of expanding insurance coverage. Bush officials tried to use waivers as backdoor block grants.

On balance, however, waivers during the Clinton, Bush, and Obama period emerge in a more positive light from the perspective of Medicaid's durability. The atrophy of formal evaluation should not be blown out of proportion. There is a tenuous relationship between knowledge derived from social science and policymaking. It remains unclear whether more commitment to well-funded evaluations of the demonstrations would have strengthened Medicaid. Though seldom rigorously assessed, many of the demonstrations produced the kind of "ordinary knowledge" that could assist policymakers seeking to strengthen Medicaid. At times, they constructively contributed to policy diffusion. Nor, with occasional exceptions, did the waivers become vehicles for policy retrenchment. Whatever the exact forces at play, many states launched major coverage expansions and otherwise worked to enhance the program. To be sure, the degree to which the demonstrations enhanced the quality of care delivered to Medicaid enrollees remains an open question. Without doubt, they galvanized the movement of large numbers of Medicaid enrollees into managed care, which has hardly proven to be the elixir that some had hoped. Still, managed care in some states almost certainly fueled greater access to suitable care than the old fee-for-service system.

In theory, waivers are supposed to be budget neutral—costing no more than if the regular Medicaid program continued in place. Hence, they might appear to constrain prospects for expanding investment in the program. But the White House and federal administrators have long resisted pressures from the GAO and others to define the exact methodology used to determine budget neutrality when they approve waivers and subsequently monitor their costs. If federal officials have substantive and political reasons to approve and sustain a waiver, they can bend over backward to give states the benefit of the doubt on cost neutrality. For example, a federal administrator during the early 1990s indicated that he strongly suspected that the cost-neutrality estimates submitted by Tennessee to obtain a demonstration would not pan out.[36] Nonetheless, the Clinton administration approved the waiver. Despite the cost-neutrality stricture, expenditures on Medicaid have probably been greater than they would have been in the absence of the demonstrations.

Ultimately, the implications of the Section 1115 waivers for Medicaid's durability go well beyond their substance. They also involve political and policy feedback from administrative action. Researchers have stressed how the passage of legislation can alter cognitive mindsets and reconfigure the political dynamics surrounding a program, at times enhancing its durability (e.g., Patashnik 2008). *The case of demonstration waivers suggests how the use of administrative tools to achieve reinvention can generate feedback that fortifies a program.* Medicaid narrowly dodged major retrenchment in 1995, when President Clinton vetoed legislation that would have converted the program to a block grant. The proliferation of waivers made it harder to open that policy window again. The critical role of the nation's governors as Medicaid's power brokers helps account for this. In 1995 an easing of Medicaid's budget increases, unhappiness with the federal bureaucracy's stringency in reviewing their waiver requests, and the ideological fervor of the moment prompted many Republican governors to back a block grant. The devolution that Medicaid waivers helped unleash did much to sap interest in this approach. Through the Medicaid waiver process, governors could increasingly have it both ways. They gained impressive new power to shape their state programs without having to forgo the federal government's open-ended funding commitment. Governors could often gain more political credit for going to Washington and successfully battling for a waiver than they could if they had to shape program specifics under a block grant. Ironically, the George W. Bush administration's continued embrace of demonstration waivers probably undercut its efforts to rally support from Republican governors for a block grant proposal in 2003. In essence, Medicaid demonstration waivers have bolstered the program's durability by providing an administrative outlet for pressures from the states—especially from their governors—for greater flexibility.

The ACA has changed the playing field for Medicaid demonstration waivers and may also undermine this supportive dynamic. Republican policymakers in fiscally strapped states have increasingly voiced concerns reminiscent of the early 1990s—that the federal government has stripped them of the flexibility they need to control state budgets and manage their Medicaid programs. As I discuss in the next two chapters, proposals to convert Medicaid into a block grant have resurfaced with a vengeance.

Notes

1. Some of the information and themes of this chapter were covered earlier by Thompson and Burke (2007).

2. Projecting costs is, of course, far from an exact science. Federal administrators can be more or less stringent in reviewing the cost estimates embedded in a waiver proposal. They can decide whether or not to give states the benefit of a doubt concerning the estimates. The efficacy of budget neutrality also depends on the willingness of federal officials to penalize states if their spending exceeds the estimates contained in the waiver. Here, too, federal executives have substantial discretion to determine the vigor of their monitoring and enforcement.

3. Frustrated with her inability to get a Medicaid waiver approved in Oregon, Governor Barbara Roberts (D) (1992) wrote the editorial.

4. See CMS, "Waivers," www.cms.hhs.gov/MedicaidStWaivProgDemoPGI/MWDL/list.asp.

5. The data in this paragraph come from www.statehealthfacts.org/comparabletable.jsp?ind=217&cat+4&sub=56&yr=1&typ=2. The percentages enrolled in comprehensive, fully capitated managed care organizations are smaller. The cited numbers reflect recipient exposure to some form of managed care for at least some services.

6. In addition to capitation, Medicaid managed care stresses the role of a primary care physician in providing a medical home and serving as a gatekeeper to specialists; it also strives to standardize treatment protocols without micromanaging physicians. The degree to which managed care under Medicaid succeeds in implementing these provisions varies. See, e.g., Sparer (2008, 40–41, 46) and Peterson (1999).

7. These data are available in the table "Enrollment by County, March 2012," New Jersey FamilyCare, www.njfamilycare.org/enroll/enroll_chart.html.

8. It also deserves note that Oregon ranked near the top of the second quartile in its growth rate for spending per poor person; see table 2.2.

9. These enrollment data come from a fact sheet provided by the Kaiser Commission on Medicaid and the Uninsured in October 2011.

10. Prior authorization requires providers to seek approval from an insurance company before initiating a certain treatment. It typically targets more expensive procedures.

11. A key staff member noted that Governor Bush was skeptical about the likely performance of the managed care organizations. He did, however, believe that the right kind of competition could make them responsive. He hoped that the provider service networks would serve that purpose (interview 23, December 14, 2010). In turn, leaders of the managed care organizations resented that these networks received special treatment from the state—less regulation and more flexible capitation rates. They did not believe that competition was on a level playing field (interview 19, December 13, 2010; interview 21, December 13, 2010). The demonstration generally secured certain financial concessions for hospitals to encourage their support.

12. Interview 8, September 24, 2010.

13. Associated Press, January 9, 2009, www2.turnto10.com/jar/news/local/local_govt politics/article/carcieri_urges_lawmakers_to_.

14. The Georgetown University Health Policy Institute, the Center for Budget and Policy Priorities, and the National Senior Citizens Law Center were among the think tanks expressing concern. For an overview, see the Poverty Institute at Rhode Island College, www .povertyinstitute.org/matriarch/MultiPiecePage.asp_Q_PageID_E_121_A.

15. This is from a letter dated January 13, 2009, from senators Jack Reed and Sheldon Whitehouse and representatives Jim Langevin and Patrick J. Kennedy, posted on the website of the Poverty Institute at Rhode Island College (see the URL in note 14).

16. "Federal–State Healthcare Reform Partnership (F-SHRP)," April 27 2005, www .health.state.ny.us/health_care/managed_care/partner/operatio/docs/chapter_27.pdf.

17. The briefing paper also called for modernizing the state's health care system through electronic medical records, e-prescribing drugs, and supporting regional health information organizations.

18. For a discussion of additional research obstacles, see Nathan (2000, 59).

19. These were forerunners of the Medicare prescription drug law in 2003. They sought to aid dual eligibles in obtaining prescriptions.

20. Though I focus on adoption by the states, diffusion could also occur if the federal government applies lessons from the demonstrations to programs it more directly administers (e.g., to Medicare).

21. For an overview of the law's provisions, see Fossett (1998, 122–24).

22. This section draws heavily on Thompson and Burke (2007, 995–98).

23. If HCFA rejected a state's process for soliciting public comment, that state could win federal approval by publishing a waiver notice in the newspaper with the widest circulation in each city with a population of at least 100,000. In the event that a state had no city of this size, it could meet the requirement by publishing the notice in the newspaper with the largest circulation.

24. See Subtitle B, Part 1, Section 10201 of the ACA.

25. Before Mitt Romney, Governor William Weld (R) of Massachusetts had also promoted a waiver; see McDonough (2000, 250–71).

26. Karl Kurtz of the National Conference of State Legislatures provided me with data on the relative professionalism of state legislatures in 2008. See also Kousser (2005, 15).

27. This study found the legislative branch in Texas, one with medium capacity, to be highly involved in waiver processes.

28. This description draws on Iric Nathanson, "Bipartisanship in the 1990s Delivered Health-Care Reform in Minnesota," *Minnpost*, www.minnpost.com/irienanathanson/2009/07/29/10546/bipartisanship_in_the_1990s.

29. Interview 16, October 4, 2010; interview 18, November 15, 2010.

30. Interview 8, September 24, 2010.

31. The Democrats in Minnesota lost control of the Senate to the Republicans in the 2010 election.

32. Among other things, Governor Bush had favored legislation that afforded greater discretion to the executive branch to define the specifics of the demonstration during its implementation. The Florida Senate bill was more directive on several matters than the governor's office preferred. For example, the senate required an uncommonly rigorous evaluation of the demonstration by an independent research unit based at the University of Florida (interview 19, December 13, 2010; interview 23, December 14, 2010). For an example of legislative involvement in the waiver process in Massachusetts, see McDonough (2000, 254–70).

33. My search for such a comprehensive survey came up dry.

34. See also Gusmano, Burke, and Thompson (2012).

35. Interview 5, September 2, 2010.

36. Interview 1, July 15, 2009.

CHAPTER SIX

Reform

The Politics of Polarization

On March 23, 2010, President Barack Obama signed the Patient Protection and Affordable Care Act—an epic breakthrough to expand health insurance in the United States. This new law, commonly called the Affordable Care Act, or ACA, culminated a century of effort to insure all Americans. Theodore Roosevelt championed universal coverage when he ran for president on the Bull Moose ticket in 1912. The idea received serious consideration during the New Deal under Franklin Roosevelt, and President Harry Truman proposed a comprehensive plan after World War II. Sweeping proposals also surfaced during the presidencies of Richard Nixon, Jimmy Carter, and Bill Clinton. But all these bold initiatives came to naught. Against this backdrop, the success of President Obama and Congress in forging the ACA stands as a rare and remarkable policy achievement.

The ACA was also noteworthy in another sense. Historically, leading health reformers had slighted Medicaid in their proposals. Many saw the program as a politically feeble, down-at-the-heels second cousin to Medicare. They assumed that Medicaid would fade away with the arrival of universal coverage based on an employer mandate, a single-payer approach akin to Medicare, or some other mechanism. Instead, Medicaid became the pivotal platform on which the ACA rested. Of the 32 million individuals who were projected to gain coverage under the new law, Medicaid was to enroll half of them.

On the surface the ACA augurs well for Medicaid's durability. Medicaid stands poised to become an even larger pillar in the American health insurance system, surging to new heights in expenditures and enrollees. But the program's expansion and enhanced effectiveness are far from assured. States may decline to participate in the Medicaid expansion. Program administrators in the states that do participate face serious challenges in implementing the ACA, and failure to master them could open a chasm between policy promise and program performance.

Even more fundamentally, the passage of the ACA has thrust Medicaid into a political maelstrom that could greatly damage the program. And its passage illuminates the degree to which partisan polarization permeates American politics, reaching levels unseen in many decades. Republican Senator Jim DeMint of South

Carolina captured the partisan ferocity of the congressional debate over health reform in July 2009 when he proclaimed that if Republicans "are able to stop Obama on [health reform], it will be his Waterloo. It will break him" (Jacobs and Skocpol 2010, 85). Republican leaders in Congress decried the reform effort and tenaciously worked to obstruct it at every turn. The ACA prevailed with no Republican votes in Congress. Meanwhile, it became a lightning rod for anger and intense ideological attacks by the Tea Party, its allies at Fox News, and many Republicans. This coalition vowed to fight for the repeal of what they derisively called "Obamacare." Partisan polarization also suffused the response to the ACA in the states. Immediately after its passage, Republican attorneys general raced to the federal courts in an effort to get the law declared unconstitutional. Many Republican governors and state legislators denounced the new law. Tensions between the states and the federal government over Medicaid returned to levels not seen since the early 1990s.

Against this backdrop of partisan polarization and intergovernmental tension, this chapter probes the dynamics leading to Medicaid's central involvement in health reform and also the challenges of survival and implementation that lie ahead. I open by assessing Medicaid's role in the birth of major health reform in Massachusetts in 2006. The Massachusetts model became the template for reform efforts in Washington and represents a case of bottom-up policy diffusion. The chapter then focuses on the policy processes that led to Medicaid's insertion in the ACA. It assays the jockeying between federal and state policymakers over how much funding states would need to contribute to the expansion of Medicaid coverage and also congressional sparring over the program's more general role in health reform. After describing the Medicaid provisions that made it into the ACA, I turn to the aftermath of reform. The ways in which Medicaid factored into the lawsuits brought by state attorneys general against the ACA come under the microscope, as does health reform's role in the 2010 congressional elections. The chapter then analyzes key challenges that Medicaid will face if the ACA escapes repeal and stays on track for implementation. I conclude by assessing the implications of the chapter for Medicaid's durability.

Massachusetts Leads the Way

On April 12, 2006, a fife-and-drum corps accompanied Massachusetts governor Mitt Romney (R) into Boston's historic Faneuil Hall for a signing ceremony. A large throng had come to this colonial-era setting to signal support for the law that Romney had come to sign—one that assured access to health insurance for nearly all the state's residents. The press reported that the ceremony was "staged with a near-presidential attention to theatrics and slogan-bearing banners." Many of the speakers at the event drew on metaphors from the American Revolution, with Senator Edward Kennedy (D) affirming that Massachusetts "may well have fired a shot heard round the world" (Farenthold 2006). Whatever notice the world paid, the Massachusetts plan clearly attracted the attention of policymakers and think tanks across the United States. Reform advocates and policymakers in many states sought information about the plan and weighed whether it could be customized to fit their jurisdictions. Ultimately, the Massachusetts plan did not trigger the adoption of similar approaches in other states. Instead, it became a template for bottom-up diffusion as the federal government approved health care reform in 2010.

Medicaid figured prominently in the shaping of the Massachusetts health reform effort, both as a spur to action and as a major component of the initiative. Intergovernmental bargaining over a waiver was at the heart of this development. When the Clinton administration announced a new receptivity to state-initiated demonstrations, Massachusetts responded by submitting a waiver proposal called MassHealth. The waiver was crafted during the administration of Governor William Weld (R), and it won federal approval in April 1995. Implementation commenced two years later. Like many Section 1115 waivers of this period, MassHealth expanded eligibility for Medicaid while requiring many beneficiaries to enroll in managed care.[1] In 2001 federal administrators approved a three-year extension of the waiver with little negotiation.

When state officials again moved to renew MassHealth in 2004, however, the George W. Bush administration signaled that it wanted significant changes in the waiver as a condition for its continuation. In particular, federal officials wanted to redirect MassHealth monies that subsidized institutions toward coverage expansions for the uninsured. Massachusetts had long been one of a handful of states that had aggressively subsidized hospitals under Medicaid's Disproportionate Share Hospital program (DSH).[2] States could use DSH dollars to shore up hospitals and related institutions that served large numbers of Medicaid enrollees and the uninsured. In 2000 Massachusetts ranked ninth among states in DSH expenditures per poor person, spending at least twice as much on this metric as thirty-six other states.[3] Under the waiver the state directed the bulk of these funds to two major providers—the Boston Medical Center and the Cambridge Health Alliance (McDonough et al. 2006, w429). The Bush administration now wanted to terminate federal support for this DSH subsidy.

The assertiveness of the federal government in the waiver process mingled with other elements in the political stream to open a policy window for major reform. After he was elected in 2002, Governor Mitt Romney searched for ways to expand insurance coverage while avoiding the approach the Clinton administration had proposed in the early 1990s. In 2004 he assembled a team of advisers and drew on ideas offered by a conservative think tank, the Heritage Foundation, to forge a proposal for submission to the legislature. His plan featured an individual mandate—a requirement that all citizens obtain insurance. Lower-income residents without insurance would either be on Medicaid or receive a subsidy from the state to enable them to purchase coverage through an insurance exchange. The leaders of the two houses of the legislature, both with huge Democratic majorities, touted alternative reforms. Led by Speaker Salvatore DiMasi, the Massachusetts House of Representatives favored expanding Medicaid and imposing a fee on employers that failed to provide insurance. For his part, the president of the Massachusetts Senate, Robert Travaglini, backed reforms that did little to reduce the number of uninsured people (McDonough et al. 2006, w427–28).

The significant differences between the governor and legislative leaders raised the prospect that the quest for health reform would end in gridlock. However, three factors encouraged a compromise. First, the state risked losing $385 million in Medicaid funds if it could not come up with a creative alternative to subsidizing the Boston Medical Center and the Cambridge Health Alliance. Responding to this prospect, Governor Romney and Senator Kennedy negotiated an agreement with federal administrators to retain these monies if MassHealth shifted them from institutional to individual subsidies by July 1, 2006 (McDonough et al. 2006, w429). Second, Kennedy urged the Democrats in the Massachusetts legislature to take Romney's proposal seriously as an innovative model for health reform. And third, the ability of a coalition of advocates, religious leaders, and other stakeholders to exploit the state's initiative process galvanized action. Massachusetts permits citizens who secure enough signatures on a petition to place policy proposals on the ballot for voter consideration. By early 2006 volunteers had gathered enough signatures to put a proposition on the ballot in November that would go beyond existing proposals in taxing business to pay for a coverage expansion. Faced with this threat, key members of the business community went along with the reform model that the legislature had been negotiating with Governor Romney—one that imposed a fee on employers that failed to insure their workers (Belluck 2006a).

Propelled by these and related forces, health reform passed both houses of the Massachusetts legislature with only two dissenting votes in early April 2006. Federal administrators promptly approved an amendment to the MassHealth demonstration that allowed the reform to take effect in January 2007. Under the waiver individuals with incomes up to 300 percent of the poverty line could enroll either in Medicaid (MassHealth) or receive a subsidy to purchase coverage from an insurance exchange called "the connector" (Commonwealth Care). The demarcation between eligibility for MassHealth and Commonwealth Care was not based on a simple income cutoff. For instance, the reform called for Medicaid to insure all children up to 300 percent of the poverty line, pregnant women up to 200 percent, and parents up to 133 percent. Uninsured families and individuals with incomes above 300 percent of the poverty line would purchase coverage from the "connector" with pretax dollars (McDonough et al. 2006, w425–26).[4]

For those committed to comprehensive health reform, the Massachusetts plan had considerable appeal for two overarching reasons. First, the plan seemed to work. To be sure, Massachusetts officials faced persistent implementation challenges. Many newly insured people had a hard time obtaining timely access to primary care practitioners. So, too, the complexities of administering a means-tested enrollment system (discussed in chapter 3) led to some churning of the rolls and gaps in coverage as income fluctuations caused people to move between Medicaid and the connector (Pryor and Cohen 2009). Above all, rising health care prices and the deep recession starting in 2007 left policymakers struggling to find ways to sustain the program—whether through enhanced revenues, benefit cuts, new provider payment methodologies, or other means. But the program endured. The individual mandate, Medicaid expansion, and Commonwealth Care helped reduce the proportion of uninsured people in Massachusetts to the lowest of any state in the nation.[5] In 2008 the federal government approved another three-year extension of the waiver.

The second reason for the considerable appeal of the Massachusetts plan was that it appeared to offer a political blueprint for those seeking major health reform (McDonough et al. 2006, w431). During a period of intense political polarization at the national level, the plan garnered bipartisan support. Republican governor Romney, who was contemplating a run for the presidency in 2008, provided indispensable leadership in developing the plan and building a supportive coalition. At the time of the bill's passage, Romney expressed pleasure that it was "95 percent of what I proposed" (Belluck 2006a). Capturing the spirit of the moment, he observed: "People ask me if this is conservative or liberal, and my answer is yes. It's liberal in the sense that we are getting our citizens health insurance. It's conservative in that we are not getting a government take-over" (Belluck 2006b). The requirement that people have health insurance resonated with the conservative theme of individual responsibility. At the same time, the Massachusetts plan seemed moderate in that it did not appear to disturb people's current coverage. Although it represented a policy breakthrough in expanding health insurance, its methods appeared highly incremental.

In crafting and rallying support for health care reform, the president and key members of Congress often pointed to the Massachusetts experience (Jacobs and Skocpol 2010, 90). At a hearing in late June 2009, for instance, Representative Edward Markey (D) of Massachusetts opened his questioning of a panel of witnesses with the following: "This is an historic time, and we are very proud in Massachusetts that we adopted a new law that puts us in the same role, as revolutionaries, that our State has historically played . . . except we are not any longer talking about Minutemen but MinuteClinics . . . and not Red Coats but the white coats of doctors." He then asked the panel for their views on the Massachusetts model. While noting various limitations, the three panelists praised the plan (US House Committee on Energy and Commerce 2009a, 105–10). To be sure, Congress heard from other witnesses who were sharply critical of the Massachusetts approach. Among other things, they charged that it failed to control costs and provide timely access to high-quality care.[6] But supporters of reform discounted these criticisms. Although the health insurance model embedded in the ACA differed in some respects from the Massachusetts plan, it featured its three most essential building blocks: the mandate that individuals obtain coverage or pay a penalty, the creation of exchanges where uninsured individuals could purchase coverage, and a Medicaid expansion. Shortly after the passage of the ACA, President Obama noted in an interview on the *Today Show* that the new law incorporated many Republican ideas: "I mean, a lot of commentators have said . . . 'this is sort of similar to the bill that Mitt Romney passed in Massachusetts'" (Buchanan 2010).

As attractive as the Massachusetts plan looked in 2006 as a harbinger for bipartisan compromise, however, it ultimately became a lesson in the degree to which partisan polarization afflicted national policymaking. In the face of intense Republican and Tea Party opposition to the ACA, Romney openly opposed the new law. Although he continued to defend the Massachusetts plan, he stressed that "this is a federalist nation. . . . States should be able to solve their own problems" (Stein 2010). He faced the irony that his most impressive policy achievement as governor became one of his biggest political liabilities in the Republican presidential primaries of 2012.

In focusing on state solutions, Romney's observation slights a critical point. The Massachusetts plan was not just a state idea and initiative. In key respects it was a creature of Medicaid and executive federalism. My point here goes well beyond the fact that without federal Medicaid monies, the reform would not have germinated. It also transcends the major role a Medicaid coverage expansion played in the Massachusetts model. Instead, it underscores the degree to which reform sprang from a highly discretionary decision within the federal executive branch. No congressional action required the Bush administration to shift its position on the contents of the Massachusetts waiver in 2005. The Centers for Medicare and Medicaid Services could have continued the waiver in its current form. Instead, federal officials stood their ground in promoting a new perspective on Medicaid waivers that had taken root in the Bush administration. This perspective stressed that these waivers should as a rule subsidize insurance for individuals rather than funnel DSH payments to institutions. This shift in the exercise of federal administrative discretion was probably a necessary, if not sufficient, condition for the birth of Massachusetts health reform. In sum, Massachusetts is a relatively rare case of bottom-up policy diffusion where federalism lived up to its billing for nurturing policy laboratories. But this diffusion also stemmed from a top-down decision in the federal executive branch. The continuation of the reform also depended on the willingness of federal administrators to renew the waiver.

In considering the intergovernmental dynamics in the Massachusetts case, I do not mean to imply that the federal bureaucracy can easily impose its will on the states. If Governor Romney and Senator Kennedy had gone to the mat in fighting the federal decision to disapprove Medicaid funding for the Boston Medical Center and the Cambridge Health Alliance, they might well have prevailed. Indeed, in Florida Governor Jeb Bush (R) successfully fought off federal pressures to disallow direct subsidies to hospitals in a major demonstration waiver at about the same time.[7] Instead, the Massachusetts episode illuminates how opposition to business as usual in the waiver process by federal administrators can prompt policymakers to become more creative in considering new and promising policy alternatives.

Medicaid: A Platform for the ACA

The 2008 election placed Barak Obama in the White House and buttressed Democratic majorities in both houses of Congress. Despite the reservations of Vice President Joe Biden, Chief of Staff Rahm Emanuel, and other key advisers, the president made health reform a top legislative priority. In early November 2009 the House passed health reform; the Senate approved a somewhat different version in late December. The unexpected election of Republican Scott Brown in Massachusetts to assume the seat of the late Senator Edward Kennedy in January 2010 meant that Senate Democrats no longer had the votes to surmount a Republican filibuster. This meant that passage of the ACA depended on the willingness of the House to approve the Senate version of the bill. In late March 2010 the House did so. Both chambers then passed a "sidecar" reconciliation measure not subject to the filibuster that revised portions of the ACA in ways House Democrats wanted.

Others have dissected the contentious politics leading to the approval of the ACA.[8] Rather than replicate their work, I focus on the politics that shaped the ACA's Medicaid provisions. From the outset policymakers assumed that Medicaid would be part of health care reform. (When I asked a key congressional staff member whether the house had ever considered a reform that did not rely so heavily on Medicaid, he responded: "Yes, for about five minutes.")[9] The large role for Medicaid mirrored the Massachusetts model. It squared with the president's desire not to disturb the insurance people already had. It meant that federal policymakers could rely on an administrative infrastructure already in place at the state level. But above all it reflected fiscal concerns. Thanks largely to the Bush tax cuts of the early 2000s, wars in Iraq and Afghanistan, plummeting federal revenues brought on by the worst recession since the Great Depression, and the cost of a major stimulus package, the federal deficit soared to $1.4 trillion in fiscal 2009, about triple that of the prior year (OMB 2010). Against this fiscal backdrop, President Obama stressed that the new health plan, through savings and new revenues, could not add one dime to the deficit. In this regard, any bill would have to pass muster with the official scorekeeper on such matters, the nonpartisan Congressional Budget Office (CBO).

Concerns about CBO scoring eventually shaped congressional decisions on how high up the income ladder to extend Medicaid. Initially, Senator Max Baucus (D-MT) and other key policymakers proposed that Medicaid cover all poor people. Those with incomes above 100 percent of the poverty line would obtain private insurance through newly created exchanges. The problem was, however, that private insurance plans cost more than Medicaid; these plans paid providers at higher rates and had greater administrative costs. To hold down the ACA's price tag, Congress eventually decided to expand Medicaid coverage to all those people with incomes up to 133 percent of the poverty line (McDonough 2011, 148–49). Cost concerns also shaped congressional deliberations over what the federal match should be for those who gained Medicaid coverage under reform. Should it be 100 percent, and thereby absolve the states of any new costs? Or should the federal match be lower, and thereby reduce the fiscal burden on the federal government but shift some costs to the states? Deliberation over these questions sparked intense expressions of concern from the governors.

Picking Up the Tab for Reform: The Intergovernmental Struggle

By early 2009 key members of the House of Representatives resolved to minimize reform's fiscal burden on the states. But the Senate Finance Committee held out hope that the states could do more. An initial proposal called for the federal government to absorb all the costs of new Medicaid enrollees for five years or so but then to apply the regular match rate. This would eventually leave states with about 43 percent of the expansion's costs. The Senate Finance Committee also discussed the possibility that states might be able to float bonds (i.e., borrow money) to cover their share of health reform's costs during economic downturns (Sack and Pear 2009).

The prospect that Medicaid would be a key component of health reform kindled great concern among the nation's governors. The NGA responded by setting up a bipartisan task force of twelve governors to forge a general position on reform. A smaller executive committee within the task force worked to build a consensus. But partisan forces proved disruptive. The White House obtained drafts produced by the NGA committee and cautioned Democratic governors not to sign on to any compromise that might complicate congressional deliberations over reform. Meanwhile, Republican governors became increasingly aware that opposition to reform was becoming a signature initiative of their party. These pressures thwarted compromise, and the NGA task force failed to produce a position statement.[10] The governors were, however, in full agreement on one principle: that the federal government should absorb 100 percent of the costs of any Medicaid expansion. The deep recession had made the governors all the more sensitive to the strains that Medicaid placed on their budgets. When the secretary of Health and Human Services, Kathleen Sebelius, and a key federal Medicaid administrator, Cindy Mann, appeared at the NGA's summer meeting in July 2009, the governors strongly opposed any measure that would boost state Medicaid costs. Governor Phil Bredesen of Tennessee (D) expressed alarm that Congress was considering a Medicaid expansion that would impose "the mother of all unfunded mandates" on states. The governors dismissed the idea that states could float bonds to meet Medicaid costs, with one likening it to "taking out a mortgage to pay the grocery bill" (Sack and Pear 2009).

Outside the NGA, governors pressed their fiscal case in Congress and garnered some support. For instance, Senator Michael Enzi (R-WY) of the Senate Finance Committee declared that the federal government should cover 100 percent of the tab for a Medicaid expansion (Pear and Herszenhorn 2009). So, too, Senator Dianne Feinstein (D) of California warned that her state was facing a "financial catastrophe" and that imposing new Medicaid costs on it would be a "deal breaker" for her (Weisman 2009). Still other senators sought to exempt their particular states from any additional Medicaid costs. Senate Majority Leader Harry Reid (D) pursued this goal for Nevada. More famously, Senator Ben Nelson (D) made exemption of Nebraska from any new Medicaid costs a condition for his support of the reform bill. Republicans pounced on this "Cornhusker Kickback" to reinforce the public's negative views of the legislative politics of health reform. (The final reform legislation deleted this provision.)

In addition to pressing the case that the federal government ought to pay the full cost of reform, governors from more liberal states sought fiscal relief on another front. Early drafts of the legislation applied the more generous federal Medicaid match solely to the population that would gain coverage under reform. States that had used highly restrictive eligibility criteria in the past would thereby receive larger federal subsidies than states that had historically been more generous. For instance, Texas had never extended Medicaid benefits to many poor adults, whereas New York had. Now it appeared that Texas would receive a greatly enhanced Medicaid match to expand coverage, whereas New York would continue to insure the same group at its regular federal match of 50 percent. If allowed to stand, this disparity would yield the ironic political effect of rewarding those states that Obama had failed to carry in the general election while penalizing those states that had supported him. Democrats in Congress resolved to correct this disparity.

By the fall of 2009 most Democratic governors believed that they had made sufficient progress in advancing their views in Congress to back the legislation under consideration. In early October 2009 twenty-two of the twenty-six members of the Democratic Governors Association sent a letter to House and Senate leaders endorsing health reform (Murray 2009). For the most part, Republican governors joined their partisan colleagues in Congress in opposing the legislation. Governor Haley Barbour (MS), chairman of the Republican Governors Association, denounced the Medicaid expansion as a "huge unfunded mandate" that would place pressure on states to raise taxes (Murray 2009).

Ultimately, the ACA took significant strides toward reducing the fiscal burdens of health reform on the states. The new law called for complete federal funding of the Medicaid expansion for three years starting in 2014. In 2017 the federal match rate of 100 percent would gradually decline, until it leveled off at 90 percent in 2020. Liberal states, which had been ahead of the curve in covering poor adults, also won concessions. The ACA guaranteed states that had insured certain adults before health reform that by 2019 they would have the same federal matching rate for this cohort as states that were now covering them for the first time. Health reform also sweetened the pot for CHIP. It affirmed that, starting in 2015, states would receive a 23-percentage-point increase in the federal match for the program up to 100 percent. Large numbers of states would thereby pay little or nothing out of their own treasuries for CHIP.

The federal government's willingness to absorb the lion's share of the costs for the Medicaid expansion eased but did not extirpate state fiscal concerns about the ACA. In part these concerns were intermingled with partisan polarization. Most Republican governors disliked the new law on ideological grounds. They resented any pressure to spend more on Medicaid, whatever its contribution to reducing the ranks of the uninsured. At times, their opposition to the ACA led them to endorse exaggerated claims about the costs to states of the Medicaid expansion. But fiscal concerns did not stop with Republicans. A top staff member at the NGA believed that the CBO and others had underestimated the costs of the ACA and that over time Medicaid would "eat education" and other important functions in state budgets.[11] Whatever their precise origin, cost concerns heightened tensions over Medicaid between the federal government and the states to a level not seen since the late 1980s and early 1990s.

Congressional Sparring over Medicaid

The politics of Medicaid and the ACA went beyond the intergovernmental struggle over how much of the tab the federal and state governments would pay. As various congressional committees deliberated on health reform, Medicaid issues occasionally surfaced. Democratic leaders, for instance, made sure that Medicaid supporters appeared at hearings. In late June 2009, for instance, a subcommittee of the US House of Representatives' Committee on Energy and Commerce (2009a, 2009b) heard testimony praising Medicaid from two major national advocates for families and children and also from a New Jersey legislator who had strongly backed Medicaid and CHIP expansions in his state.[12]

For their part, congressional Republicans at times targeted Medicaid in their overall effort to kill reform. A Senate Finance Committee session in September

2009 to consider amendments to the health reform bill illustrates certain of their themes. By this time committee Democrats had drafted legislation that contained most of the components that the ACA would eventually incorporate. During the session Republicans raised four Medicaid issues. First, they joined the Republican governors in criticizing the Medicaid expansion as an unfunded mandate. Senator Charles Grassley (IA) claimed that the burden on the states would be $33 billion, and his colleague, Senator John Cornyn (TX), placed the figure at $20 billion for his state alone.[13]

Second, Republican senators introduced amendments linking Medicaid to one of their favorite health care proposals: malpractice reform. A key Republican tenet holds that much of the excess cost in the health care system springs from the ability of lawyers to extract huge settlements in court from physicians convicted of malpractice. Faced with this threat, doctors allegedly practice defensive medicine to a fault, ordering endless procedures of little or no value in order to protect themselves legally. Praising Texas and the other states that had capped malpractice awards, Republicans sought to use Medicaid to galvanize diffusion of such reform. In this vein Senator Cornyn offered an amendment that would require "any state receiving funds under Medicaid" to "limit total economic damages in a medical malpractice case to $1 million or less" (US Senate Committee on Finance 2009, 322). Alternatively, Senator John Ensign (R-NV) proposed that states enacting medical liability reform receive an enhanced federal Medicaid match. To fund his amendment, Ensign sought to cut the subsidy for individuals slated to purchase insurance from the exchanges to be created by the ACA. Democrats believed that those people living at up to 400 percent of the poverty line should receive some federal aid to buy insurance; Ensign wanted the eligibility reduced to 275 percent (US Senate Committee on Finance 2009, 315, 320).

Third, Republicans on the committee criticized provisions in the health reform bill that cut Medicaid funding for the DSH program. Since 1981 DSH had funneled Medicaid dollars to hospitals and other institutions that served large numbers of the uninsured and Medicaid enrollees. Democrats were eager to contain the costs of the ACA, so, drawing on the Massachusetts model, they reasoned that they could reduce DSH funding because hospitals would treat fewer uninsured patients. Two Republican senators objected. Senator John Kyl of Arizona underscored that his state had a large immigrant population that was likely to be ineligible for coverage under the new law and that the DSH cuts would harm the state's safety net. For his part Senator Orrin Hatch of Utah claimed that rural hospitals in his state, which "are already struggling to survive," would be adversely affected (US Senate Committee on Finance 2009, 376–78, 386).

Fourth, Republican senators trumpeted a theme that liberal critics of Medicaid might applaud: that the program offered coverage inferior to that of private insurance and Medicare.[14] In their view this stemmed from "lousy" Medicaid payment rates that limited physicians' participation in the program.[15] Senator Cornyn cited research indicating that Medicaid reimbursement was only 72 percent of that provided by Medicare and claimed that the percentage would be even lower compared with private insurance. Referring to a 2002 study, Senator Enzi said that 40 percent of doctors would not see Medicaid enrollees (US Senate Committee on Finance 2009, 361, 407). Senator Cornyn also bemoaned the quality of care that Medicaid enrollees received. He observed: "Numerous studies have documented the poor patient outcomes in the Medicaid program relative to patients in private plans. For example, Medicaid patients are almost 50 percent more likely to die after coronary artery bypass surgery than patients with private coverage or Medicare" (US Senate Committee on Finance 2009, 407). Claims such as these prompted summary judgments from Republican senators that the Medicaid expansion under health reform was a "shell game" whereby policymakers would "promise folks care that we are not going to be able to deliver."[16] Or as Senator Kyl put it, the Medicaid expansion would lead to a "higher degree of this kind of subtle rationing, and it is not right" (US Senate Committee on Finance 2009, 417).

Having fired these broadsides at Medicaid, Republican senators offered two amendments. One, by Senator Grassley, required state Medicaid programs to pay pediatricians, dentists, and certain hospitals Medicare rates starting in 2014. Grassley proposed that the federal government cover the entire costs of this pay hike for two years before phasing down to the regular Medicaid match by 2019. To underwrite the costs of this measure, he sought to reduce eligibility for federal subsidies for those people who were buying insurance from the exchanges. The cutoff for federal assistance would be 300 rather than 400 percent of the poverty line. A second amendment, by Senator Cornyn, called for states to achieve a physician participation rate in Medicaid of 75 percent before the proposed expansion of the program could occur (US Senate Committee on Finance 2009, 348–49, 408–10).

None of the proposed amendments passed the committee.[17] Most aimed at slowing down the legislative process, unraveling the agreements that the Democrats had forged to obtain the votes needed for passage, and scoring points with certain constituents (doctors in the case of provider payment and medical malpractice; safety net institutions in the case of Medicaid DSH). Some amendments sought to bolster Medicaid funding by stripping subsidies from those people who would seek insurance through the exchanges. Others, such as the Cornyn amendment on physician participation rates, would have effectively blocked implementation of the Medicaid expansion.[18]

In response to the Republican critique of Medicaid, Democratic senators mounted a modest defense. They noted that an expanded Medicaid and CHIP Payment and Access Commission would evaluate barriers to access and subsequently make recommendations to Congress (US Senate Committee on Finance 2009, 354, 409–12). They challenged the view that employer insurance invariably provided superior access. In this vein, Senator Max Baucus noted that he and his wife participated in the federal employee health benefit plan, but "not a single one of my wife's doctors will take Blue Cross Blue Shield patients" (US Senate Committee on Finance 2009, 409–10; also see 354, 411–12). While offering some defense of Medicaid, however, Democrats on the Finance Committee acknowledged that Medicaid payment rates and access to providers tended to lag. (In fact, these circumstances eased passage of the ACA by lowering the CBO's estimate of its costs.)[19] Some expressed concern that the poor would receive substandard coverage. At one point in the session, Senator Ron Wyden (D-OR) went so far as to say that "the Medicaid program is this country is broken. If I had my way, we would have the poorest and most vulnerable in our society getting the same kind of choices that members of Congress have. I think we ought to make it possible in a doctor's office for the poor person to walk right by the congressperson."[20] But Wyden and his Democratic colleagues fully fathomed that the Republican criticisms of Medicaid did not rest on a commitment to providing low-income people with a more attractive insurance option. None of the Republican senators who chronicled Medicaid's limitations had endorsed a plan that would provide any kind of coverage whatsoever to the vast sea of uninsured, poor adults. Hence, for Democrats, the choice was not between Medicaid and a "first-class" option that would rally Republican support; it was a choice between Medicaid and no insurance for millions of Americans.

Key Medicaid Provisions of the ACA

As passed in March 2010, the ACA featured two vehicles for extending health insurance to 32 million Americans starting in 2014. Sixteen million people would obtain coverage through the newly created insurance exchanges or some other vehicle. Those with incomes between 133 and 400 percent of the poverty line would receive federal subsidies to purchase insurance through the exchanges.[21] In turn, Medicaid would add 16 million people to its rolls by targeting the bottom income tier—uninsured people under sixty-five years of age with incomes up to 133 percent of poverty line. (Eligibility workers could also disregard some earnings, thereby raising the threshold to 138 percent). Poor adults, especially those without offspring, would be the primary beneficiaries of the ACA, because Medicaid already covered most children in this income bracket. The law continued the exclusion of illegal immigrants from Medicaid benefits.[22] The ACA preserved CHIP but provided an escape from the enrollment caps that many states had imposed.[23] Those subject to these caps could purchase subsidized coverage through the exchanges. The ACA froze in place existing Medicaid and CHIP eligibility criteria for children until 2019, and for most adults until 2014. The ACA also provided states with one sweeping option. As of 2017 a state could apply for a demonstration waiver to opt out of the ACA and pursue an alternative approach so long as it provided coverage at least as comprehensive at an acceptable cost to the federal Treasury.

In addition to expanding insurance coverage, the new law took steps to assure that Medicaid enrollees would have access to providers. It subsidized higher reimbursements for primary care doctors for 2013 and 2014. More specifically, it required states at a minimum to pay physicians practicing family medicine, pediatrics, or general internal medicine at Medicare rates. The ACA also poured additional funds into grants for community health centers, a major provider of care for Medicaid enrollees. As of 2008 some 1,080 of these centers operated at more than 7,500 sites throughout the United States. Seventy-five percent of the patients who received services at the centers were either on Medicaid or uninsured. The ACA pledged an additional $11 billion to expand community health centers and reaffirmed the requirement that Medicaid reimburse the centers at more generous rates than it typically paid providers. Analysts projected that the number of patients served by centers would mushroom from 19 million in 2009 to 50 million in 2019 (Rosenbaum et al. 2010, 2, 3, 7). The ACA also expanded the role of the Medicaid and CHIP Payment and Access Commission, which the legislation reauthorizing CHIP in early 2009 had created. The commission would now be responsible for reviewing and advising Congress on barriers to access affecting not only children but also adults.

The ACA addressed Medicaid in other ways as well. It further pared Medicaid DSH funding and took modest steps to hone the targeting of these monies among and within states.[24] It authorized Medicaid demonstrations to explore the utility of various payment alternatives and took further steps to tamp down fraud and abuse. The ACA also set up two new organizational units within the Centers for Medicare and Medicaid Services to enhance Medicaid's performance. One, an Innovation Center, was charged with testing reimbursement methods and finding ways to improve the cost-effectiveness of Medicaid and Medicare. The other, the Federal Coordinated Health Care Office, sought to improve the integration of services for those people who were simultaneously enrolled in both Medicaid and Medicare. As discussed in chapter 4, the ACA gave states more options and incentives to pursue home and community-based services for the elderly and people with disabilities.

Through these provisions the ACA envisioned Medicaid as a key platform for moving the United States toward health insurance for all. But this outcome was far from assured. Medicaid still faced storm clouds on two overlapping fronts. First, key Republicans at the national and state levels made repeal of the ACA a top priority. Second, the ACA faced serious implementation challenges, even if these efforts at repeal failed.

Medicaid and the Republican Fight for Repeal

The struggle to pass health reform ignited sharp resistance among Republican policymakers at the state level. Legislators in at least forty states proposed measures to signal their disapproval. The Virginia legislature, for instance, enacted a law specifying that no resident should be required to have a health insurance policy (Cauchi 2011). These initiatives helped mobilize and respond to a Republican and Tea Party base angered by the push for health reform. But these steps could not, per se, block the ACA's implementation. To accomplish that end, the law's opponents turned to the federal courts and electoral politics.

The Court Challenge

Myriad opponents of the ACA filed suit in federal district courts around the country to derail health reform. Republican attorneys general led the way. The activism of these officials reflects a central development in state government during the past two decades: the rise of attorneys general as major political players. These officials are elected to office in forty-three states, and they have emerged as important policy entrepreneurs who place issues on the federal and state legislative agendas, block federal initiatives, win major financial settlements by suing private corporations, and undertake many more initiatives. Many of them use their activism as stepping-stones in the quest for higher political office (Provost 2003). Consistent with this trend, twenty-one attorneys general—all but one Republicans—initially joined in lawsuits to invalidate the ACA. In doing so, they did not always reflect the preferences of the governors of their states. For instance, Attorney General Rob McKenna (R) of Washington participated in the suit over the objection of Governor Christine Gregoire (D).

The Republican attorneys general had high hopes that two pending lawsuits would pave the way for eviscerating health reform. The most important of these was a case filed immediately upon passage of the ACA by Florida attorney general Bill McCollum (R). McCollum, who made an unsuccessful run for governor later in the year, pursued the time-honored tactic of seeking a court likely to be sympathetic to his arguments. Even though his office in Tallahassee was six blocks from a federal district court, he filed the suit 200 miles away in Pensacola. The partisan backgrounds of the judges in the two courts shaped his decision. President Clinton had appointed the judge in Tallahassee. In contrast, President Reagan had selected the judge in Pensacola, who also has a reputation for hewing to conservative political positions in his rulings. Eventually twenty-five other attorneys general joined the Florida suit.[25] Attorney General Kenneth Cuccinelli (R) of Virginia brought a second legal challenge in a federal district court in Richmond.

Substantively, both the Florida and Virginia suits targeted the ACA's mandate that all individuals obtain health insurance. The issue here that garnered the most attention and debate centered upon whether the US Constitution permitted the federal government to impose such a mandate (e.g., see Jost 2010; Shapiro 2010). Though less salient, the suits also targeted the Medicaid provisions of the reform law via two legal arguments—one based on claims of federal commandeering and the other on nonseverability. The Florida, but not the Virginia, suit made the case for *commandeering*. Courts have long held that the federal government can impose requirements on the states as a condition of their receiving federal grants. The reasoning runs that if a state finds the federal mandates onerous, it can withdraw from the grant program. In the case of Medicaid, however, the Florida attorney general challenged this view, arguing that states "cannot effectively withdraw from participating in Medicaid, because Medicaid has, during the more than four decades of its existence, become customary and necessary for citizens throughout the United States." States realize that coverage of "tens of millions of residents can only be accomplished by their continued participation in Medicaid." Going further, Attorney General McCollum claimed that the ACA "converts what has been a voluntary federal–state partnership into a compulsory top-down program" that violated the Tenth Amendment to the Constitution.[26] Hence, the new law illegally commandeered states to do the federal government's bidding (Rosenbaum 2010).

The second line of legal attack on the ACA's Medicaid provisions, one embedded in both the Florida and Virginia suits, stressed the issue of *nonseverability*. This view contended that the many components of the ACA represented an intricate, tightly coupled, highly interdependent model for health reform. This model could not be decomposed without undermining the entire approach. In essence, this view saw the ACA as a house of cards; remove any one of them and the whole edifice would collapse. If judges ruled against the individual mandate, therefore, the entire ACA, including its Medicaid provisions, should be discarded.

The initial decisions of the two politically conservative judges in Florida and Virginia, along with the rulings of three appellate courts, provided early clues about Medicaid's legal prospects. The commandeering argument (considered only in Florida) fared poorly. Though siding with the state plaintiffs on most matters, Judge Roger Vinson in Pensacola rejected their argument that they had no choice but to participate in Medicaid.[27] The Eleventh Circuit Court of Appeals in Atlanta—a conservative court widely expected to be sympathetic to opponents of the ACA—agreed with Vinson in rejecting state claims of commandeering.

Nor did the issue of nonseverability gain much traction in the lower courts. The Florida and Virginia judges differed on the matter. Judge Henry Hudson in Virginia chose to "hew closely to the time-honored rule" to sever "any problematic portions" of the law "while leaving the remainder intact."[28] Hence, the Medicaid provisions of the ACA remained in effect despite his ruling that the individual mandate was unconstitutional. In contrast, Judge Vinson in Florida assumed a more activist judicial posture, declaring that the individual mandate was the "essential piece" in "a finely crafted watch." In ruling against the mandate, therefore, he voided the entire ACA.[29] But Vinson's position on nonseverability did not survive a review by the Eleventh Circuit Court of Appeals. In August 2011 a three-judge panel in this circuit found the individual mandate to be unconstitutional, but left the rest of the ACA intact.

By the fall 2011 the Eleventh Circuit was the only appellate court that had found any provision of the ACA unconstitutional. Courts in the Sixth and District of Columbia circuits upheld the entire law, with certain judges appointed by Republican presidents joining in these decisions. In late September 2011 the Obama administration decided to bring matters to a head by asking the Supreme Court to hear its appeal of the Eleventh Circuit's ruling against the individual mandate. In mid-November the Supreme Court agreed. As Medicaid advocates anticipated, the court announced that it would weigh the issue of nonseverability. To the surprise and concern of these advocates, however, the court also scheduled time to hear arguments that the Medicaid expansion amounted to federal coercion of the states (Aizenman 2011).

The Supreme Court's ruling in late June 2012, in fact dealt a blow to the Medicaid expansion. To be sure, a 5 to 4 court majority handed a victory to the Obama administration on several fronts. The majority opinion crafted by Chief Justice John Roberts upheld the ACA's individual mandate on grounds that the constitution gives Congress to the right to "lay and collect taxes." It construed the penalty the new law imposed on people for failing to purchase health insurance as a tax. To the surprise of many legal scholars, however, the court curbed the federal government's ability to sanction states that failed to implement the Medicaid expansion. In securing compliance with mandates attached to grants, federal administrators have long relied on an important, if seldom used, tool—the ability to withhold federal monies from noncompliant states. The presence of this tool meant that, at least in theory, states would expose their existing Medicaid programs to fiscal penalties if they refused to cover the new categories of enrollees designated by the ACA. The Supreme Court decided that this went too far in tilting the balance of intergovernmental power toward the nation's capital. It ruled that the ACA had so enlarged and transformed Medicaid that leaving this administrative weapon in the federal arsenal would inappropriately coerce the states. It would be a "gun to the head" of state officials that would permit the federal government to engage in the "economic dragooning" of state budgets. Hence, the court ruled that federal officials were "not free to penalize States" that declined to participate in the ACA "by taking away their existing Medicaid funding" (US Supreme Court 2012b: 51–52, 55).

The court decision dramatically altered the implications of the ACA for Medicaid. It essentially converted the law's Medicaid expansion from a mandate to a state option. The degree to which Medicaid would grow apace in the wake of the ACA depended more than ever on the preferences of state policymakers. The political drama associated with state decisions on whether to participate might well play out over several years.

The Political Stream Turns Negative: The 2010 Elections

Republican opponents of health care reform also committed themselves to repealing the law by recapturing control of the federal government. In the 2010 elections they took a major step in this direction. Nearly all Republicans running for House and Senate seats in that year called for repeal of the ACA. Many Republicans seeking office at the state level voiced similar views. The election yielded a stinging defeat for Democrats. At the national level, Republicans gained six Senate and sixty-three House seats. Now in control of the House of Representatives, Republican leaders made a vote to repeal the ACA one of their first orders of business in January 2011. Democrats also suffered a shellacking in state elections. The number of Republican governors grew from twenty-three to twenty-nine, and the Republicans gained more than seven hundred seats in state legislatures (Campbell 2010, 1). As January 2011 dawned, Republicans controlled the governor's office and both houses of the legislature in twenty states, up from nine the year before; in contrast, the Democrats had unified control of the three branches in nine states, down from sixteen in 2010. Hence, those officials who were charged with implementing the ACA at the national and state levels faced a new constellation of political masters who were often unsympathetic to their efforts.

The degree to which opposition to the ACA in general, let alone its Medicaid expansion, prompted voters to side with Republicans remains an open question. Other factors, such as high unemployment rates and a sluggish economy, also loomed large. Data from a tracking poll conducted shortly after the election found the general public about evenly divided on the merits of the ACA (Kaiser Family Foundation 2010b). However, of critical importance, most voters opposed the law. Among all voters, health reform ranked fourth among the factors influencing their decisions, with 17 percent noting its importance. Those who backed Republicans cared more about the issue, with 21 percent identifying it as a key motivator compared with 13 percent among those voters who were supporting Democrats. Eighty-two percent of Republican voters viewed the ACA unfavorably, whereas 77 percent of their Democratic counterparts assessed it positively. Eighty-four percent of those people voting Republican wanted all or parts of the law repealed, compared with 24 percent of those backing Democrats. It deserves emphasis, however, that negative views of the ACA do not automatically translate into a lack of support for its Medicaid provisions. Indeed, Kaiser tracking polls before and after the 2010 election found that more than two-thirds of respondents (not just voters) consistently said they were very or somewhat favorable to "expanding the existing Medicaid program to cover low-income, uninsured adults regardless of whether they have children." To be sure, support for the Medicaid expansion differed by party, with 83 percent of Democrats positive compared with 47 percent of Republicans. But independents backed the Democratic view, with two-thirds of them favorable to the Medicaid expansion.[30]

The triumph of the Republicans in the 2010 election did not portend the immediate demise of the ACA. But it sparked a federal budget battle that would have serious implications for health reform and Medicaid's durability. (I illuminate aspects of this struggle in chapter 7.)

The Implementation Challenges

Whether or not the ACA survives, it deserves note that the health reform law presented Medicaid with several pressing implementation challenges.[31] The Supreme Court ruling on the ACA left federal administrators with a plethora of complex, thorny issues to interpret as they carried out the law. Beyond these issues, five overlapping challenges loom especially large: provider network adequacy; enrollment of the eligible; government fiscal stress; the degree of state commitment; and the problem of large, lagging states.

Provider Network Adequacy

Congressional deliberations concerning the ACA highlighted the problem of whether those people who were gaining Medicaid coverage would have adequate access to a full network of providers offering primary and specialty care. Issues of provider payment, which had long bedeviled Medicaid, in part drove this concern. Although they have varied from state to state, Medicaid reimbursement rates have typically trailed those of Medicare or employer insurance, especially for physicians. Moreover, some evidence suggests that Medicaid physician fees in inflation-adjusted dollars declined in the period from 2003 to 2008 (Zuckerman, Williams, and Stockley 2009). And because of these low reimbursement rates, many doctors do not participate in the program or greatly restrict the number of Medicaid patients they treat. In response, Medicaid enrollees have often flocked to hospital emergency rooms. The degree to which the movement of most Medicaid enrollees to managed care has shored up provider payments and fostered network adequacy is unclear. In fact, the rise of managed care has made it more difficult to track Medicaid payment trends because these organizations view the information as proprietary. Although managed care plans must document to state Medicaid officials that they have signed up enough providers to assure adequate access to quality health care, other stakeholders often complain that managed care contractors promise much more than they deliver. Emergency room use often remains high. The efforts of state Medicaid administrators to evaluate the extent of access to high-quality services provided by managed care networks often fall short.

In addition to perennial problems with provider payments, concerns about network adequacy spring from the anticipated surge in demand relative to the supply of primary care providers. The reform experience in Massachusetts rang warning bells in this regard. As demand increased in the wake of that state's coverage expansion, complaints increasingly surfaced about inadequate access to primary care practitioners. Many doctors declined to take on new patients, and wait times for appointments tended to increase. Despite a significant decline in the ranks of the uninsured, the number of Massachusetts residents reporting regular access to a personal doctor failed to increase (Zhu et al. 2010).

As noted above, the ACA made some effort to bolster network adequacy. The law requires Medicaid to pay certain primary care doctors at Medicare rates in 2013 and 2014. Unless these physicians believe that this enhanced reimbursement will continue after 2014, however, many may be reluctant to take on new patients only to face subsequent fiscal pressures to drop them. The expansion of community health center sites under the ACA will also facilitate access. But unless the federal government targets the new sites in medically underserved areas, many Medicaid enrollees will continue to face access problems. Federal officials have a long road to traverse in this regard. As of 2007 a total of 43 percent of medically underserved areas did not have a community health center. The Midwest region faced a particular deficit, with 60 percent of underserved areas lacking sites (GAO 2009a).[32] It also deserves note that neither the temporary boost in primary care payment nor the expansion of community health centers addresses a chronic problem for Medicaid enrollees: inadequate access to specialists.

The Enduring Take-Up Challenge

As noted in chapter 3, an enrollment labyrinth blocks many people who are entitled to Medicaid benefits from receiving them. The passage of the ACA did not solve this take-up problem. As their incomes ebb and flow, many people will be eligible for Medicaid (or CHIP) at one point and for the insurance exchanges created by the ACA at another. For instance, one study found that 40 percent of adults who qualified for Medicaid would lose eligibility after six months due to income increases that put them above 133 percent of the poverty line. In turn, 30 percent who started out with subsidized insurance from the exchanges would drop below 133 percent of the poverty line and become eligible for Medicaid during that period (Sommers and Rosenbaum 2011, 230). States will need to display uncommon administrative acumen to avoid a churning of the rolls, with individuals being uninsured as they transition from one source of coverage to another. As successful as the Massachusetts reform has been in achieving near-universal coverage, the administrative processes it employs to monitor changes in enrollee income and redetermine eligibility have caused some beneficiaries to experience bouts of being uninsured (Pryor and Cohen 2009).

The ACA contains provisions and funding to help states cope with this enrollment challenge (Morrow and Paradise 2010). The law's requirement that individuals obtain insurance may well motivate many to pay the transaction costs needed to sustain eligibility for Medicaid or other insurance. Beyond this, the ACA calls on states to create a "no wrong door" enrollment system supported by a website that facilitates "one-stop shopping."[33] This system would foster simultaneous assessment of whether an individual meets the criteria for enrollment in Medicaid, CHIP, or the exchange. It also requires states to reduce the need for applicants and enrollees to track down and submit information that is pertinent to determining eligibility by developing electronic interfaces with other data systems (e.g., tax returns) "to the maximum extent practicable." The ACA provides grants to the states and an enhanced federal match to develop these client-friendly enrollment systems. But these and related ACA provisions do not guarantee state success. Although the individual mandate will probably bolster take-up, the large majority of those people who are eligible for Medicaid will be exempt from penalties for failure to comply (Holahan and Headen 2010, 5). Furthermore, some states may lack the capacity or commitment to establish seamless enrollment systems designed to maximize take-up.

The degree to which states tame Medicaid's enrollment labyrinth will significantly affect the ACA's impact, as an analysis performed for the Kaiser Commission on Medicaid and the Uninsured illustrates (Holahan and Headen 2010, 10–11). This analysis probed two implementation scenarios for the enrollment of adults living below 133 percent of the poverty line, assuming that all fifty states participated. The standard participation scenario relies on the official assumption of the CBO that states will achieve a relatively modest 57 percent participation rate among adults newly eligible for Medicaid. This scenario predicts that Medicaid will acquire nearly 16 million new enrollees and reduce the number of low-income uninsured adults by 45 percent.[34] A second model assumes that states will enhance outreach and adopt more client-friendly enrollment processes to achieve a 75 percent take-up rate. Under this simulation Medicaid enrollments would rise by nearly 23 million and the ranks of uninsured low-income adults would drop by 70 percent. Medicaid enrollment gains could, of course, fall below the projections of both scenarios if state implementation efforts prove inadequate or states decline to participate in the expansion.

The Fiscal Challenge

The challenges of take-up and network adequacy intersect with more general problems related to state fiscal stress. To the extent that state policymakers find it harder to fund their share of Medicaid costs, they may decline to participate in the ACA's coverage expansion. If they do participate, fiscal constraints may well fuel implementation problems. States may lag in establishing the administrative infrastructure needed to carry out the ACA. Among the factors elevating state fiscal stress in the period following passage of the ACA, three stand out. First, the deep recession starting in December 2007 and ending in June 2009 precipitated declines in state government revenues that greatly exceeded those of other recessions during the past three decades (Oliff 2011). Stubbornly high unemployment rates and related factors may well cause state revenues to respond more slowly to economic recovery than in earlier downturns. Second, some state governments increasingly have come under fiscal pressure from prior decisions on pension and health benefits for their retired employees. Ideally, a state routinely sets aside the monies it needs to fund these commitments. But many states have failed to do so. Estimates of the unfunded pension liabilities of state and local governments range from $700 billion to $3 trillion; health insurance commitments to retirees of these governments are approximately $500 billion. Some state governments have far greater problems on this front than others. Certain highly populated states with relatively generous Medicaid programs face some of the most acute fiscal pressure from this source. These include California, Illinois, New Jersey, and Pennsylvania (Lav and McNichol 2011, 2–3).

Third, the growing federal deficit and debt could well undermine compensatory federalism—the principle that the federal government should increase its share of Medicaid costs during economic hard times. Although the ACA shifts a much higher share of the Medicaid tab to the federal government, states will continue to cover most enrollees under the long-standing federal formula. Unless the federal government ups the match during recessions, state Medicaid programs will tend to erode. During the past decade, Congress has increased the match rate in response to economic downturns in 2003, 2009, and again in 2010. But massive federal deficits ($1.5 trillion in fiscal 2011) and debt ($14 trillion) seem sure to weaken congressional resolve to assist state governments when their economies slump (Herszenhorn 2011). Although many states have continued to struggle economically, the enhanced federal match in the Obama stimulus program expired in July 2011.

Given these sources of fiscal stress, the question of how much the ACA will actually cost states looms large. These cost estimates vary greatly. Much of this variation depends on the assumptions studies make about take-up rates under the ACA not only for the newly eligible but for those people who qualify under the state's current Medicaid program. With respect to the latter, some believe that the individual mandate and general publicity about insurance under the ACA will fuel a woodwork effect.[35] It will encourage those people who qualified for Medicaid in the past but failed to enroll to now sign up for the program. Any such effect has financial implications for the states because they would receive their ordinary federal match for covering "woodwork" enrollees rather than the 90 percent match for the newly eligible.

Predicting the future Medicaid costs of the ACA is an inexact science. Arguably, the most sophisticated and comprehensive projection comes from a study released by the Kaiser Commission on Medicaid and the Uninsured (Holahan and Headen 2010, 42, 46). This simulation indicates that the Medicaid expansion will cost states an additional $21 billion from their own sources in the 2014–19 period if they achieve a 57 percent participation rate among newly eligible adults (the official rate projected by the CBO). Assuming that all fifty states participate, this represents a modest 1.4 percent increase over the states' projected Medicaid expenses if the ACA had failed to pass. If, however, states achieve a 75 participation rate among the newly eligible, the tab to the states will be $43 billion, more than double the 57 percent scenario. This would amount to a 3 percent increase over projected state expenditures on Medicaid without the ACA.

It deserves emphasis that these aggregate cost figures mask substantial variation among states. Some states—such as Maine, Massachusetts, and Vermont—are projected to spend *less* on Medicaid than would have been the case without the ACA. Others, such as Arkansas, will spend appreciably more than the average for all states.[36] In general the ACA imposes the least new costs on states that have historically had more generous Medicaid programs and lower rates of uninsured residents. This means that states in the Northeast will face less additional cost than those in the South. (By the same token, however, southern states will also have the greatest percentage increases in the infusion of federal Medicaid dollars.)

A balanced assessment of future Medicaid costs for the states should also take into account the savings to be realized from the coverage expansion. These savings will accrue from such factors as a reduced need for state and local governments to pay hospitals for treating the uninsured. Some studies suggest that in the aggregate, savings from various sources will offset the new costs of the ACA, though the ability of particular states to realize these savings will vary (Dorn and Buettgens 2010; Bovbjerg, Ormond, and Chen 2011, ix).

Not surprisingly, state assessments of the ACA price tag appear at times to reflect the partisan ideologies of their elected policymakers. Analyses performed for officials in Florida and Texas, for instance, projected that the ACA and Medicaid would cost so much as to impose an onerous, unsustainable fiscal burden on them. However, the Florida analysis assumed that Medicaid take-up rates would be 100 percent and the Texas study 94 percent. Participation rates of this magnitude are highly unlikely. So, too, these studies did not consider the savings that the ACA might yield to offset the price of reform (Bovbjerg, Ormond, and Chen 2011, 8–11).

State Commitment and Retrenchment Options

The implementation fortunes of Medicaid under the ACA depend not only on the fiscal and administrative capacities of the states. They also hinge on the commitment of states to the program—the degree to which dominant political coalitions within them wish to preserve and expand Medicaid. Such commitment manifests itself in many ways. One involves a willingness to bolster Medicaid through greater tax effort. Some states are more willing than others to consider this option. Where Republicans dominate state government, the emergence of the Tea Party and its appeal to shrink government has reinforced antitax sentiment. Aside from revenue enhancements, states can divert money from other policy areas to subsidize added Medicaid costs. Many policymakers, however, strongly oppose such transfers because they believe that Medicaid has already crowded out investments in other important functions, especially education. It deserves note that states vary appreciably in the share of their budgets devoted to Medicaid. About the time of the ACA's passage, Medicaid consumed about 22 percent of total state expenditures (including intergovernmental transfers from the federal government). But this share ranged from a low of 7 percent in Wyoming to a high of 34 percent in Missouri. Ten states spent less than 16 percent of their total budgets on Medicaid (National Association of State Budget Officers 2011, 11). For this cluster, some increase in Medicaid effort may well be possible without inflicting a serious toll on other public services.

In the absence of increases in state revenues—either from economic growth or tax hikes—policymakers can turn to a number of retrenchment options. By far the most dramatic is withdrawal from Medicaid. In the year following the ACA's passage, prior to the Supreme Court's ruling, policymakers in at least six states (Colorado, Nevada, South Carolina, Texas, Washington, and Wyoming) weighed this option. Withdrawal would, of course, free them from any federal Medicaid requirements. But it would also terminate a vast infusion of federal dollars. In this vein, a report produced for Wyoming state officials acknowledged that the ACA would heighten state costs, but that "the strain that will ensue should Wyoming determine to opt out of participating in Medicaid without a solid plan to replace it is truly immeasurable." Among other things, the report noted that Medicaid accounted for 63 percent of nursing home revenues in the state (Adamy and King 2010). None of the states considering withdrawal pursued it. The Supreme Court's ruling on the ACA in 2012 negated the need for states to consider complete withdrawal. Now they could opt out of the Medicaid expansion without jeopardizing federal funding for their existing programs.

It deserves note that, regardless of whether states expand coverage under the ACA, they can turn to other items on the retrenchment menu in fiscally troubled times. As noted above, states can target provider payment. In 2010, for instance, the sluggish economy prompted thirty-nine states to cut providers' reimbursements for Medicaid (Sack 2011b). Federal legislation and court decisions in the late 1990s and early 2000s made it harder for providers to sue state officials for better payment.[37] Subsequent developments, however, threatened the autonomy of the states on this front. In 2008 and 2009 California providers persuaded the federal court of appeals in the Ninth Circuit to overturn that state's reductions in Medicaid reimbursement. California officials promptly appealed this ruling to the Supreme Court. Fearing that the decision would open the floodgates to other litigation over provider payments, twenty-two states filed a brief with the Supreme Court urging it to overturn the appellate court's decision. The Supreme Court agreed to hear the case but in February 2012 declined to rule and instead remanded the case back to the court of appeals for further deliberation.[38]

The traditional retrenchment menu also features the paring of optional services. For instance, upon taking office in 2011 Georgia governor Nathan Deal (R) proposed to terminate Medicaid coverage for dental, vision, and podiatry treatments for most adult enrollees. More dramatically, Arizona governor Jan Brewer (R) and the Republican-controlled legislature passed a law eliminating Medicaid reimbursement for certain transplants of the heart, liver, lung, pancreas, and bone marrow. (Responding to a public outcry, Arizona policymakers suspended the policy six months after it took effect.) At times policymakers seek to cap the amount of services that enrollees can receive rather than abolish the benefit. In this vein, Governor Jerry Brown (D) of California sought to limit certain Medicaid enrollees with more acute health problems to ten physician visits and six prescriptions per year in early 2011 (Sack 2010a, 2011b).

Finally, state policymakers have often retrenched by reducing the number of enrollees. One variant of this approach involves reshaping eligibility criteria so that fewer people can qualify. The ACA attempted to foreclose this option through a mandate that required states to preserve their existing eligibility criteria until the law took full effect in 2014. This maintenance-of-effort requirement sparked vehement opposition from Republican governors. In early January 2011, for instance, thirty-three sitting and newly elected Republican governors sent a letter to Congress and the White House calling for the repeal of this provision (Adamy 2011).

Although the ACA constrained states from reducing enrollments, it did not completely tie their hands. The law allowed states under fiscal duress to petition the federal government to drop coverage for certain adults. The waiver process also offered some hope of relief. In 2010, for example, the administration of Governor Jan Brewer sought to end a demonstration waiver that Arizona had obtained in the early 2000s to cover certain low-income adults. Termination of the waiver would allow the state to remove some 250,000 childless adults and 30,000 parents from the Medicaid rolls. In February 2011 the Obama administration affirmed that Arizona could abandon the waiver when it expired in September of that year

(Sack 2011b, 2011d). In more subterranean fashion, states can also tamp down enrollment by limiting outreach and increasing the transaction costs of application and renewal processes for those people who are seeking Medicaid benefits. The ACA sought to staunch this form of erosion by requiring states to maintain their current enrollment practices. In response, states have generally preserved their formal rules with respect to eligibility processes (Heberlein et al. 2011). But this formal adherence does not eliminate the possibility of less energized implementation. Declines in administrative capacity (e.g., personnel layoffs or furloughs) may undercut vigorous enrollment practices. Moreover, street-level workers and managers in administrative agencies where state policymakers openly oppose the law may well sense a tacit endorsement of less welcoming take-up practices.[39] Officials in these states may place a low priority on establishing the seamless, streamlined systems designed to reduce churning and foster take-up when the insurance exchanges open in 2014.

The Potential Problem of Large, Lagging States

The ACA initially promised to reduce the vast variation among states in the generosity of their Medicaid programs (see chapter 2). All states would now cover children and nonelderly adults up to 133 percent of the poverty line. But the Supreme Court's ruling on the ACA means that the anticipated reduction in state variation will likely be much less. Some states will participate in the Medicaid expansion and others will not, at least over the short term. This issue looms especially large in the case of certain populous states with heavy concentrations of uninsured people. If these states lag in their Medicaid effort, the numbers gaining coverage via the ACA will dip below the projected 32 million people. In considering this possibility, Florida and Texas deserve particular attention. These two states are slated to insure nearly one-fifth of those people who would gain Medicaid coverage under the ACA (Holahan and Headen 2010, 10–11).[40] To illuminate the possible issues that large, lagging states may pose, I examine the political characteristics, health care profiles, and past Medicaid performance of Florida and Texas.

Florida: Do The Minimum

As the nation's fourth-largest state, with a population of just under 19 million, Florida ranks third among states in the proportion of residents without health insurance, at 21 percent.[41] The state's high proportion of uninsured people fits a general profile of lagging achievement in the health arena. For instance, a scorecard on state health system performance released by the Commonwealth Fund places Florida in the bottom quartile of states.[42] If Florida achieved the projected participation rate of 57 percent under the ACA, it would add more than 950,000 people to its Medicaid rolls and reduce the number of uninsured adults living under 133 percent of the poverty line by 44 percent. If the state achieved a more robust 75 percent take-up rate, it would gain 1.4 million Medicaid enrollees and trim the ranks of its low-income uninsured by 70 percent (Holahan and Headen 2010, 10–11).

At the time of the ACA's passage, Florida devoted 30 percent of its overall state spending to Medicaid—8 points above the national average. But Florida has long ranked relatively low on indicators of Medicaid effort, falling into the bottom quartile of states on both expenditures and enrollees per poor person.[43] Medicaid eligibility criteria constrain enrollment growth. Florida's CHIP effort extends coverage to children in families with incomes up to 200 percent of the poverty line but caps enrollment. Among nondisabled adults below the age of sixty-five years, the state has extended optional coverage only to certain parents up to 53 percent of the poverty line (Artiga 2009b; Heberlein et al. 2011, 29). Florida officials have promoted some user-friendly take-up practices for children. For instance, they do not require a face-to-face interview, an asset test, or paper documentation of income. But as of 2010 they had not adopted "express lane eligibility," which the federal government has touted as a vehicle for maximizing participation rates.[44] Nor have they adopted continuous eligibility for one year for children enrolled in Medicaid (Heberlein et al. 2011, 46–47, 54). On balance, the state has not proven highly efficacious in take-up efforts for children under Medicaid and CHIP. Nationally, 17 percent of children at or below 200 percent of the poverty line remained uninsured as of 2008, even though many qualified for public coverage; in Florida, 30 percent of these children lacked coverage.[45]

Florida's challenges do not flow from a political culture inimical to competent public administration. To the contrary, the state has often been a leader in certain "good government" practices, such as those related to due process and transparency. The staffs within both the executive and legislative branches tend to be experienced and professional. State agencies have not infrequently won national recognition for innovation. In 2007, for instance, the state received an Innovations in American Government Award from the John F. Kennedy School of Government at Harvard University for developing a Web-based system for applications to Medicaid and other social programs. But the unwillingness to raise revenues has generally muted the impact of creative policy and administrative initiatives. As two observers note, the state government's health initiatives tend to feature "making do on the cheap" and a resulting "innovation with little follow-through" (Weissert and Weissert 2008a, 357, 379).

Although Florida voters favored Barack Obama in the 2008 election, conservatives have dominated state politics and policy. Slightly more than 20 percent of the state's residents who identify with a political ideology consider themselves liberals, whereas nearly 40 percent style themselves as conservatives (Parker and Toner 2008, 37). Republicans have controlled the governor's office and both houses of the legislature since 2001. In the 2010 election Rick Scott (R) won the governorship with Tea Party backing. Policymakers of both parties have exhibited a strong aversion to raising taxes, and the state is one of the few not to impose an income tax.

Key Florida Republican policymakers have strongly opposed the ACA. As noted above, the state's attorney general led the court challenge to the law immediately after its passage. The Republican-controlled legislature also fired a shot across the bow of administrative agencies concerning implementation. In this vein, the House speaker designate, Dean Cannon (R), sent a letter to the governor's office in October 2010 complaining that state agencies had been implementing the ACA "without waiting for clear and comprehensive guidance from the Legislature." The letter demanded that the executive branch submit a complete inventory of activities taken to implement the ACA. It insisted that agencies launch any new implementation activities "only after notification and consultation with the Legislature."[46] After a federal district court judge in Florida ruled against the ACA in early 2011, newly elected governor Rick Scott (R) announced: "We are not going to spend a lot of time and money with regard to trying to get ready to implement [the law] until we know exactly what is going to happen" (Sack, Herszenhorn, and Pear 2011). The governor and key legislators vowed to do the minimum to implement the law even if it involved turning down federal monies (Sack 2011c). In the meantime, the state legislature moved ahead with proposals to cut Medicaid payment rates to hospitals, nursing homes, and health maintenance organizations.

The governor and top legislators also moved to build on the demonstration waiver launched by Governor Jeb Bush in a handful of counties (see chapter 5). Legislation to request a waiver that would shift nearly all Medicaid enrollees to managed care (including the elderly and many people with disabilities) won approval. This legislation also took the unprecedented step of imposing a premium on Medicaid enrollees regardless of income, including those people living below the poverty line. Applying a model developed by the Urban Institute, analysts predicted that the new premium would cause take-up rates in Florida to plummet, precipitating a decline in Medicaid enrollment of more than 800,000 adults and children. In August 2011 more than a hundred organizations in the state, including the Florida Medical Association, urged the Centers for Medicare and Medicaid Services to reject the waiver request.[47] As of May 2012 it remained unclear whether federal administrators would approve the waiver proposal. Finally, after the Supreme Court ruling in late June 2012, Governor Scott announced that Florida would not implement the ACA's Medicaid expansion.

Texas: Opposition and Steps to Surmount an Enrollment Debacle

As the nation's second-largest state, with a population of more than 25 million, Texas leads the country in the proportion of residents without insurance, at 26 percent.[48] Like Florida, the Commonwealth Fund ranks Texas in the bottom quartile of states on overall health system performance.[49] The ACA offers Texas a major opportunity to pare the ranks of its uninsured. Under the standard participation scenario, featuring a 57 percent take-up rate, Texas would add 1.8 million to its Medicaid rolls and reduce uninsured low-income adults by 49 percent. If the state ramped up implementation to attain a 75 percent participation rate, it would have 2.5 million new Medicaid enrollees and the number of uninsured adults living below 133 of the poverty line would drop by 74 percent (Holahan and Headen 2010, 10–11).

Like Florida, Texas ranks low among the fifty states on Medicaid effort—forty-eighth for both expenditures and enrollees per poor person. In fiscal 2009 it devoted about 25 percent of total state expenditures to Medicaid—about 3 points above the national mean.[50] Consistent with these rankings, Texas has long imposed restrictive eligibility criteria. Among nondisabled adults under sixty-five years of age, only certain parents in the direst fiscal straits (26 percent of poverty) can qualify for Medicaid (Artiga 2009b, 2). Texas extends CHIP coverage to children up to 200 percent of the poverty line but caps enrollment. The state has adopted some practices to reduce transaction costs for applicants and beneficiaries—for instance, twelve months of continuous eligibility for CHIP. Still, there is much to commend the view of one advocate that the Texas enrollment system features officials "encircling themselves in complexity" to make it hard for people to obtain and retain eligibility.[51] Texas is one of only two states that requires children on Medicaid to apply for renewal every six months—a cumbersome practice that fuels a churning of the rolls and depresses the take-up rate. It also imposes an asset test for children—a criterion imposed on families in only two other states (Heberlein et al. 2011, 29, 46, 54). Given these practices, it is not surprising that 29 percent of Texas children living below 200 percent of the poverty line lack insurance, compared with a national rate of 17 percent.[52]

Take-up challenges also emanate from ongoing issues of administrative capacity. The issue here does not revolve primarily around the experience and competence of state civil servants. Indeed, stakeholders tend to praise the professionalism of the state workforce.[53] Texas agencies have at times been innovative. For instance, the state was a pacesetter in establishing "Money Follows the Person"—a Medicaid initiative that provides incentives for the elderly and people with disabilities to leave institutions and receive community-based services.[54] Rather than workforce competence, capacity problems tend to derive from inadequate investments in administrative infrastructure and other missteps by state policymakers. The approach the state took with respect to enrollment systems for Medicaid and related social programs offers a vivid example. Although some states depend on counties to process Medicaid applications and renewals, Texas relies on its own administrative agencies in Austin and across the state. In the 2000s top policymakers moved to privatize the enrollment system while simultaneously downsizing the number of state eligibility workers. Between 1996 and 2006, the number of these workers dropped from some 13,000 to slightly more than 5,000.[55] Meanwhile, the private contractor hired to upgrade enrollment processes foundered. Many of the new employees it hired off the street to process applications lacked pertinent knowledge. Moreover, the contractor's efforts to design a new software package for enrollment went awry. Eventually, the state terminated the contractor. But problems continued as staffing within the state bureaucracy continued to lag. The ongoing problems with enrollment software meant that front-line eligibility workers in many areas had to use two computer systems to process applications.

Texas's limited Medicaid effort partly reflects its status as one of the most politically conservative states in the country. A leading text on the state's government describes its political culture as marked by "extreme individualism deriving from the myth of the frontier" mingled with "social Darwinism." Anglo Texans have "seen themselves as self-sufficient pioneers who need no help from anyone and are not obligated to support other people with their taxes" (Kraemer, Newell, and Prindle 2005, 21). During the last fifteen years, the Republican Party has dominated state politics. Democrats have not held the governorship since 1994, and Republicans have also increasingly controlled both houses of the legislature. With Tea Party support, Governor Rick Perry (R) defeated a more moderate Republican in the 2010 primary election and went on to win a third term. Not surprisingly, Texas ranks near the bottom of all states in tax effort and, like Florida, has no income tax (Kraemer, Newell, and Prindle 2005, 399).

Top policymakers in Texas strongly opposed the ACA; Governor Perry characterized the new law as "socialism on American soil" and vowed to fight it "on every front available" (Sack 2010c). The state's Republican attorney general promptly joined Florida's suit to have the ACA declared unconstitutional. Even before its passage, the Texas legislature had directed the state bureaucracy to prepare a report assessing the impact of withdrawing from Medicaid. A report jointly prepared by the Texas Health and Human Services Commission and Texas Department of Insurance (2010) persuaded policymakers that withdrawal was not a viable option. The attention of elected officials thereby turned to more incremental modes of retrenchment. With tax increases off the table, the magnitude of the cuts in part hinged on how much the governor would permit policymakers to withdraw from the state's ample "rainy day" fund. Governor Perry grudgingly allowed the use of some of these monies over the short term, but he announced that they were off limits as a source of relief in the coming fiscal year. As a result the legislature approved significant cuts in Medicaid provider payment and benefits. In an effort to save money, it also authorized the state to pursue two demonstration waivers. One would expand Medicaid's managed care. The other would "block grant" Medicaid, with the state accepting a capped global allotment from the federal government in exchange for greater flexibility to shape the program. On another front, Governor Perry indicated that he would not sign legislation creating an insurance exchange before a definitive court ruling on the ACA's constitutionality. The creation of an exchange is a necessary step toward establishing a seamless enrollment structure under health reform. After the Supreme Court upheld the key provisions of the ACA, Governor Perry announced that Texas would not create an exchange or pursue the Medicaid expansion.

Although the actions of elected officeholders in Texas hardly augur well for a smooth transition under the ACA, state administrators did work diligently to remedy some of the earlier damage to the Medicaid enrollment system. In particular, Thomas Suehs, the chief executive of the Health and Human Services Commission, prioritized repair of this system. Suehs, who was appointed by Governor Perry in September 2009, had extensive experience in top leadership roles in the state bureaucracy. To improve the enrollment system, Suehs recruited a skilled administrator from Michigan known for his expertise in dealing with computer-based processes for eligibility determinations. He also reached out to hard-pressed eligibility workers in local offices throughout the state. He traveled to many of these offices, where he praised front-line workers for their contribution and promised improvements that would make their tasks less onerous and frustrating. He also persuaded the legislature to authorize the hiring of additional eligibility workers. Officials of the Health and Humans Services Commission estimated that the reformed computer system would be in place throughout the entire state in 2012. The system would, among other things, facilitate Web-based applications to Medicaid and eliminate the necessity for eligibility workers to bridge two computer systems. Suehs's efforts won praise from across the spectrum of Medicaid stakeholders in Texas.[56] This repair of the enrollment system will not, however, be the elixir for take-up, especially if policymakers leave in place the eligibility criteria discussed above or fail to fund additional intake workers. But the administrative improvements clearly provide a better launching pad for an eligibility expansion under the ACA.

In sum, the political characteristics, health care track records, and Medicaid legacies of Texas and Florida suggest that they will severely impede efforts to expand insurance coverage for people up to 133 percent of the poverty line. To be sure, the data presented in chapter 2 suggest that their Medicaid effort may well improve over time. Medicaid expenditures and enrollees per poor person grew in both states from 1992 through 2008. But despite this growth, Texas and Florida made little headway in closing the gap between themselves and the leading Medicaid programs.

Implications for Program Durability

The ACA vividly testifies to Medicaid's prominence and political strength. The program had come a long way since 1995, when it narrowly escaped conversion to a diminished block grant. The ACA now established it as the platform for comprehensive reform. Medicaid would no longer offer patchwork coverage to the poor with great variation from one state to the next. Instead, Medicaid programs in every state would guarantee insurance to those people with incomes up to 133 percent of the poverty line. It would also, though with more variation across states, continue to subsidize services to the elderly, people with disabilities, and some CHIP enrollees. Medicaid expenditures and enrollees seemed destined to grow appreciably.

The Supreme Court's ruling in 2012 took considerable wind out of the sails of the Medicaid expansion envisioned by the ACA. States obtained the option to exit from the expansion without penalty to their existing Medicaid programs. At least over the short term, several governors vowed to pursue this option. Even if the great majority of states ultimately participate in the expansion, difficult challenges will linger. Nagging problems of how to maximize take-up in a means-tested social program persisted. If states (especially populous and growing ones like Florida and Texas) lacked the will or capacity to establish client-friendly outreach and enrollment practices, Medicaid coverage would fall below projections. Moreover, the perennial problem of assuring adequate provider networks continued to loom. Temporary increases in payment for primary care physicians and the proliferation of community health centers would help some. But a significant risk remained that, as Medicaid rolls swelled, beneficiaries would face more difficulties than ever in obtaining timely access to care. The ACA also pushed Medicaid in the direction of being a program for the poor. To be sure, eligibility for Medicaid would be more divorced than ever from that for welfare. Moreover, Medicaid would continue to reach to the middle class through benefits offered to the elderly and people with disabilities. But the program would eventually lose many of its working enrollees with incomes above the poverty level to the insurance exchanges. This departing cohort had helped create a more positive social construction of Medicaid. Now a greater proportion of the program's beneficiaries would be at the bottom of the economic barrel and less socially attractive.

Beyond these challenges, Medicaid in the context of the ACA became increasingly ensnared in the partisan polarization that permeated American politics. No matter that the ACA drew from a bipartisan Massachusetts model and contained many ideas previously endorsed by Republicans, the repeal of "Obamacare" became a rallying cry for the Republicans. Furthermore, the rise of the Tea Party pushed the Republicans toward even more strident opposition to health reform. Energized by the Tea Party, Republicans scored impressive gains in the 2010 election based not just on a repudiation of the Democrats and the Obama administration, but on a rejection of how Republicans had governed during the George W. Bush years. Hence, the substantial durability that Medicaid exhibited throughout the Bush administration may not be replicated if the Republicans again gain the presidency and dominate both houses of Congress. Clearly, the prospects for compensatory federalism with higher federal match rates during tough economic times have dimmed.

The ACA also brought back more fractious federalism—heightened tensions between the federal government and the states over Medicaid, much of it along partisan lines. The health reform law reversed a trend that had been unfolding smoothly for nearly two decades to devolve more discretion to the states to shape Medicaid. Instead, the ACA imposed an array of new Medicaid mandates concerning coverage and other matters. In response Republican attorneys general banded together in an unprecedented fashion to fight health reform in the courts. Republican governors also joined the fray. Despite a relatively generous federal match for new enrollees, nearly all of them denounced the new law. The maintenance-of-effort requirements for those people who are currently eligible for Medicaid sparked gubernatorial opposition from both parties. The limits on state discretion to reshape eligibility criteria and enrollment processes until 2014 came at a time when many of them faced acute fiscal stress. Maintenance of effort heightened the political costs to elected officials of Medicaid retrenchment. Rather than cut eligibility for relatively powerless low-income groups, they faced the prospect of incurring the wrath of politically well-connected hospitals and nursing homes by paring their payments. In this context, open endorsement of greater flexibility via a Medicaid block grant, an idea that had fallen out of political favor after the government shutdown in 1995, again surfaced among Republican governors.[57]

Hence, the expansion of Medicaid promised by the ACA may become a symbol of the program's fragility rather than its durability. Republican control of the presidency and Congress after the 2012 election would probably prevent Medicaid's great leap forward from commencing in 2014. If the ACA can survive until 2014 and the uninsured finally begin to benefit, the outlook for Medicaid's durability improves. At this point the ACA will begin to generate supportive policy feedbacks that fortify it against repeal. Growing numbers of states may respond to the law's generous federal subsidy by participating in the Medicaid expansion. Even in this case, however, Medicaid will remain vulnerable to decline, especially if health care costs maintain their upward trajectory, and the federal deficit and debt continue to grow.

Notes

1. The demonstration committed MassHealth to covering all uninsured children up to 200 percent of poverty. The waiver increased the number of Medicaid enrollees in managed

care and launched the Insurance Partnership program, which provided premium subsidies to small employers and their low-income employees to obtain private health insurance.

2. DSH was created in 1981, and Congress capped the amount of funds states could spend on DSH a decade later. By that time Massachusetts had become one of about ten high-DSH states that allocated substantial sums to institutions (Gusmano and Thompson 2012).

3. The Kaiser Commission on Medicaid and the Uninsured provided these data.

4. That is, the premiums could be deducted from their incomes for tax purposes.

5. Some have estimated the proportion of uninsured in Massachusetts to be less than 3 percent (see Goodnough 2009); the US Census Bureau (2011) placed the proportion not covered for all of 2010 at 5.6 percent.

6. See, e.g., the testimony of Dr. John Goodman of the National Center for Policy Analysis (US House Committee on Energy and Commerce 2009b, 18–19).

7. Interview 23, December 14, 2010.

8. See especially Jacobs and Skocpol (2010), McDonough (2011), and Starr (2011). Alter (2010) also casts light on the initial politics of reform.

9. Interview 29, January 28, 2011.

10. Interview 6, September 2, 2010.

11. Ibid.

12. Those testifying were Marian Wright Edelman of the Children's Defense Fund, Ron Pollack of Families USA, and Senator Joe Vitale of New Jersey.

13. These figures come from US Senate, Committee on Finance (2009, 365, 422, 424). A committee staff member subsequently corrected Senator Cornyn's estimate.

14. On the liberal critics of Medicaid, see, e.g., Olson (2010).

15. Senator John Cornyn used the adjective "lousy" (US Senate Committee on Finance 2009, 414).

16. Senator Cornyn used the phrase "shell game." The other quotation comes from Senator John Kyl (US Senate Committee on Finance 2009, 411, 416).

17. A version of Senator Grassley's proposal to boost payment for primary care physicians did make it into the ACA.

18. Though precise data are unavailable, the evidence suggests that few, if any, states achieve participation rates of 75 percent.

19. Interview 6, September 2, 2010.

20. US Senate, Committee on Finance (2009, 414). Before the Obama administration, Senator Wyden had crafted the Healthy Americans Act. This plan proposed to achieve near-universal coverage through federal subsidies to individuals and businesses (based on ability to pay) to purchase private insurance. The plan eliminated the Medicaid program.

21. This subsection's description draws heavily on a useful summary document released by the Kaiser Family Foundation (2010d). Subsidies to individuals living at between 133 and 400 percent of the poverty level were to be made on a sliding scale, with those earning more receiving less federal assistance.

22. The law continues to bar most legal immigrants from Medicaid enrollment during their first five years in the United States (Kaiser Family Foundation 2010d, 4).

23. Some members of Congress wanted to "mainstream" CHIP enrollees in the insurance exchanges. However, opponents noted that CHIP beneficiaries would face much steeper cost sharing if lawmakers took this step (McDonough 2011, 154).

24. For a discussion of the limits to targeting in the current DSH program, see Gusmano and Thompson (2012).

25. See Sack (2010b) Some Republican attorneys general joined the suit after they won election in 2010.

26. Case 3:10-cv-00091-RV-EMT of document 1, p. 5, obtained from the website of the attorney general of the State of Florida, http://myfloridalegal.com.

27. Case 3:10-cv-00091-RV-EMT, document 150, filed January 31, 2011, US District Court for the Northern District of Florida, pp. 6–13.

28. Case 3:10-cv-00188-HEH, document 161, filed December 13, 2010, US District Court for the Eastern District of Virginia, p. 40.

29. Case 3:10-cv00092-RV, document 150, filed January 31, 2011, US District Court for the Northern District of Florida, p. 73.

30. I am indebted to Mollyann Brodie, Claudia Deane, and Sarah Cho of the Kaiser Family Foundation for sharing these data with me.

31. Some of the discussion in this section is also given by Thompson (2011).

32. To reinforce this point, 61 percent of uninsured low-income adults under sixty-five years of age resided in officially designated Health Professional Shortage Areas in the 2005–7 period (Hoffman, Damico, and Garfield 2011, 4).

33. Joel Ario, director of the federal Office of Health Insurance Exchanges, used this phrase (Lotven 2010).

34. Holahan and Headen (2010, 10) estimate that about 70 percent of the new Medicaid enrollees will be uninsured. The remainder will switch to Medicaid from other types of insurance.

35. Some advocates believe that the "woodwork effect" carries a negative connotation and prefer the phrase "welcome-mat effect" (interview 38, March 18, 2011). I continue to use "woodwork" because it is a widely understood term among Medicaid stakeholders, many of whom are strong supporters of enhanced take-up.

36. Assuming a 57 percent participation rate, Arkansas costs would increase by nearly 5 percent relative to a baseline trend (Holahan and Headen 2010, 10–11).

37. The Balanced Budget Act of 1997 undercut the ability of providers to win concessions in court by repealing the Boren Amendment. Rosenbaum (2009) also stresses the importance of the Supreme Court's 2002 ruling in *Gonzaga v. Doe* as a vehicle for undermining claims by providers and enrollees that they had federally enforceable rights under Medicaid.

38. Unlike most prior litigation, the California providers based their claim on the Supremacy Clause of the US Constitution—the principle that federal laws take precedence over state statutes (Rosenbaum 2009). See also Baker (2010) and US Supreme Court (2012a).

39. For example, Fossett and Thompson (2006) find that gubernatorial leadership affects state take-up practices for Medicaid and CHIP.

40. California ranks well ahead of both Florida and Texas in terms of the numbers projected to gain Medicaid coverage. But California has consistently exerted more Medicaid effort, and its top policymakers have expressed support for the ACA.

41. The rate reflects a two-year average for 2008–9 and comes from the US Census Bureau, *Current Population Survey, Annual Social and Economic Supplement*, 2007–10.

42. See McCarthy et al. (2009, 9). This study analyzes indicators clustered under five dimensions: access, prevention and treatment, avoidable hospital use and costs, equity, and healthy lives. It deserves note that Florida achieves a somewhat higher ranking—around the median among states—on the healthy lives dimension. In this regard Florida has relatively low, age-adjusted death rates for breast and colorectal cancers. However, it ranks in the bottom quartile on infant mortality and mortality rates amenable to health care (McCarthy et al. 2009, 91).

43. See National Association of State Budget Officers (2011, 11) and table 2.4 in the present volume.

44. This option permits states to use data and eligibility findings from other public programs when assessing the eligibility of children for Medicaid and CHIP.

45. The author obtained these data from the US Census Bureau, *Current Population Survey, Annual Social and Economic Supplement*, 2007–9. They reflect a three-year average for 2006–8.

46. Interviewee 23 (December 14, 2010) gave me a copy of the letter, dated October 19, 2010.

47. See Davis (2011) and www.miamiherald.com/2011/08/06/2347722/florida-doctors-organization-opposes.html. The data on the projected enrollment decline come from Hoadley and Alker (2011).

48. US Census Bureau, *Current Population Survey, Annual Social and Economic Supplement*, 2007–10. The percentage is a two-year average for 2008–9.

49. See note 39 for a discussion of the Commonwealth dimensions. Though Texas ranks in the second quartile of states in avoiding infant mortality, it falls in the bottom quartile on mortality amenable to health care (McCarthy et al. 2009, 91).

50. See tables 2.1 through 2.3 in the present volume and National Association of State Budget Officers (2011, 11).

51. Interview 33, March 16, 2011.

52. US Census Bureau, *Current Population Survey, Annual Social and Economic Supplement*, 2007–9. They reflect a three-year average for 2006–8.

53. Interview 38, March 18, 2011.

54. The federal government subsequently drew on the Texas experience to encourage other states to adopt Money Follows the Person (interview 30, March 16, 2011).

55. Interview 38, March 18, 2011.

56. Most of the people whom I interviewed in Austin expressed this view. I have especially relied on interview 36, March 17, 2011, and interview 38, March 18, 2011.

57. At the winter meeting of the National Governors Association in February 2011, a leading Republican governor, Haley Barbour of Mississippi, asserted that "if we could get Medicaid as a block grant with total flexibility to run the program as we see fit, I would be willing to take a cap on growth of 2 percent a year. Many governors feel that way" (Pear 2011b).

CHAPTER SEVEN

Durability, Federalism, and the Future of Medicaid

From the dawn of the Clinton administration in January 1993 to the contentious politics of divided government under Barack Obama in 2011, dramatic political and economic changes buffeted Medicaid. At various intervals the two major parties won and lost control of Congress and the presidency. The march toward asymmetric partisan polarization continued apace, with the Republican Party trending toward greater conservatism. The quest to end Medicaid as an entitlement via a block grant surged, ebbed, and surged again. Democratic policymakers scored an epic breakthrough in forging comprehensive health reform, with Medicaid as the platform, while energized Republicans vowed to achieve what would be an equally epic repeal of the law. The country enjoyed considerable prosperity through most of the 1990s and into the 2000s, only to plunge into the worst recession since the Great Depression in 2007. This downturn stoked large hikes in the federal deficit, which in turn fueled political claims that the federal government's major entitlement programs could not be sustained.

To the surprise of many, Medicaid—a program for the economically and (presumably) politically disadvantaged—expanded and proved remarkably durable throughout this period. This development partly reflected policy dynamics that led to changes in federal and state Medicaid laws. It also reflected the twists and turns of implementation, especially the rise of waivers as a policy tool.

This chapter puts Medicaid's evolution and the forces that drove it in broad perspective. First, I return to the question of how durable Medicaid was in the 1993–2010 period. Although uncertainty shrouds certain aspects of the program's performance and the evidence does not all point in the same direction, key indicators testify to Medicaid's resilience and growth. Second, I zero in on the nexus between federalism and the forces shaping Medicaid's durability. Medicaid reflects a catalytic rather than a constraining model of federalism. More specifically, the interplay of six main factors looms especially large in explaining the program's strength. Third, I turn to Medicaid's prospects in an era of austerity—one marked by mounting alarm over the federal debt—and analyze how three prominent debt reduction proposals treated the program. Two of the proposals, those offered by the Bowles-Simpson Commission and the Domenici-Rivlin Task Force, assumed the need for expenditure cuts and revenue increases. A third, sponsored by Representative Paul Ryan (R-WI), sought to stanch the flow of red ink almost completely through spending cuts. And fourth, I offer a personal perspective on caveats that should be salient as policymakers consider the future of Medicaid in America's health insurance system.

How Durable Has Medicaid Been?

This study has examined three sets of markers in an effort to gauge the Medicaid program's durability—its status as a formal entitlement, pertinent expenditure trends, and some of its outputs (especially enrollment) and outcomes. In reprising evidence with respect to these markers, an entitlement paradox stands out. Until the passage of the ACA, the 1993–2010 period featured considerable erosion in Medicaid's status as a formal legal entitlement. But simultaneously, trends in expenditures and enrollees per poor person paint a picture of Medicaid's growth and durability. In noting this paradox, it is critical to distinguish between Medicaid as a financial entitlement for the states and as a service entitlement for beneficiaries. The program withstood Republican efforts to convert it from a fiscal entitlement to a block grant in 1995 and again in 2003. If it had failed to do so, program expenditures and enrollments would surely not have evinced the patterns of growth described in chapter 2. During the Clinton and George W. Bush administrations, all fifty states increased their Medicaid expenditures and enrollees per poor person. Although the states would sporadically cut the program in response to fiscal stress, a steady ratcheting up of Medicaid benefits emerges as the dominant pattern. Although the take-up challenge continually dogged the program and kept many qualified people from obtaining services, the period witnessed considerable state progress in streamlining enrollment procedures, which abetted enrollment growth.

The expansion of Medicaid occurred as the proliferation of waivers, federal statutory changes, and certain court actions chipped away at the program as a service entitlement. Those people who could qualify for the program had a diminished legal "right" to health care. This erosion assumed several forms. Through waivers, the states won greater discretion to limit services to those living in certain areas rather than provide them statewide. Geographic inequality in the availability of certain program benefits—especially HCBS—soared. States also gained more leeway to cap Medicaid enrollments and put low-income people on waiting lists. This manifested itself most dramatically in the rationing of HCBS under the Section 1915c waivers. But it also played out in the 1997 passage of CHIP. Over time, more and more states moved away from Medicaid toward a separate CHIP grant, which allowed them to cap enrollment. In other instances, formal legislative changes offered the states the opportunity to thin coverage. The Deficit Reduction Act of 2005, for instance, allowed the states to impose additional cost sharing on Medicaid enrollees, whether through premiums or copayments. The law also gave the states permission to scale back the standard Medicaid service package for certain categories of adults.

The ability of Medicaid providers and beneficiaries to enforce their rights in the courts also ebbed. To be sure, the Supreme Court's *Olmstead* ruling in 1999 gave advocates for the elderly and people with disabilities more leverage under the Americans with Disabilities Act. They could sue state Medicaid programs for failing to move rapidly enough to rebalance long-term care from institutions to the home and community. But on other fronts, the opportunities for Medicaid stakeholders to press their case in court dimmed. Since the early 1980s, hospitals and nursing homes had used the Boren Amendment to the Medicaid statute to sue states in the federal courts over payment rates.[1] In 1997 Congress repealed this provision. The Supreme Court's 2002 decision in *Gonzaga v. Doe* further undercut prospects for court intervention to uphold the rights of Medicaid stakeholders. Although focused on issues of student privacy rights in higher education, the decision more broadly limited the circumstances under which individuals could turn to the courts for relief. In the wake of *Gonzaga*, federal appellate courts consistently ruled against petitioners who sued state governments for failing to uphold the federal Medicaid law (Rosenbaum 2009, 14).

The ACA was, of course, a remarkable reversal of fortune for Medicaid as a service entitlement. The new law mandated coverage for vast multitudes of low-income people whom the program had previously neglected. Medicaid expenditures and enrollees per person living in poverty seemed destined to rise sharply. However, the Supreme Court's ruling in 2012 gave states the option to walk away from the Medicaid expansion without fear of serious penalty. The degree to which states will seize this option remains unclear. Moreover, the service entitlement to long-term care remains limited. States can continue to use waivers to ration HCBS geographically and by the availability of funding.

Whether the growth in Medicaid spending and enrollments from 1993 through 2010 was accompanied by improvement in the access of Medicaid beneficiaries to high-quality care remains an open question. As this book has noted, serious problems persist on this front, especially with respect to Medicaid's provider networks. Although states vary appreciably, payment rates for Medicaid tend to lag behind those for Medicare and private insurers. Many physicians limit the Medicaid enrollees they will see, and access to specialists is especially problematic. Hospitals and nursing homes generally do better than physicians in extracting suitable payments, but they also complain that the program shortchanges them. In the case of hospitals, the impact of lower Medicaid reimbursement on quality partly revolves around the degree to which they shift costs to other payers. To the extent that hospitals do so, their temptation to scrimp on the quality of care delivered to Medicaid enrollees diminishes. They can recoup the money lost on Medicaid from other payers. But one recent review of the evidence finds little support for "the notion that cost shifting is . . . large and pervasive" (Frakt 2010, 30). Another analysis reaches a similar conclusion, arguing that lower Medicaid rates trigger "burden sharing" in hospitals that leads to "reduced quality or intensity of services" for patients.[2] It may well be that Medicaid enrollees disproportionately suffer this quality loss relative to the other hospital patients.[3] So, too, nursing homes with higher proportions of Medicaid patients tend to have more quality deficiencies (Amirkhanyan, Kim, and Lambright 2008).

While acknowledging these limitations, however, it deserves note that three developments from 1993 through 2010 may well have enhanced access and quality for Medicaid enrollees. First, the period witnessed a great increase in the number of Medicaid beneficiaries enrolled in managed care. Proponents of this development thought it would simultaneously trim costs, foster access, and better coordinate services. Research on the efficacy of managed care under Medicaid yields mixed conclusions (see chapter 5). Although managed care has been far from a silver bullet, however, few if any Medicaid stakeholders support a return to the practices that were in place before its ascendance. At least in some states, the expansion of Medicaid managed care appears to have strengthened both access and quality.[4]

Second, there was a dramatic increase in access to HCBS for the elderly and people with disabilities. The proportion of Medicaid long-term care dollars spent on these services rather than nursing homes and related institutions increased from 15 percent to more than 40 percent.[5] Although many people remained on waiting lists for HCBS and stakeholders called for additional rebalancing, this development represented a big step forward in providing appropriate care.

Third, the access of Medicaid enrollees benefited from growth in the number of community health centers—a key component of the health care safety net. These federally supported centers almost doubled in number from 1993 to 2008. By the end of the Bush years, 1,080 centers operated at more than 7,500 sites, providing care to 19 million patients, about three-quarters of whom were Medicaid enrollees or uninsured. The ACA pledged increases in funding for these centers that would more than double the people they served during the next decade.[6] Because the federal government requires states to pay these centers more generous rates, their expansion promises significant gains in access to high-quality care for Medicaid beneficiaries.[7]

The available evidence on Medicaid from 1993 through 2010, though far from definitive, points to the program's expansion and improvement. To be sure, Medicaid continued to suffer from infirmities that distanced it from "mainstream" health care. But the story line seems best expressed as a glass that is half full rather than one that is half empty. This development naturally raises the question: What accounts for the durability that Medicaid has achieved?

Federalism and the Forces That Have Fortified Medicaid

Chapter 1 noted the conflicting perspectives embedded in the constraining and catalytic models of federalism concerning the durability of redistributive programs such as Medicaid. The constraining model sees competition among states as a brake on public-sector investment in programs that reallocate monies from the haves to the have-nots. It rests on assumptions about how firms and individuals vote with their feet, and it holds that firms faced with higher taxation to support programs like Medicaid will, all else being equal, tend to relocate to lower-tax states with more penurious social programs. Affluent individuals purportedly do the same. States with bountiful social benefits also risk becoming welfare magnets. The have-nots within their borders remain, while the disadvantaged from less generous states become tempted to join them. To avoid this development, state policymakers have an incentive to curtail the pull of the magnet by keeping social benefits low. The constraining model assumes that its dynamics will unfold not only if firms and individuals vote with their feet in this way but also if the states' policymakers *perceive* that they do. At the extreme, this model posits that interstate competition will precipitate a "race to the bottom," with a steady erosion in program benefits over time. Others, however, point to a significant but more limited effect of the model. They suggest that the metaphor of a "naval convoy" better captures the implications of interstate competition: "Just as no single ship sailing in a naval convoy during wartime can risk getting too far ahead of the other ships, or too far behind," the fifty states face pressures not to let their taxing and spending policies stray too far from the pack.[8]

Some evidence supports the constraining model. Cross-national studies suggest that federalism tends to limit government spending in countries (e.g., the United States, Canada, and Switzerland) whose states or provinces have more taxing authority and depend less on the central government to finance their activities (Rodden 2003; Sorens 2011). Other analyses affirm that in the United States increasingly mobile business firms in fact respond favorably to lower tax rates in making their location decisions (e.g., Donahue 1997, 178; Kenyon 1996, 266). So, too, some research suggests that a welfare magnet effect may be in play, whereby low-income individuals move to jurisdictions with more generous social benefits (e.g., Peterson and Rom 1990; Bailey 2005). Although these studies typically probe programs that offer cash benefits, one analysis suggests that interstate competition tends to erode state expenditures on Medicaid.[9]

In contrast to the constraining perspective, the catalytic model sees federalism as a force for government expansion and often for greater expenditures on redistributive programs.[10] The political scientist Richard Nathan (2008, 21) puts the case strongly: "The unabashedly opportunistic and dynamic character of American federalism has abetted government growth." Consistent with this view, competition between national and state policymakers to claim credit for dealing with a social problem can prompt greater overall government intervention (e.g., Volden 2005). A comparative analysis of six countries (including the United States) concludes that federalism at times stimulates social programs' growth and inhibits their erosion (Leibfried, Castles, and Obinger 2005, 308, 332). Cross-national research on federalism underscores the stimulatory effect of grants or other fiscal transfers from the central government to states or provinces.[11] These allow the states to be more generous without having to worry that their tax levels will drive away firms and affluent citizens. In essence states draw from a free "common pool" of resources. The presence of a "flypaper effect" further abets program expansion. Its presence means that states do not respond to central government subsidies by cutting taxes or reducing their own expenditures on the program. Instead, the grant monies stick like flypaper and thus spur program growth (Rodden 2003, 2006).

Given Medicaid's expansion in the period 1993–2010, the catalytic model holds out greater explanatory promise. But it uses a very broad brush, and the details matter. Coming to grips with the sources of Medicaid durability requires a finer-grained assessment of the catalytic interaction among six main factors: (1) the federal funding mechanism, (2) the increasingly positive social construction of Medicaid beneficiaries, (3) support from private interest groups, (4) governors as an intergovernmental lobby, (5) the proliferation of federal waivers, and (6) the achievement of unified party governance under the Democrats.

Funding Formula as Fiscal Stimulus

Federal grants for social programs assume myriad forms; many fail to spur sustained effort by the states and thus erode over time (e.g., see Gais 2009). In the case of Medicaid, however, certain interrelated features of its funding formula have made it a force for catalytic federalism. Above all, each level of government leverages substantial funding from the other levels when it commits money to Medicaid. For instance, federal policymakers seeking to expand Medicaid could historically count on the states overall to chip in about 75 cents for every federal dollar invested. At times, these policymakers turned to federal mandates to extract funds from the states' coffers (e.g., by requiring the states to cover all poor children). On other occasions, they gave the states new options to assist certain groups (e.g., by permitting them to extend eligibility for long-term care up the income ladder). When federal officials pursue this optional approach, their leveraging of state funds typically increases. More affluent states with a 50 percent match rate tend to be more aggressive about the optional expansions than those states with higher federal matches. In mandating Medicaid coverage expansions under the ACA, the federal government leveraged far fewer state dollars (eventually, a 10 percent state match for new enrollees). Still, Medicaid's role in health reform made the critical difference in allowing lawmakers to hold down costs and earn an acceptable score from the CBO.

Medicaid offers even greater leveraging opportunities to the states. In the aggregate, they have extracted more than $1.30 from the federal Treasury for every $1.00 in state funds that they spend on Medicaid. The poorest states claim close to an 80 percent federal match. During economic downturns, the states have often leveraged additional federal subsidies. Under the ACA the states got an extraordinary bargain for the newly eligible Medicaid population—about $9.00 in federal monies for every $1.00 they spend as of 2020. The Medicaid funding formula's status as an open-ended fiscal entitlement also advantages states. The absence of a federal budget cap means that the states determine how much the federal government will spend on the program. This feature insulates Medicaid in the competition for dollars in the federal budget process.

The leveraging and open-ended qualities of the Medicaid program's funding formula give elected officials at both levels of government copious opportunities to take political credit and avoid blame. Policymakers can win kudos from their constituents for expanding the program's coverage without enduring the political downside of having to raise taxes or raid other programs to find all the needed funds. Simultaneously, Medicaid provides policymakers at both levels a chance to deflect or dodge blame for the program's inadequacies. State officials can complain that the deficiencies reflect the federal government's failure to provide even more funding and flexibility. Federal policymakers can respond to complaints by blaming the states for not living up to their potential for program delivery.

The particulars of the Medicaid funding formula fuel spending. But it lacks one feature that would make it even more stimulative: automatic increases in the federal match when the GDP shrinks and unemployment rises.[12] The inevitability of economic cycles and the political costs of cutting benefits prompt some states' policymakers to hedge uncertainty by limiting Medicaid coverage in good times. To be sure, the success of governors in lobbying for temporary hikes in the federal match has to some extent offset the absence of a countercyclical provision in the formula. But governors and others cannot count on the success of their lobbying, especially in austere times. Nor can they easily predict the exact amount of the enhanced federal contribution. Certainty that the federal match would increase by a particular amount in response to deterioration in specified economic indicators would, all else being equal, further propel Medicaid's expansion.

Toward a Positive Social Construction

The movement toward a more favorable social construction of Medicaid enrollees has also been integral to catalytic federalism. This began in the period before the Clinton years, but it picked up steam in the 1990s and early 2000s. "Social construction" refers to the "cultural characterizations or popular images" of a program's beneficiaries and can be positive or negative.[13] These constructions vary in the degree to which they are widely held and change over time. They manifest themselves in such sources as political speeches, legislative hearings, media coverage, and opinion surveys. At times, a contentious politics flourishes between competing factions over the appropriate images of program beneficiaries. Active maneuvering among partisans to make their characterizations dominant in public debate persistently occurs.

In Medicaid's early years, its image as welfare medicine prevailed. To be sure, providing health care to welfare mothers and their children tended to carry less public stigma than cash payments (e.g., Cook and Barrett 1992, 62). But this did not free Medicaid enrollees from a negative construction. Many found it easy to blame welfare mothers for their health care needs, whether they were the result of pregnancy out of wedlock or unhealthy behaviors (e.g., smoking, eating too much, substance abuse). So long as Medicaid remained joined at the hip to welfare, its public image would suffer. From 1993 to 2010 several developments attenuated this link.

As described in chapter 3, the welfare reform law of 1996 and other measures increasingly divorced eligibility for Medicaid from that for cash assistance. To be sure, individuals receiving Temporary Assistance to Needy Families and those who met the old income criteria for Aid to Families with Dependent Children still qualified for Medicaid. But their numbers declined sharply in the wake of welfare reform, and they constituted a smaller share of enrollees. Moreover, the diminished value of welfare as an election issue after 1996 suppressed public consciousness of the remaining link to Medicaid. Thanks to steady implementation of mandates approved before Clinton, low-income children increasingly became eligible for Medicaid regardless of whether their parents received any other social benefits.[14] At another level, the actions of the National Association of State Medicaid Directors symbolized the drive toward delinkage. This group had long been associated with the American Public Human Services Association, an assembly of administrators representing an array of social programs including Temporary Assistance to Needy Families and food stamps. In 2010 the state Medicaid directors withdrew from this association and affiliated with the National Governors Association.

Medicaid also increasingly became a program for working families. Social notions of deservingness depend substantially on whether program beneficiaries work.[15] Hence, the growing proportion of Medicaid enrollees who held jobs benefited its image. This development played out against the backdrop of deterioration in employer-based health insurance for low-wage workers. Many employers offered no insurance. Others, whether McDonald's or Walmart, offered very thin coverage that did little to provide for the workers' other family members. Hence it became harder to portray working people on Medicaid as freeloaders who had access to generous insurance from their employers.

Federal policymakers also moved to brand Medicaid as a program that is off-limits to undocumented residents. In 2005 a Republican Congress approved citizen documentation requirements for enrollees. The Democrats followed suit when they controlled Congress, cutting off benefits for the undocumented when they reauthorized CHIP in 2009 and passed the ACA in 2010. These measures probably did less to boost the image of Medicaid than save it from deterioration. A significant majority of Americans see illegal immigration as a very serious problem. Conservatives, such as those active in the Tea Party, feel even more strongly about the issue and tend to portray illegal immigrants (especially Hispanics) as having come to the United States to secure education, health care, and other public benefits (Williamson, Skocpol, and Coggin 2011, 34). Although many conservatives believe that these undocumented immigrants obtain benefits anyway, the formal elimination of their Medicaid rights gave the program some political cover.

Finally, and probably most important, Medicaid increasingly garnered recognition as a middle-class benefit. This development manifested itself with children, the elderly, and people with disabilities. The advent of CHIP and the growing use of waivers meant that children in families with incomes well above the poverty line received public health insurance. Change also occurred with respect to the elderly. For decades, of course, Medicaid had essentially served as long-term care insurance for older people and their families. Middle-class people who had worked all their lives and never needed public assistance frequently depleted their assets after they entered a nursing home and became dependent on Medicaid. The program benefited not only the enrollees but also their spouses and other family members who would have otherwise faced pressure to cover the costs of care. What distinguished the 1990s and early 2000s was greater effort by the Democrats to brand the program as a kind of middle-class benefit. In fighting the Gingrich block grant proposal, for instance, President Clinton publicly stressed that it would impoverish spouses with loved ones in nursing homes. The 1996 Democratic Party platform also played on this theme. In pursuing this initiative, Democratic leaders felt confident that their sympathetic view would triumph over one portraying the elderly as "greedy geezers" whose families ought to be responsible for their care.

A similar dynamic applies to people with disabilities who are under the age of sixty-five years. The rise of the disability rights movement in the 1970s, the passage of the Americans with Disabilities Act in 1990, and other forces kindled a more positive image of this group. People with intellectual impairments (a major cluster of Medicaid enrollees) became less stigmatized than they had been at any point in the country's history. Part of their success came from changing the language used to describe them. Having vanquished such labels as "imbecile," "idiot," and "moron" at a much earlier point, they now made progress in replacing "mental retardation" with "intellectual disabilities" in policy discourse and law. Those who had acquired crippling physical disabilities as adults also won new respect for their ability to contribute to society. The view gained sway that people with disabilities should not be shunted off to institutions but should instead be assisted to live with dignity in their homes and communities. In this context Medicaid functions as disability insurance for the middle class. It assures parents who give birth to children with intellectual or other developmental disabilities that their offspring will receive care for life. It is a safety net for adults who became disabled through accidents. Although many people in this cohort qualify for Social Security and Medicare, these programs do not provide them with the personal assistance they need to function in the community. Medicaid often fills this gap, at least partially.

The importance to Medicaid of its positive image as a middle-class benefit becomes all the more crucial in light of the trend toward diminished trust in government. This trend manifests itself in the view that the government cannot be counted on to act in the interests of ordinary citizens, and pessimism about the government's ability to deliver programs efficiently and effectively. This diminished trust has more adverse implications for public attitudes toward social programs for poor people than those benefiting the middle class (Hetherington 2005). For instance, even though Tea Party members want to slash government spending, they tend to support programs that benefit themselves, such as Medicare and Social Security (Williamson, Skocpol, and Coggin 2011). To the degree that Medicaid gains public recognition as a middle-class benefit, it stands more chance of weathering the bias toward retrenchment incubated by low levels of government trust.

Supporters: Providers and Advocates

The degree to which a program stimulates private groups to emerge and support it also affects its durability. The effect can be particularly catalytic when these groups lobby in both the national and state policy arenas. Positive policy feedbacks can thereby buttress a program at two governmental levels. The political weakness of programs for the disadvantaged presumably stems largely from a dearth of potent groups to support them in the policy process.

Unlike many redistributive programs, however, Medicaid has long benefited from provider groups that lobby on its behalf in Washington and in state capitals. Nursing homes, which depend on Medicaid for more than 40 percent of their revenues and about 70 percent of their residents, have a huge stake in the program

(Kaiser Commission on Medicaid and the Uninsured 2011, 11). Located in almost every legislative district in the country, they work through the state affiliates of the American Health Care Association and other venues to support Medicaid long-term care, devoting particular attention to payment rates. Hospitals, especially those that play a large role in the safety net, also lobby aggressively on Medicaid reimbursement. More than a hundred of these hospitals belong to the National Association of Public Hospitals and Health Systems. These institutions are typically located in urban areas, and they disproportionately serve Medicaid enrollees and the uninsured. About one-third of these institutions' net revenues derives from Medicaid, a figure that greatly exceeds that for hospitals in general (Zaman, Cummings, and Spieler 2010). In addition to pressing for higher payment rates for emergency room, obstetrics, and other services, these hospitals have often fought hard to preserve and enhance Medicaid payments under the Disproportionate Share Hospital Program—direct program subsidies that flow to safety net institutions.[16] In the period of this study, managed care organizations also developed a substantial stake in Medicaid as states increasingly channeled enrollees to them. In many states, such as Florida, these organizations maintain a significant presence in state capitals. Many affiliate with a larger trade association called America's Health Insurance Plans to promote their interests at the national level. Increasingly, they have touted the virtues of expanding managed care under Medicaid beyond children and their parents to the elderly and people with disabilities.

In a few states unions representing workers for hospitals, nursing homes, HCBS, and other health care providers have been formidable advocates for Medicaid. In New York, for instance, leaders of the Service Employees International Union 1199 have been particularly aggressive in defending Medicaid. Legislators in the state assembly, which Democrats have controlled for decades, have been especially mindful not to incur the union's displeasure on Medicaid. So have most governors, regardless of political party.

Medicaid's beneficiaries also have advocates. At the national level, groups such as Families USA and the Children's Defense Fund promote Medicaid as a vehicle for expanding health insurance to more low- and moderate-income adults and children. In doing so, they can draw on sophisticated and timely evidence-based analyses from think tanks—especially the Center for Budget and Policy Priorities, the Kaiser Commission on Medicaid and the Uninsured, and the Urban Institute. These think tanks loom large in providing the intellectual underpinnings for the policy positions that advocates adopt. (Conservatives, in turn, draw more on reports and issue briefs from the American Enterprise Institute and Heritage Foundation.)

As noted in chapter 4, advocates for the program's middle-class constituents—the elderly and people with disabilities—tend to be more potent than those for poor adults and children. They are more likely to be a force in both the halls of Congress and the corridors of state capitols. It is no accident that more than 70 percent of Medicaid expenditures on these cohorts are "optional"—that is, not mandated by federal law. In contrast, only about a third of spending on nondisabled children and adults under sixty-five years of age is optional (Courtot and Artiga 2011). The myriad groups representing people with diverse disabilities typically set the pace for advocacy, often working hand in glove with the providers who serve them. In contrast to people with disabilities, advocates for the elderly have been less systematic and vigorous in the Medicaid policy arena. At the national level, for instance, AARP only belatedly sounded concerns about the Medicaid block grant proposal in 1995. In the 2000s it has been somewhat more aggressive.[17] When another proposal to convert Medicaid into a block grant surfaced in early 2011, AARP strongly opposed the measure (Dixit 2011). At the state level AARP typically ranks behind advocates for people with disabilities in the vigor of its Medicaid advocacy.[18] To a significant degree nursing homes and providers of HCBS provide the primary voice for the elderly on the states' decisions related to Medicaid.

The Intergovernmental Lobby: Governors to the Fore

Although private interest groups help bolster Medicaid, the program's durability at the federal level more markedly reflects the importance of the intergovernmental lobby. In essence, the catalytic interaction between key government actors at two levels of the federal system does much to shape Medicaid's fortunes. It deserves note that this intergovernmental relationship supports theories of government-centered or state-centered politics. These theories place less emphasis on the role of private interest groups and public opinion in shaping policy and more on the "political, ideological, and strategic motivations" of policymakers within government. This perspective highlights the considerable "autonomy" of government actors in the policy process.[19]

Among the panoply of state officials shaping federal Medicaid policy, governors stand front and center. Chapter 2 described some of the power resources that governors possess in the federal policy process. Whether through their own offices in Washington, their formal partisan associations, the NGA, their personal relationships with federal policymakers, or some other vehicle, governors command the attention of Congress and the White House on Medicaid. As much as any interest group, governors have the capacity to monitor the twists and turns of the federal policy process affecting Medicaid. More than any other actors, they can claim to offer a comprehensive, realistic perspective on how changes in federal Medicaid law will play out when implemented. In addition to their expertise, governors have other resources. To a greater degree than private lobbyists or other clusters of state officials, they have access to the media. Some governors enjoy the added stature of being seen as major players in American politics—often as potential presidential candidates. Hence, the opposition of governors to a proposal heightens the political costs to federal policymakers of enacting it.

The political assets of governors do not assure that they can place a Medicaid proposal on the congressional policy agenda for action. Nor do these resources mean that a majority of governors will prevail when Congress weighs changes to Medicaid. But the governors' assets do mean that national policymakers bent on altering Medicaid value the political cover and legitimacy that governors can provide. A consensus endorsement from the NGA is the biggest prize. But short of that, winning the backing of at least some governors helps. To this end, members of Congress and the White House typically try to rally governors to endorse their Medicaid proposals. They stand ready to make some concessions to these state executives to garner their support.

The importance of governors in the Medicaid policy arena at the federal level does not automatically augur well for the program's durability. Governors can be fickle allies of Medicaid, and some of them have promoted major program retrenchment efforts. But during the "ordinary" political times that marked much of the 1993–2010 period, gubernatorial lobbying tended to buttress the program. By "ordinary" I mean those times where incremental pragmatism tends to prevail. These times stand in contrast to periods when Medicaid becomes enmeshed in ideological, partisan debates. During ordinary times governors have favored preserving Medicaid as a fiscal entitlement for the states. They look for ways to increase the federal share of Medicaid costs, and they lobby to boost the federal match during economic downturns. But even during these "ordinary" times, the fiscal incentives in Medicaid have their limits. To the degree that governors believe that federal laws, regulations, and procedures handcuff them and engulf them in red tape, they become tempted to trade off the open-ended fiscal entitlement for flexibility. Their willingness to support a block grant increases, and the prospects for Medicaid's erosion grow. Hence, all else being equal, gubernatorial support for Medicaid tends to depend on the extent to which federal policymakers devolve key Medicaid decisions to the states. It hinges on whether policymakers in Washington are willing to tolerate considerable variation in the states' Medicaid efforts.

The support governors provided for Medicaid during the 1993–2010 period partly reflects their success in obtaining more flexibility. A more permissive federal stance on waivers expanded opportunities for states to reshape their programs. The processes involved in applying for HCBS waivers became increasingly routine—almost like applying for the renewal of a driver's license. Federal legislation also increased the states' options. The states gained more discretion to set provider payment rates in the wake of congressional action in 1997.[20] In the case of CHIP, they won the authority to expand coverage through Medicaid, a capped block grant, or a hybrid. So, too, the Deficit Reduction Act of 2005 increased the states' options to impose cost sharing on Medicaid enrollees. This law, as well as the ACA, also granted the states discretion to design HCBS for the elderly and people with disabilities in ways that had previously been possible only through waivers. To be sure, the governors suffered some setbacks. In the early 2000s, for instance, Congress imposed new reporting requirements to weed out eligibility and reimbursement errors along with new rules governing citizen documentation. Subsequently, a Democratic Congress required the states to follow more elaborate procedures for public notice and comment when they submitted waiver requests. But on balance, the states gained considerable flexibility.

The instrumental balancing act between state flexibility and political support from governors tends to prevail in the states during ordinary political times. But this calculus tends to fall by the wayside when proposals to reshape Medicaid become enmeshed in defining ideological struggles between the parties. During such times, the identities of governors as members of a broad partisan coalition tend to trump their more instrumental Medicaid preferences.[21] To some degree this pattern occurred in initiatives to convert Medicaid into a block grant. The support of Republican governors for this step in 1995 partly reflected frustration that they lacked discretion to shape the program. But they also got swept up in the partisan momentum generated by the decisive Republican victory in the 1994 election and the quest to foster a "devolution revolution" in the federal system. Subsequently, the George H. W. Bush administration recruited a few Republican governors to push for its version of a block grant. But this initiative did not proceed under the banner of a grand conservative vision to reshape the federal government's role. It attracted little gubernatorial support.

The process of gaining approval for the ACA also underscores the potential role of partisan ideology in shaping orientations toward Medicaid. The new law piled many new mandates on the states that markedly restricted their discretion. Yet even given the reservations the Democratic governors had about this law, they endorsed it. In turn, the vast majority of Republican governors followed congressional leaders from their party in defining the debate over the ACA as a great contest between socialistic and market-based approaches to health care. Thus most opposed the ACA and its Medicaid provisions, even though in many cases it would at limited cost bring great health care benefits to the residents of their states. In such a polarized context, the NGA had limited significance as a vehicle for representing state interests. The question looms: Will the nation's growing partisan polarization increasingly link debates over Medicaid to broad ideological concerns rather than the instrumental ones that shaped the actions of the intergovernmental lobby during most of the 1993–2010 period? If so, it would imply greater party cohesion across levels of the federal system in future Medicaid debates. The ability of the NGA to forge a common position on Medicaid among its members would further diminish; it would fade in significance as partisan organizations of governors became more important in Medicaid politics. The degree to which the intergovernmental lobby functioned as a catalyst for program growth would depend largely on which party dominated the nation's capital and elected the most governors.

Executive Action: The Contribution of Waivers

The story of catalytic federalism also revolves around the primacy of executive branch action and the use of waivers. Chapters 4 and 5 describe how the Clinton administration used this policy tool to profoundly alter the Medicaid playing field. Its willingness to throw open the doors to state initiatives via waivers of Section 1115 and Section 1915c of the Social Security Act fueled an outpouring of state efforts to reinvent Medicaid. The willingness of the Bush administration to continue the use of waivers reinforced this transformation. On balance, waivers have strengthened Medicaid. To be sure, they have undercut the program as a legal entitlement. Moreover, the Bush administration signaled its willingness to approve waivers that would erode Medicaid. But by and large, states did not seize this retrenchment opportunity. Furthermore, as noted in chapter 4, freeing the states from certain entitlement provisions may well have done more to enable the states to expand HCBS to the elderly and people with disabilities than they would have in the absence of waivers. For their part, the demonstration waivers kindled appreciable coverage expansions in many states, most dramatically in Massachusetts. The waivers also became vehicles for bottom-up vertical policy diffusion. Drawing on state experience with the 1915c waivers, Congress passed statutory revisions that made it easier for states to offer HCBS through the regular state plan process. Facilitated by a demonstration waiver, the Massachusetts plan of 2006 became the template for the ACA in 2010.

The experience with Medicaid waivers points to a need for revision of conventional thinking about American governance and policy change. Consider, for instance, the implications for presidential leadership. The separation of powers built into the US political system has long prompted leading scholars to assert that such leadership above all involves the "power of persuasion" (Neustadt 1964). This perspective portrays presidents as working to sustain their public prestige and professional reputation while deploying myriad strategies to coax Congress to approve their initiatives. More recently, however, the politics of direct presidential action—a kind of "power without persuasion"—has garnered attention. In this view presidents increasingly take unilateral action through executive orders, proclamations, directives, and other tools of the "administrative presidency." The chief executive sets policy, and his or her opponents must pay the heavy transaction costs of getting Congress or the courts to reverse it. For some observers, these direct actions "constitute the distinguishing mark of the modern presidency."[22] Scholarly proponents of this "unilateral-action" perspective have, however, paid scant attention to waivers as a presidential tool. This study demonstrates the need to remedy this omission in future assessments of presidential and executive branch leadership.

Medicaid waivers possess distinctive features as tools of presidential leadership. In comparison with executive orders, formal changes in the *Code of Federal Regulations*, or other directives (e.g., official letters from the Centers for Medicare and Medicaid Services), they tend to expedite changes that are much larger in scope. Their authorization in the Social Security Act makes them harder to challenge in court, as does the fact that they reflect an alliance between the federal government and a particular state. To be sure, presidents can turn to other executive tools to reshape Medicaid substantially. As described in chapter 3, the George W. Bush administration relied on a letter to state Medicaid directors that imposed a stringent Medicaid take-up requirement for children that would have greatly curtailed state initiatives to extend CHIP coverage to higher-income families. But unlike the experience with waivers, these moves came under fire from Congress, the GAO, and the states. The prospect loomed that the federal courts would intervene to overrule the measure. Eventually the Bush administration abandoned this initiative.

Ultimately, of course, it takes two to tango. Presidential administrations can use waivers to invite the states to dance. But the states must decide whether to accept. In the case of Medicaid, many states were willing partners, especially for waivers that expanded coverage. The Clinton administration realized many of its preferences in this way. In contrast, the Bush administration felt disappointment that the states generally did not pursue backdoor block grants or other vehicles that would thin Medicaid coverage. In this sense, waivers may well seem to deviate from other forms of unilateral action, such as executive orders, whereby a president can more explicitly provide direction. But this difference can be overdrawn. As one study of presidential executive orders and proclamations notes, "when it comes to [their] implementation, . . . the power modern presidents wield very much depends on their ability to persuade" (Howell 2003, 22). The same applies to the federal executive in its dealings with states over Medicaid waivers.

The more permissive federal stance on waivers has altered the states' policy processes. It has expanded the array of problems that state policymakers can use Medicaid to address. In essence, it has enriched the stream of Medicaid policy "solutions" (e.g., managed care, coverage expansions). Greater federal receptivity to waivers has opened new policy windows for top state officials. Governors, top administrative officials, and, at times, legislators sense more opportunity to be policy entrepreneurs in the Medicaid arena and thus to win political credit for their initiatives. In these and other ways, the waivers have served as a catalyst for action at the state level.

Waivers are in a sense a policy tool for our times. The growing partisan polarization has exacerbated the probability of legislative gridlock. By elevating the importance of executive branch action, waivers provide a flexibility and capacity for decision making in the political system that would otherwise be difficult to achieve. They permit the federal government and the states to play off against each other much more rapidly than would otherwise be the case. This intergovernmental back-and-forth helped bolster Medicaid's durability in the 1993–2010 period.

At a more basic level, making it easier for states to get waivers (especially for the demonstration projects) engendered beneficial political and policy feedback. It signaled to governors and other state policymakers that they need not exchange their fiscal entitlement for a block grant to gain more flexibility to shape Medicaid. It reinforced their political support for the program. Observers have noted how the passage of legislation can enhance a program's durability by transforming the political dynamics surrounding it. Among other things, it can expand the set of actors who sense they have a stake in the program, and it can reconfigure the values, perceptions, and beliefs of key stakeholders. The Medicaid waivers testify to how a shift in the exercise of administrative discretion without major changes in the law per se can fuel similar reinforcing feedbacks.

However, the catalytic role of waivers in fostering Medicaid's durability from 1992 to 2010 need not automatically continue in the future. During a debate with other candidates for the Republican presidential nomination in September 2011, for instance, Mitt Romney affirmed that one of his first acts as president would be to "put out an executive order granting a waiver from Obamacare to all 50 states" (Turner 2011, 1). Whatever the legal viability of such a step, it illustrates how future presidents may double down on the initiatives of the Bush administration to invite waivers that would retrench Medicaid. The catalytic role of waivers described in this book substantially rested on two underlying conditions: the absence of acute fiscal stress; and a pragmatic, rather than ideologically charged, approach to Medicaid among elected state officials. In a climate of intensified austerity and polarized ideologies, the states' policymakers may come to see waivers as a convenient tool for retrenchment. And if they do so, this policy tool will cease to fuel catalytic federalism.

A Fleeting Period of Dominant Party Governance

As important as waivers have been, they take us only so far in understanding Medicaid's policy evolution. As the ACA vividly illustrates, the capacity for catalytic federalism to play out as bottom-up vertical policy diffusion leading to a dramatic policy change requires congressional action. In this regard the story of Medicaid's durability intersects with a rare episode of unified and dominant party governance. The American political system tends to yield divided government. Such division prevailed in ten of the eighteen years from 1993 through 2010. The Democrats controlled the presidency, while the Republicans dominated both houses of Congress from 1995 through 2000. A Republican president presided while the Democrats controlled at least one house of Congress in the years 2001–2 and 2007–8. The remaining years were evenly divided between unified Democratic (1993–94, 2009–10) and Republican governance (2003–6).

Some political scientists have pointed to the potential for significant legislative breakthroughs during periods of divided government (e.g., Mayhew 1991). But this did not occur in Medicaid's case. Divided government yielded no major Medicaid retrenchment. The Republicans' success in getting Congress to approve a Medicaid block grant in 1995 foundered when President Clinton vetoed the measure. On one occasion, the passage of CHIP in 1997, Republicans and Democrats joined to augment coverage for low-income children. By the time CHIP came up for renewal in 2007–8, however, the forces of polarization dominated. President George W. Bush vetoed the initiatives of a Democratically controlled Congress to expand the program.

Prospects for major changes in Medicaid increase during times of unified party governance. Partisan polarization has enhanced the ability of congressional leaders to achieve party cohesion in votes on major policy initiatives. Nonetheless, presidents cannot be sure that members of their own party in Congress will back their proposals. Thus, the Bush administration failed to rally sufficient Republican support to approve his proposal for a Medicaid block grant in 2003. The Republicans in Congress at this point remained sensitive to the ways in which the Democrats had taken political advantage of the issue in 1995 and 1996. After winning reelection in 2004, Bush spent his political capital seeking to privatize Social Security rather than resurrecting the effort to retrench Medicaid. In contrast, unified party control under the Democrats had major implications for Medicaid. The Democrats pursued major health care reform in both the periods 1993–94 and 2009–10. The failed reform initiative under Clinton assigned Medicaid a minor role. In contrast, in 2010 the ACA resulted in the largest expansion of Medicaid since its creation in 1965. Here, a critical intervening factor beyond unified party governance deserves emphasis. In an era marked by intense polarization, the margin of party control also matters greatly, largely because it takes sixty senators to prevent the opposition from filibustering a bill to death. From 1993 to 2010 such *dominant party governance* occurred only in 2009, when the Democrats controlled sixty senate votes (with fifty-eight Democrats and two independents). This was a necessary, if not sufficient, condition for the passage of health reform.

The Enduring Relevance of the Constraining Model

In sum, the catalytic model of federalism better depicts the pattern of Medicaid's durability from 1993 through 2010 than the alternative constraining model. Medicaid drew strength from the special characteristics of its federal funding formula, from movement toward a more positive social construction of its beneficiaries, from lobbying by providers and advocates, from the support of governors as part of the intergovernmental lobby, from a greater use of waivers, and from the Democrats' ephemeral dominance of the federal government in 2009. These factors interacted in complex ways to fuel a dynamic relationship between the federal government and the states vis-à-vis Medicaid. Each level of government responded to the actions of the other in ways that frequently strengthened the program. The absence of any of these conditions would have subtracted from Medicaid's durability.

Although these factors fueled catalytic federalism, the constraining model of interstate competition maintains some explanatory relevance in at least two ways. First, though states certainly did not race to the bottom in their Medicaid effort, their pattern of variation tends to be consistent with what this model predicts. With all else being equal, the model hypothesizes that less wealthy states with more disadvantaged people will have less generous Medicaid programs (Peterson 1995). In this way these states will avoid becoming magnets for the needy. In this vein table 7.1 presents correlations between two measures of state Medicaid effort (expenditures and enrollees per poor person) and three indicators of state economic well-being (the percentage of the population living in poverty, per capita income, and total taxable resources). As a proxy for need (or problem acuity) it also relates Medicaid effort to the percentage of people without health insurance. In general, the data support the hypothesis (especially for expenditures) that less affluent states will tend to exert less Medicaid effort. They also reinforce the proposition that Medicaid effort will tend to be less in states with greater numbers of uninsured residents. These findings do not, of course, cast light on the causal underlying mechanisms.[23] The relationship between the states' incomes and poverty rates with other potential explanatory variables awaits further explication.[24] But in the absence of additional research, the explanatory relevance of the constraining model for the states' Medicaid effort should not be dismissed.

Second, the pertinence of the constraining model partly stems from its centrality to the Republicans' ideology and strategy in an era of heightened polarization and high unemployment. A key Republican tenet is that less government and lower taxation create jobs and a more vibrant economy. This perspective has prompted some governors to trumpet their faith in a model of interstate competition that rewards low taxation. When Democratic policymakers in Illinois boosted taxes in 2011, for instance, the Republican governors of Indiana, New Jersey, and Wisconsin staged media events announcing that this would make it easier for them to attract firms and jobs from Illinois. The Wisconsin governor, Scott Walker, even announced a major marketing campaign in Illinois to attract business. Meanwhile, he promised further tax cuts in Wisconsin and announced his support for a severe retrenchment of Medicaid through a block grant.[25] In a similar vein Texas governor Rick Perry, in his run for the Republican presidency in 2011, stressed that his state's success in creating new jobs stemmed from its commitment to keeping taxes

Table 7.1 Relationship between Medicaid Effort and State Wealth

Aspect of Relationship	*Medicaid Expenditures per Poor Person, 2009*	*Medicaid Enrollees per Poor Person, 2008*
Percent living in poverty (2009, 2008)	−0.54**	−0.34*
Per capita income (2009, 2008)	0.66**	0.27
Total taxable resources (2009, 2008)	0.51**	0.26
Percent uninsured (2008, 2007)	−0.51**	−0.37**

*Correlation is significant at the 0.05 level (2-tailed). ** Correlation is significant at the 0.01 level (2-tailed). Results are Pearson correlation coefficients for the fifty states.

Sources: Data on persons living in poverty are from the US Census Bureau, "Table 21: Number of Poor and Poverty Rate, by State: 1980 to 2009," www.census.gov/hhes/www/poverty/data/historical/hstpov21.xls. Data on uninsured persons are from the *Current Population Survey*, "Table HIA-4: Health Insurance Coverage Status . . . 1999 to 2009," www.census.gov/hhes/www/hlthins/data/historical/index.html. Data on per capita income are from the US Bureau of Economic Analysis, "SA1-3 Personal Income Summary," www.bea.gov. Data on total taxable resources are from the US Department of the Treasury, "TTR Estimates," www.treasury.gov/resource-center/economic-policy/taxable-resources/Pages/Total-Taxable-Resources.aspx.

low and creating a business-friendly climate. Meanwhile, Texas ranks near the bottom in Medicaid effort and in the proportion of its residents with health insurance. In these and other ways, the Republican governors have become proselytizers for the constraining model of federalism. To the degree that they can convince policy elites and the informed public of the validity of this model, they can more readily cut Medicaid and other social programs under the banner of economic development. The political pronouncements that firms will flee states with higher taxes may also become a self-fulfilling prophecy by encouraging firms to leverage more tax breaks from states in making their location decisions.

Polarization and the Debt: Will the Medicaid "Beast" Be Starved?

Whether the dynamics of catalytic federalism that bolstered Medicaid from 1993 through 2010 can be sustained is highly uncertain. The Supreme Court's anticipated ruling in 2012 could vitiate these dynamics. Beyond this possibility, trends with respect to the federal debt and health care prices matter greatly for Medicaid's future. Since the last time the federal budget was balanced in 2001, the federal debt had mushroomed from 33 to 62 percent of the GDP (National Commission on Fiscal Responsibility and Reform 2010, 10). The sea of red ink seemed destined to grow. The CBO (2011, 3, 6) offered two scenarios. One "extended-baseline" version assumed no changes in current law; it projected that the debt as a percentage of the GDP would be 74 percent in 2030 and 84 percent in 2040. But this version assumed that Congress and the president would do such politically unpalatable things as letting the Bush tax cuts expire at the end of 2012. Hence, the CBO also provided a less optimistic alternative scenario that took into account "several changes to current law that were widely expected to occur."[26] Under this scenario the debt would explode to 146 percent of GDP in 2030 and 233 percent in 2040. No one knew for sure what percentage would trigger a debt crisis that would wreak havoc on the economy. But virtually everyone agreed that the debt needed to be well below these projections for the US economy to prosper.

Medicaid and Medicare figured prominently in the considerations of those seeking ways to significantly reduce the nation's debt. The two entitlement programs made up 21 percent of federal spending (excluding interest on the debt) in 2010, and they were projected to grow to 31 percent by 2020 (Debt Reduction Task Force 2010, 44). The growing numbers of baby boomers reaching retirement age would fuel the demands on these programs. Of even greater importance, the tendency for health care prices to rise more rapidly than the general inflation rate threatened their viability. From 1993 to 2010 the Consumer Price Index rose by an annual average of 3 percent while its health care component increased by 5.5 percent.[27]

How these fiscal pressures will play out for Medicaid remains unclear. If policymakers can work in a bipartisan way to raise revenues and cut programs, Medicaid could conceivably emerge relatively unscathed during the next decade. Consider, for instance, a proposal emanating from the bipartisan National Commission on Fiscal Responsibility and Reform, which was established by President Obama in early 2010 and cochaired by Erskine Bowles (White House chief of staff during the Clinton administration) and Alan Simpson (a former Republican senator from Wyoming). The commission's eighteen members included twelve members of Congress, equally divided between Republicans and Democrats. Ultimately, the commission failed to achieve the fourteen votes it needed to endorse an official blueprint for debt reduction. But in late 2010 it did release a document, *The Moment of Truth*, that was supported by eleven members.

Whereas *The Moment of Truth* called for the lion's share of debt reduction to be achieved through federal budget cuts rather than revenue enhancements, it proposed modest changes to Medicaid. The Bowles-Simpson Commission preserved the ACA while endorsing four steps to achieve Medicaid savings of $58 billion through 2020 (see table C.1 in appendix C). First, it recommended the elimination of certain federal reimbursement practices that the states had exploited to inflate the federal government's share of Medicaid costs.[28] Second, it endorsed placing the dual eligibles—again, those elderly and people with disabilities who simultaneously enroll in Medicare and Medicaid—in managed care plans. Although Medicaid had made great strides in enrolling more beneficiaries in managed care during the 1990s and 2000s, the elderly and people with disabilities largely remained outside these plans. Third, the commission recommended that the federal government achieve certain administrative savings. And fourth, it backed an expedited waiver process for well-qualified states that wanted to pursue cost containment and quality enhancement. More generally, the commission endorsed a global budget target for all federal health care spending (including Medicaid) that held growth in such outlays to the percentage increase in the GDP plus 1 percent. But it proposed no mechanism to enforce this cap (National Commission on Fiscal Responsibility and Reform 2010, 39–41).

Bipartisan initiatives that seek to achieve debt reduction need not, of course, do as much as Bowles-Simpson did to spare Medicaid. Under great pressure to reduce the debt, the Democrats might agree to a significant restructuring of and cuts in Medicaid. A proposal from the Bipartisan Policy Center, which attracted considerable media attention, illustrates how this might occur. With private funding, four former Senate majority leaders—two Republicans and two Democrats—created this think tank in 2007 to engage stakeholders in the "art of principled compromise."[29] In 2010 it sponsored a Debt Reduction Task Force cochaired by former senator Pete Domenici (R-NM) and the economist Alice Rivlin, who had served in key federal fiscal positions (including director of the Office of Management and Budget under President Clinton). The task force soon released a report called *Restoring America's Future*. Unlike Bowles-Simpson, this proposal espoused major steps to restructure and retrench Medicaid (for the details, see table C.1 in appendix C). It endorsed doing away with the federal matching formula that had been such a catalytic force for Medicaid's expansion. Instead, the task force recommended that a process be set in place "to determine the optimal allocation of program responsibilities" between the two levels of government." This sorting-out process was to be budget neutral and to "divide up responsibility" between the federal government and the states for "fully financing different components of the Medicaid program." By making each level of government "fully responsible for the future growth of the components under its direct control," each would presumably have more incentives for cost containment and the growth of Medicaid spending would slow. Through these steps, the Domenici-Rivlin Task Force estimated that Medicaid savings would total $202 billion from 2012 through 2025, considerably more than that sought by Bowles-Simpson (Debt Reduction Task Force 2010, 60, 64).

It is not surprising that in a time of intense, asymmetrical partisan polarization, both the Bowles-Simpson and the Domenici-Rivlin proposals failed to win much support among federal policymakers. However, if one party were to gain control of the federal government, the need would lessen to achieve a bipartisan compromise on how to reshape Medicaid. The partisan outcome of future elections thereby constitutes another important factor shaping the future of Medicaid's durability. If the Republicans were to regain control of the presidency and Congress, they would be unlikely to squander the opportunity to retrench Medicaid. Escalating concern about the federal debt could well give them the opportunity to downsize the program appreciably, even without a filibuster-proof majority in the Senate.

In the year following the 2010 elections, the Republican leaders pulled no punches about their desire to significantly retrench Medicaid. The major Republican candidates for president, including Mitt Romney, endorsed converting the program to a block grant. The top Republicans in Congress also backed major Medicaid cuts. By far the most dramatic retrenchment plan came from Representative Paul Ryan (R-WI), whom many Republican elites touted as one of their intellectual leaders and who chaired the House Budget Committee. A more detailed sketch of the Ryan plan appears in table C.1 in appendix C. For present purposes, suffice it to note that Ryan sought to repeal the ACA and turn Medicaid into a block grant starting in 2013. The grant would grow each year to reflect hikes in the Consumer Price Index and population growth.[30] This meant that federal allocations would not keep up with more rapidly rising health care prices. The proposal gave states vast new flexibility to shape the specifics of their Medicaid programs. It slashed expenditures on Medicaid by $771 billion through 2022—many times the reductions embedded in the Bowles-Simpson or the Domenici-Rivlin proposals. An analysis performed for the Kaiser Commission on Medicaid and the Uninsured concluded that the Ryan plan would precipitate severe declines in Medicaid enrollment and "dramatic increases in the number of uninsured" (Holahan et al. 2011, 13).

The budget resolution containing the Ryan plan passed the House of Representatives on a party-line vote, with nearly all Republicans supporting it. Although the resolution met defeat in the Senate, it captured all but five Republican votes in that body (Steinhauer 2011). (Not a single Democrat in the House or Senate voted for the Ryan proposal.) To assuage concerns that the proposal might have harmful health outcomes, claims began to surface from those affiliated with conservative think tanks that "Medicaid is worse than no coverage at all."[31] At its core, the Ryan plan reflected the long-standing Republican bet that a starve-the-beast strategy could massively shrink the federal government. During recent decades this strategy had featured a one-two punch: One, cut taxes with little regard for the impact of such action on the deficit—a practice particularly evident during the George W. Bush years. Two, rigidly insist that belated efforts to bring down the deficit could succeed only through spending cuts with no revenue increases.

Ryan and the House Republicans showed no signs of softening their call for Medicaid cuts when they passed a subsequent budget resolution early in 2012. This resolution essentially parroted the contents of the prior year's proposal (US House Committee on the Budget 2012). It remains an open question whether the Ryan plan will be the template for Medicaid restructuring if the Republicans gain control of the presidency and Congress in 2012. Thus, much depends on developments with respect to another pivotal factor shaping the future of Medicaid's durability: the stance of the Republican governors. If many of these governors see themselves as part of a grand ideological venture to slash government at all levels, they may well join their partisan colleagues in Congress and the White House in support of major Medicaid retrenchment. But if they sustain some sense of the pragmatic, incremental approach to the program that they have frequently exhibited in the past, they may well temper Medicaid cuts. As much as many governors complain about Medicaid, its revenue stream has become a big part of their budgets. Certainly, reductions of the magnitude proposed by Representative Ryan would put these governors in a stressful political position. A majority of the public opposes major cuts to the program, and it provides indispensable services to many middle-class constituents (Altman 2011). Some signs of caution about Medicaid surfaced among the Republican governors, even as their counterparts at the national level championed major retrenchment. A report with thirty-one Medicaid "solutions" that the Republican Governors Association submitted to Congress in late August 2011 did not specifically endorse the Ryan plan. Though allowing that a "block grant" might be appropriate, the report did not criticize Medicaid as a fiscal entitlement for the states.[32]

As America moved closer to the 2012 presidential election, Medicaid found temporary refuge in partisan gridlock. By late July 2011 the Republican budget strategy boiled down to an unprecedented threat not to raise the nation's debt ceiling unless the Obama administration and Senate Democrats agreed to make severe budget cuts with no tax increases. Last-minute bargaining averted a debt crisis and led to passage of the Budget Control Act of 2011. This law established a Joint Select Committee consisting of six Democrats and six Republicans equally divided between members of the House and Senate. The bill charged this "supercommittee" with devising a proposal that would slash spending by $1.5 trillion between 2012 and 2021. If a majority of the committee could not reach an agreement that Congress and the president would approve, automatic cuts ("sequestration") amounting to $1.2 trillion would occur over ten years.[33] Of central importance to Medicaid, the Democratic lawmakers succeeded in making sure that the Budget Control Act exempted the program from sequestration. Subsequent negotiations found both the Republicans and Democrats on the supercommittee envisioning cuts to Medicaid as a significant part of a "grand bargain" over debt reduction. But the forces of partisan polarization prevailed, and the committee failed to produce a proposal. The resulting sequestration process set the stage for a new round of budget politics. At least over the short term, partisan gridlock shielded Medicaid from retrenchment.

Medicaid and Health Reform: What Is to Be Done?

The preservation and enhancement of Medicaid is hardly an end in itself. One can easily imagine a health insurance system that achieves universal coverage and reasonable standards of access, quality, and cost containment without Medicaid.

Perhaps, at some point in the future, a policy window will open for this option. At present, however, proponents of universal coverage have made Medicaid central to their efforts. Hence, the question naturally rises: What should be done to sustain and enhance Medicaid? In this vein I offer three general recommendations.

First, illuminate and challenge common austerity principles when analysts and stakeholders apply them to Medicaid. Pundits, policy analysts, and groups committed to bipartisan solutions for reducing the federal debt have at times offered general austerity principles to guide their efforts. Two in particular deserve note in the context of Medicaid. One austerity principle is "shared sacrifice"—that the "hurt" of cuts "should be spread widely and fairly" (Brooks 2011). This contention naturally links to countless political claims that *all* the major federal entitlement programs must undergo significant retrenchment—not only to significantly reduce the debt but also to fight waste and price escalation in the medical sector. In considering the sacrifice to impose on Medicaid, however, certain caveats appropriately command attention. Thanks in part to its low provider payment rates and embrace of managed care, Medicaid has done better than other components of the health insurance system in constraining cost escalation. Program spending per enrollee has, for instance, risen more slowly than premiums for employer-sponsored health insurance (Holahan et al. 2011, 2). Nor, as noted above, can one blame Medicaid for the rising costs of Medicare and private insurance plans. Limited cost shifting has occurred as a result of Medicaid's lower reimbursement rates.

Policymakers can probably wring some savings out of Medicaid under the banner of pursuing efficiency. Efforts to fight fraud and abuse may well yield some benefits. So, too, initiatives to place all Medicaid enrollees, including the elderly and people with disabilities, in capitated managed care may prove cost-effective. (The managed care organizations will, however, need to build their capacity far beyond current levels to achieve this end.) Although these and other measures could yield some savings without major damage to Medicaid, proposals to impose proportionately equal cuts in Medicaid relative to the other pillars of American's health insurance system would surely vitiate the health benefits for society's most vulnerable population. At the end of the day the fact remains: Medicaid is on the whole a bare-bones program for people who live on the economic margin. The options available for cutting costs in Medicare and employer health insurance plans frequently do not exist for Medicaid. Perhaps, for instance, the affluent can pay more for Medicare through higher premiums or other means. But cost sharing for the poor will most likely prompt them to become uninsured or otherwise forgo needed care.

The second austerity principle that has received some attention from analysts is to "trim from the old to invest in the young" (Brooks 2011). In this vein the economist C. Eugene Steuerle (2010, 876, 878) has cautioned that the federal budget promotes "fiscal sclerosis" through its excessive commitment to consumption for the elderly at the expense of investments in children, education, and work supports.[34] If one accepts this principle—and some experts do not—the wisdom of shrinking Medicaid becomes all the more suspect.[35] About half of all Medicaid beneficiaries are children, and another quarter are adults, most of whom work. Implementation of the ACA will increase the proportion of adult beneficiaries still further. To be sure, only one of every three Medicaid dollars provides services to this younger cohort of beneficiaries. Taking this into account, the program might seem ripe for retrenchment under the second austerity principle. But the single most expensive Medicaid cohort is not the elderly but people under the age of sixty-five years with disabilities. This group alone accounts for from 40 to 45 percent of Medicaid expenditures. Many of the most costly of these enrollees were born with acute intellectual or other developmental disabilities. The second austerity principle fits uneasily with this fact. The moral arguments concerning society's obligation to help younger people with disabilities differ sharply from those concerning the elderly at advanced stages of life. They engage not just liberals, who naturally assign a broad role to government in helping society's least fortunate, but also social conservatives, who place a premium on eliminating abortions and assuring the right to life. In the case of adults with disabilities, Medicaid at times provides support that enables these individuals to work and remain active in the community.

Finally, austerity principles need to be placed against the backdrop of the tax effort. The United States ranks last among the major industrial democracies in total government revenues as a share of the national economy (i.e., GDP).[36] Austerity partly reflects the multiple forces that make it so politically difficult to raise government revenues even incrementally. Pressures to cut and thin health insurance would be evident in the absence of the antitax movement due to rising health care prices, the aging of the population, and other factors. But the sense of scarcity would be considerably less. The Bowles-Simpson plan exemplifies an approach that takes serious strides toward reducing the federal debt without imposing major sacrifices on Medicaid or a crushing tax burden on Americans.

My second general recommendation focuses on the balance between national purpose and state discretion: *Stakeholders should be alert to the instrumental and political benefits of sustaining and at times enhancing the fifty states' flexibility over Medicaid.* As this book has delineated, federal policymakers at times seek to impose their preferences on Medicaid through mandates or other directives that reduce the states' discretion. These mandates at times do much to meet health care needs. For instance, the mandates entitling all poor children to Medicaid have bolstered their access to health care in several states, including populous ones such as Texas. Had not the Supreme Court intervened, the ACA's requirement that Medicaid cover all those living below 133 percent of the poverty line would have enhanced health services for many uninsured adults. Viewed more broadly, federal mandates can mute the constraining forces of competitive federalism. They can take certain forms of retrenchment off the table as states compete for firms and the affluent. They can give credence to the view that Americans as members of a national community have certain basic standards of social justice that must be met.

But mandates and restrictions on the states' discretion also have a downside. They at times make it impossible for the most innovative and progressive states to pursue more cost-effective approaches to Medicaid. Administrative rules at times increase transaction costs for state officials to the point where they represent the triumph of process over purpose. Beyond policy substance, mandates can undermine political support for Medicaid, especially among the states' governors.[37] Although federal policymakers may prevail over the intergovernmental lobby, actions that kindle broad opposition from the governors bode poorly for Medicaid's durability over the longer term. They incline the governors to be more receptive to the periodic calls to retrench Medicaid in exchange for flexibility.

A case exists that the ACA in its interim measures departed too sharply from the devolutionary spirit that had animated Medicaid policy from 1993 to 2010. Consider, for instance, the ACA's requirement that the states maintain their eligibility criteria for all cohorts of Medicaid beneficiaries until at least 2014. This mandate came at a time when the global financial and economic crisis of 2008–9 had left many state governments struggling to balance their budgets. Moreover, it occurred when federal policymakers had declined to extend the enhanced match rate embedded in the Obama stimulus bill. So it was little wonder that even in a polarized age, Republican and Democratic governors found common ground. The NGA sent a letter to Congress in January 2011 urging repeal of the ACA's maintenance-of-effort provisions.[38]

These provisions have proven particularly galling for many governors in light of other forces working to constrain the states' discretion with respect to provider payments. In mid-2011 the Obama administration proposed an administrative rule that would place a greater burden of proof on states to show that their payment levels afford enrollees adequate access to care.[39] The proposal sparked sharp complaints from Medicaid directors in states with both Democratic and Republican governors. One complained that the Obama administration had gone "overboard" and another termed the proposal a "power grab" (Pear 2011c). Clearly, penurious provider payments significantly undermine the value of Medicaid coverage in many states. They damage service to the least fortunate. But unless the federal government can boost its share of Medicaid costs in hard economic times, shutting one door after another to the states' cost savings will significantly strain intergovernmental relationships at a time when the program needs all the political support it can muster. Moreover, the federal government may go too far in essentially compelling states to invest in Medicaid relative to other important functions, such as education.[40]

In striving for a balance between federal direction and state flexibility, waivers can play a critical role. This study has shown that waivers are valuable as a tool not only for galvanizing policy innovation and accommodating diverse preferences but also for engendering political support. To its credit, the ACA incorporates new waiver authority. The law establishes the Center for Medicare and Medicaid Innovation and provides significant new funding to evaluate various delivery system and payment models designed to contain costs while preserving and enhancing quality. In 2017 states can apply for waivers that allow them to sponsor major alternatives to the ACA so long as these demonstrations sustain coverage and benefit levels and do not increase the federal deficit. Congress would be well advised to move this date up so that states may seek these waivers before that time. In this regard, senators Ron Wyden (D-OR) and Scott Brown (R-MA), with the endorsement of President Obama, have proposed legislation that would advance the date for these waivers to 2014.[41]

To note the benefits of state flexibility is not to gainsay that the Supreme Court's 2012 decision may well have gone too far in restricting the use of mandates to extend Medicaid coverage. To be sure, the seven justices who supported this part of the ruling declared that the restriction would not have applied to more incremental Medicaid mandates enacted in the past, such as those requiring states to cover pregnant women and poor children (US Supreme Court 2012b, 55). But the ruling clearly undercuts the ability of Congress to launch dramatic expansions in insurance coverage via Medicaid mandates in the future. Even with a generous federal subsidy, for instance, it is unlikely that a law requiring states to cover all persons up to 300 percent of the poverty line could withstand a court challenge.

My third recommendation takes advantage of the work of others: *Stakeholders should be vigilant in monitoring for political opportunities to draw on the vast reservoir of good ideas about how to improve Medicaid.* There is no shortage of thoughtful recommendations for making Medicaid better (e.g., Sparer 2009). Analysts have pointed to an array of reform foci. Some have stressed improving the Medicaid funding formula so that it better targets those states with the greatest need for assistance and responds automatically and rapidly to states' conditions during economic slumps.[42] Others have zeroed in on ways to improve the coordination of medical and long-term care for dual eligibles enrolled in both Medicare and Medicaid—a cohort that tends to have the most acute and costly health problems.[43] (To this end, the ACA created a new Federal Coordinated Health Care Office.) Yet others have suggested ways to speed up the rebalancing of Medicaid long-term care away from institutions and toward HCBS (e.g., Smith et al. 2005). Various proposals also seek to enhance and calibrate Medicaid provider payments to foster greater cost-effectiveness while also promoting more aggressive outreach for prenatal care to reduce inpatient hospital admissions (e.g., Grannemann and Pauly 2010, 80–101, 250–68). So, too, chapter 3 has highlighted steps to streamline enrollment and retention procedures to bolster take-up. Progress in enacting this spectrum of reforms would do much to enhance Medicaid. But this progress will depend on keeping these Medicaid "solutions" afloat in the policy stream. It will depend on seizing the time to enact these reforms when political circumstances open a policy or administrative window.

Conclusion

Not long ago, a colleague only half facetiously remarked that the study of American politics had replaced economics as the new "dismal science."[44] Clearly, there is cause for concern about the health of American governance. Well-functioning democracies possess an array of attributes. One of them is an ability to aggregate interests effectively—to forge coherent, theoretically plausible policy that establishes priorities among competing demands and, when necessary, imposes losses on certain groups to promote the general good. In the absence of this quality, governments run the risk of being "overwhelmed and bankrupted" (Weaver and Rockman 1993, 10). The growing partisan polarization in the United States and the roughly even division of voters among the two parties has vitiated the federal government's capacity to meet this standard. Rather than moderate their positions in an appeal to the median voter, Republican members of Congress increasingly seek to head off primary opposition by accommodating the politically engaged members of their party who tend to be very conservative.[45]

To be sure, polarization has an upside. It presents voters with clear choices at election time. It motivates a greater proportion of the electorate to become politically engaged. But when melded with the fragmented, anti-majoritarian institutions of American governance, productive policy compromise becomes much more difficult. As political scientist Paul Abramowitz (2010, 168) has observed: "Politically engaged partisans believe, in all sincerity, that those on the other side are wrong, if not immoral, and that therefore the solution to partisan gridlock is for those on the other side to simply surrender." For those who support a positive role for government in the health arena, polarization has an additional downside. The intense partisan discord in Congress lowers public approval ratings for this body, which in turn further saps trust in government and support for redistributive health programs (Hetherington and Rudolph 2008, 504, 507).

The prevailing pattern of polarization bodes poorly for the federal government's ability to cope sensibly with two major problems that will shape Medicaid durability—growing public debt and the escalation of health care prices. To be sure, the ACA tried to address or at least not add to either problem. The CBO scored the new law as budget neutral. The ACA also introduced an array of sensible provisions designed to bend the cost curve. Whether these measures or related developments succeed has major implications for Medicaid even if other debt reduction initiatives leave the program relatively unscathed. If health care prices continue to mount more rapidly than the general inflation rate, the prospects for Medicaid erosion become almost certain.

The current political pattern is not, of course, set in concrete. Perhaps one of the two parties will gain control of the presidency and Congress for sufficient time to enact or preserve its health policy agenda without the need for significant compromise. Or perhaps leaders of both political parties will rise to the occasion and forge constructive bipartisan compromises in spite of the ideological gulf that divides them. So too, Republicans may pull back from a vision that severely reduces the federal government's role in assuring access to health care, especially for society's least fortunate.[46] This vision calls for driving the United States much further down the road toward inequality in health care benefits, with market forces increasingly rationing services to lower-income citizens and many in the middle class. It would introduce cost sharing and other market mechanisms, hoping that they would miraculously weed out wasteful and inappropriate care while preserving access to quality services.[47] Is this vision sustainable politically? Or will Republicans over time acquire a renewed appreciation for the pragmatic approaches to coverage expansions embraced, for instance, by many of the party's governors in the 1990s and 2000s? I obviously have no crystal ball to predict this. But, as befits democracy, the ballot box will matter. Upcoming elections may well be the most important for the future of America's health insurance system since 1964, when Lyndon Johnson's landslide victory led to the birth of Medicaid and Medicare.

Notes

1. Providers persuaded some courts that a law (Title 42, Section 1983, of the US Code) that was passed after the Civil War to protect the federal rights of those living in former Confederate states also applied to institutional payments under Medicaid. This statute created liability for anyone who, acting on behalf of state government, infringed upon the federally guaranteed rights of Medicaid stakeholders.

2. See Grannemann and Pauly (2010, 221); they further elaborate that in the burden-shifting model "the hospital maximizes profit in the private market but takes the prices set in the public sector and then adjusts quality to break even."

3. In this vein, Jha, Arav, and Epstein (2011) found that the "worst" hospitals (based on a set of process measures) tend to have disproportionate numbers of Medicaid enrollees.

4. States have launched many initiatives to monitor and enhance the quality of services provided by Medicaid managed care organizations. For instance, sixteen states require them to undergo accreditation by independent groups committed to fostering high standards of access and care (Gifford et al. 2011, 33–42). Research suggests that some managed care organizations with Medicaid enrollees—especially provider-sponsored plans rather than the large commercial companies—have performed well on quality and consumer experience measures (McCue and Bailit 2011, 5).

5. See Thompson and Burke (2009, 29) and table 4.2 in the present volume.

6. These data come from Rosenbaum et al. (2010, 3,7) and the National Association of Community Health Centers (2009, figure 2.3).

7. For instance, research by Rothkopf et al. (2011, 1338) found that Medicaid enrollees receiving care from community health centers were less likely to have preventable hospital admissions and ninety-day hospital readmissions than beneficiaries who obtained care from private providers.

8. Kenyon (1996, 255) attributes this metaphor to John Shannon.

9. See Bailey and Rom (2004), who focused on state Medicaid costs per capita (excluding the federal match) in constant dollars adjusted for state-level differences in the cost of living from 1975 through 1998. They found no erosion in the case of two other measures of Medicaid generosity—recipients per poor person and annual average expenditures per recipient.

10. Brown and Sparer (2001) have also used the term "catalytic model" to capture how federal and state governments in the United States play off of one another to expand coverage. It deserves emphasis here that the catalytic model implies growth. A theory of a race to the bottom could conceivably be portrayed as catalytic retrenchment as states lower benefits in response to each other. For present analytic purposes, I treat this as a separate constraining model.

11. For an assessment of other circumstances that abet government growth under federalism, see Obinger, Leibried, and Castles (2005) and Sorens (2011). For instance, the latter contends that federal systems with fewer states or provinces mute the downward pressure of competition to keep taxes low. Lower numbers means fewer competitors in the "federalism market."

12. Various analysts have recommended this kind of automatic adjustment in the Medicaid formula. See, e.g., Thompson (1987, 98) and Grannemann and Pauly (2009, 42).

13. Schneider and Ingram (1993, 334); this paragraph generally draws on the insights of their article.

14. The ACA made all adults living at up to 133 percent of the poverty line eligible for Medicaid coverage. But this group has not enjoyed as positive a social construction as children, the elderly, and people with disabilities.

15. For an overview, see Williamson, Skocpol, and Coggin (2011, 32).

16. Gusmano and Thompson (2012) provide an overview of Medicaid DSH.

17. AARP departed from this pattern when it aggressively supported legislation in 2003 that expanded Medicare coverage for prescription drugs (Brandon and Alt 2008, 390).

18. This conclusion stems primarily from interviews in Florida, Minnesota, and Texas.

19. See Oberlander (2003, 148); he found substantial support for state-centered theories in his analysis of Medicare politics. For a more general perspective on the "autonomy of the state," see Nordlinger (1981).

20. The Balanced Budget Act of 1997 repealed the Boren Amendment, which had been the provenance for provider suits in federal court; see note 1.

21. For a discussion of this phenomenon in a cross-national context, see Rodden (2006, 119–39).

22. See Howell (2003,175, and generally). The concept of the administrative presidency comes from Nathan (1981).

23. Causal inference is particularly problematic in interpreting the relationship between Medicaid effort and the percentage of uninsured residents. Though I lag the measures of Medicaid effort by one year relative to the data point for the uninsured, I cannot confidently judge the degree to which states lower their Medicaid effort in response to concerns about being swamped with applicants.

24. It deserves note that the two measures of state Medicaid effort do not correlate significantly with the percentage of a state's population that is either black or Hispanic. Focusing on redistributive spending more generally, Peterson (1995) finds certain political variables significant in explaining state variation. His findings on state wealth are generally consistent with those discussed here.

25. This description of the governors' actions draws from Bauer (2011), Gibson (2011), *Huffington Post Chicago* (2011), and Walker (2011).

26. These changes included extension of the Bush tax cuts, relief from the alternative minimum tax, and increases in discretionary spending that matched the growth rate of the GDP.

27. For medical care, see http://data.bls.gov/pdq/querytool.jsp?survey+cu-CUUR0000SAM; and for all items, see http://data.bls.gov/pdq/querytool.jsp?survey+cu-CUUS0000SAO.

28. For an overview of state practices, see Gusmano and Thompson (2012).

29. The four former senators were Howard Baker (R-TN), Tom Daschle (D-SD), Robert Dole (R-KS), and George Mitchell (D-ME).

30. More specifically, the plan based the adjustment on changes in the Consumer Price Index–Urban, a measure of inflation in metropolitan areas.

31. See Scott Gottlieb (2011), who is an affiliated researcher with the American Enterprise Institute. Gottlieb cherry-picked a few studies dealing with major medical procedures to support this claim, but he ignored other studies that pointed to Medicaid's positive health effects. For a critique of his perspective, see Frakt et al. (2011).

32. See Republican Governors Policy Committee (2011, esp. 8).

33. The Budget Control Act required both houses of Congress to have an up-or-down majority vote without amendments on the proposal emerging from the supercommittee.

34. In addition to economists, analysts from other academic disciplines have supported this view. See, e.g., Callahan and Nuland (2011).

35. See, e.g., Henry Aaron (2010); he notes that the United States tends to have less generous programs for the elderly than many European countries.

36. These 2008 data come from the Organization for Economic Cooperation and Development. See Center for Budget and Policy Priorities (2011).

37. In contrast leaders of state Medicaid agencies at times support the mandates out of commitment to their programs and a sense of how mandates enhance their leverage in the budget process (see, e.g., Posner 1998, 79, 83–84, 137).

38. The letter was signed by the NGA's chair, Governor Chris Gregoire (D-WA), and its vice chair, Dave Heineman (R-NE) (Everstine 2011).

39. Under the Obama administration the Justice Department had earlier shown some sensitivity to state concerns on this front. It sided with the states in their appeal to the Supreme Court that providers cannot sue them in federal court over reimbursement rates (Pear 2011a).

40. E.g., Peter Orszag (2010) argues that Medicaid spending has helped fuel a steady decline in state support for higher education.

41. See Starr (2011, 256). Senator Wyden had tried to insert a provision in the ACA that would have permitted states to apply for comprehensive demonstration waivers as early as 2014. But the CBO resisted this provision on the grounds that it would be difficult to score. In essence, pressures on Congress to win a favorable cost estimate for the ACA prompted them to delay the date for the waiver applications (McDonough 2011, 45).

42. See especially Grannemann and Pauly (2010) and Smith et al. (2005).

43. See Smith et al. (2005) and Birnbaum and Halper (2009).

44. My thanks to Bert Rockman for permitting me to quote him.

45. For documentation of this development, see especially Abramowitz (2010, 104, 141–42).

46. This vision features the boldest attack on America's health insurance regime in half a century. It calls for repeal of the ACA, major retrenchment of Medicaid, and a thinning of Medicare benefits under a premium support program that would massively shift costs to health care beneficiaries. The CBO (2011, 21) estimated that by 2030 a typical sixty-five-

year-old would pay well over twice as much for the private insurance as he or she would spend for Medicare.

47. There is good reason to be skeptical that this approach would increase the cost-effectiveness of the health care system. As David Mechanic (2006, 46) observes, cost sharing "is a very crude barrier to care that filters out both trivial and useful care. People don't necessarily know when they could benefit from treatment. . . . This deficiency is most likely to be experienced by persons with less education and income, who have more illness but less health knowledge and sophistication."

Appendix A
Medicaid Expenditures

Table A.1 Medicaid Expenditures, 1992–2008

Year	*Billions of Dollars*	*% Change*	*Billions of Constant 2008 Dollars*	*% Change*	*2008 Dollars per Person Living in Poverty*	*% Change*
1992	115.6		176.8		4,651	
1993	128.2	10.92	191.0	8.02	4,864	4.58
1994	138.0	7.68	200.2	4.79	5,259	8.11
1995	152.2	10.23	214.5	7.19	5,890	12.00
1996	155.7	2.30	213.3	–0.60	5,838	–0.89
1997	161.5	3.78	216.5	1.50	6,085	4.23
1998	169.6	5.01	223.9	3.45	6,495	6.74
1999	182.1	7.36	234.9	4.92	7,165	10.31
2000	198.6	9.06	248.3	5.68	7,862	9.73
2001	220.0	10.74	268.3	8.08	8,155	3.72
2002	249.6	13.47	299.5	11.61	8,664	6.24
2003	267.2	7.07	312.7	4.40	8,719	0.64
2004	288.5	7.95	328.9	5.18	8,879	1.83
2005	305.4	5.88	336.0	2.16	9,093	2.41
2006	304.8	–0.20	326.2	–2.92	8,946	–1.62
2007	319.7	4.87	332.5	1.93	8,919	–0.30
2008	338.8	5.98	338.8	1.90	8,506	–4.63

Note: Expenditures include services plus Disproportionate Hospital Share payments.

Sources: Expenditure data are from the Kaiser Commission on Medicaid and the Uninsured and Urban Institute analysis of HCFA/CMS-64 data, 1992–2006. Data for 2007 and 2008 are from www.statehealthfacts.org/comparemaptable.jsp?ind=177&cat=4. The inflation adjustment is based on the Bureau of Labor Statistics' consumer price index calculator, www.bls.gov/data/inflation_calculator.htm. Data on persons living in poverty are from the US Census Bureau, www.census.gov/hhes/www/poverty/data/historical/hstpov2.xls.

Table A.2 Medicaid Expenditures Adjusting for Medical Care Price Increases, 1992–2008

Year	*Billions of Constant 2008 Dollars*	*% Change*	*2008 Dollars per Person Living in Poverty*	*% Change*
1992	220.7		5,807	
1993	232.0	5.11	5,909	1.76
1994	237.4	2.33	6,238	5.57
1995	251.1	5.75	6,893	10.49
1996	247.5	-1.42	6,775	-1.70
1997	250.4	1.17	7,038	3.88
1998	254.5	1.63	7,381	4.86
1999	264.1	3.78	8,053	9.11
2000	278.1	5.30	8,805	9.34
2001	292.5	5.20	8,890	0.96
2002	317.0	8.35	9,169	3.14
2003	326.0	2.86	9,092	-0.84
2004	337.5	3.53	9,113	0.23
2005	345.2	2.26	9,341	2.51
2006	329.2	-4.62	9,030	-3.33
2007	332.5	-0.99	8,919	1.22
2008	338.8	1.90	8,506	-4.63

Note: Expenditures include services plus Disproportionate Hospital Share payments.

Sources: Expenditure data from the Kaiser Commission on Medicaid and the Uninsured and Urban Institute analysis of HCFA/CMS-64 data, 1992–2006. Data for 2007 and 2008 are from www.statehealthfacts.org/comparemaptable.jsp?ind=177&cat=4. Medical care inflation adjustment data are based on the Bureau of Labor Statistics' series CUUR0000SAM. Data on persons living in poverty are from the US Census Bureau, www.census.gov/hhes/www/poverty/data/historical/hstpov2.xls.

Appendix B
Medicaid Enrollees

Table B.1 Total Medicaid Enrollees and Enrollees Relative to Persons in Poverty, the Fifty States and District of Columbia, 1992–2008

Year	*Number*	*% Change*	*Enrollees per Person Living in Poverty*	*% Change*
1992	35,754,420		0.941	
1993	38,808,182	8.54	0.988	5.08
1994	40,787,817	5.10	1.072	8.43
1995	41,677,036	2.18	1.144	6.76
1996	41,294,880	-0.92	1.130	-1.20
1997	40,590,776	-1.71	1.141	0.93
1998	40,380,879	-0.52	1.171	2.65
1999	Not available			
2000	44,279,100	9.65	1.402	19.71
2001	47,060,700	6.28	1.430	2.00
2002	51,419,500	9.26	1.487	4.01
2003	55,071,200	7.10	1.536	3.25
2004	57,586,800	4.57	1.555	1.24
2005	58,929,900	2.33	1.595	2.58
2006	58,714,800	-0.37	1.610	0.97
2007	58,106,000	-1.04	1.559	-3.20
2008	59,468,700	2.35	1.493	-4.22

Sources: Data for 1992–98 are Urban Institute estimates based on data from HCFA-2082 reports. Data for 2000–2008 are Urban Institute estimates based on data from the Medicaid Statistical Information System. Data on persons living in poverty are from the US Census Bureau, www.census.gov/hhes/www/poverty/data/historical/hstpov2.xls.

Appendix C
Medicaid Provisions of Key Debt-Reduction Plans

Table C.1 Medicaid Provisions of Key Debt-Reduction Plans

Plan	*Savings and Debt-Reduction Estimates*	*Main Medicaid Provisions*
Bowles-Simpson National Commission on Fiscal Responsibility and Reform	Debt reduced to 60 percent of GDP by 2023 and 40 percent by 2035 Estimated savings achieved in Medicaid through 2020: $58 billion Debt reduction targets federal revenues and expenditures at 21 percent of GDP	Eliminate state gaming of the Medicaid formula that informally increases the federal match Place dual eligibles in Medicaid managed care Reduce Medicaid administrative costs Expedite waivers in well-qualified states to provide new flexibility to control costs and improve quality Related: Establish a global budget target for all federal spending on health care (including Medicaid) that limits growth to the percentage increase in the GDP plus 1 percent; require president and Congress to make recommendations whenever average cost growth exceeds this target over the prior five years
Domenici-Rivlin Debt Reduction Task Force, Bipartisan Policy Center	Debt reduced to 60 percent of GDP by 2020 and less than that by 2035 Estimated savings achieved in Medicaid through 2020: $20 billion; through 2025: $202 billion	Place dual eligibles in Medicaid managed care Eliminate matching formula and in a budget-neutral way sort out Medicaid responsibilities between the federal government and the states; each level would fully fund the responsibilities assigned to it; federal requirements would still be in place to provide the allocated services at an acceptable level; adjustments would be necessary to assure that each state started with an adequate base Establish goal to limit Medicaid cost growth to the annual percentage increase in the GDP plus 1 percent
Ryan Plan Budget Resolution for Fiscal 2012, US House of Representatives, Committee on the Budget	Debt would be 70 percent of GDP in 2022 but fall to 48 percent in 2040 and 10 percent in 2050 Estimated savings achieved in Medicaid through 2022: $771 billion	Repeal the Medicaid expansion in the Affordable Care Act Block grant Medicaid limiting annual increases in federal aid to the increase in the consumer price index (urban areas) plus population growth States would no longer pay Medicare premiums and other cost sharing for dual eligible elderly people

Sources: Davis (2011); Debt Reduction Task Force (2010); Kaiser Commission on Medicaid and the Uninsured (2010); National Commission on Fiscal Responsibility and Reform (2010); US Congressional Budget Office (2011); US House of Representatives, Committee on the Budget (2011).

References

Aaron, Henry J. 2010. "How to Think about the U.S. Budget Challenge." *Journal of Policy Analysis and Management* 29, no. 4: 883–90.

Abelson, Reed. 2010. "Insurers Push Plans That Limit Health Choices." *New York Times*, July 18.

Abramowitz, Alan I. 2010. *The Disappearing Center*. New Haven, CT: Yale University Press.

Adamy, Janet. 2011. "GOP Governors Seek Leeway to Cut Medicaid Rolls." *Wall Street Journal*, January 7.

Adamy, Janet, and Neil King Jr. 2010. "Some States Weigh Unthinkable Option: Ending Medicaid." *Wall Street Journal*, November 22.

Agranoff, Robert, and Michael McGuire. 2004. "Another Look at Bargaining and Negotiation in Intergovernmental Management." *Journal of Public Administration Research and Theory* 14, no. 4: 495–512.

Aizenman, N. C. 2011. "Court's Review Shocks Medicaid Advocates." *Washington Post*, November 17.

Alter, Jonathan. 2010. *The Promise: President Obama, Year One*. New York: Simon & Schuster.

Altman, Drew. 2011. *A Public Opinion Surprise*. Washington, DC: Kaiser Family Foundation.

Amirkhanyan, Anna A., Hyun Joon Kim, and Kristina T. Lambright. 2008. "Does the Public Sector Outperform the Nonprofit and For-Profit Sectors? Evidence from a National Panel Study on Nursing Home Quality and Access." *Journal of Policy Analysis and Management* 27, no. 2: 326–53.

Anderson, Elizabeth. 1994. "Administering Health Care: Lessons from the Health Care Financing Administration's Waiver Policy-Making." *Journal of Law and Politics* 10, no. 2: 215–62.

Antos, Joseph. R. 1993. "Waivers, Research, and Health System Reform." *Health Affairs* 13, no. 2: 178–83.

Antos, Joseph. R., and Alice M. Rivlin. 2007. "Rising Health Care Spending: Federal and National." In *Restoring Fiscal Sanity 2007: The Health Spending Challenge*, edited by A. M. Rivlin and J. R. Antos. Washington, DC: Brookings Institution Press.

Appleby, Julie. 2006. "Judge Overturns Wal-Mart Law." *USA Today*, July 19. www.usatoday.com/money/industries/retail/2006-07-19-walmart-healthcare_x.htm.

Artiga, Samantha. 2009a. *The Role of Section 1115 Waivers in Medicaid and CHIP: Looking Back and Looking Forward*. Washington, DC: Kaiser Commission on Medicaid and the Uninsured.

———. 2009b. *Where Are States Today? Medicaid and State-Funded Coverage Eligibility Levels for Low-Income Adults*. Washington, DC: Kaiser Commission on Medicaid and the Uninsured.

Bailey, Michael A. 2005. "Welfare and the Multifaceted Decision to Move." *American Political Science Review* 99, no. 1: 125–36.

Bailey, Michael A., and Mark C. Rom. 2004. "A Wider Race? Interstate Competition across Health and Welfare Programs." *Journal of Politics* 66, no. 2: 326–47.

Baker, Sam. 2010. "States Seek Justice Dept. Help in Urging Supreme Court to Hear Medicaid Suit." July 1. http://insidehealthreform.com/1010062913344661/Health-Daily-News/Daily-News/states-see.

———. 2011. "Budget Deal Slashes Incentives for States to Boost CHIP Enrollment." April 15. http://insidehealthreform.com/201104132360791/Health-Daily-News/Daily-News/budget-deal-sla.

Banthin, Jessica S., Peter Cunningham, and Didem M. Bernard. 2008. "Trend: Financial Burden of Health Care, 2001–2004." *Health Affairs* 27, no. 1: 188–95.

Bauer, Scott. 2011. "Governor Scott Walker Uses Illinois Tax Increase to Bolster Wisconsin." January 13. www.postcrescent.com/article/20110113/APC0101/101130553/Governor-Scott.

Beer, Samuel H. 1978. "Federalism, Nationalism, and Democracy in America." *American Political Science Review* 72, no. 1: 9–21.

Belluck, Pam. 2006a. "Massachusetts Sets Health Plan for Nearly All." *New York Times*, April 5.

———. 2006b. "The Nurturing of Health Care." *New York Times*, April 6.

Birkland, Thomas A. 1997. *After Disaster: Agenda Setting, Public Policy, and Focusing Events*. Washington, DC: Georgetown University Press.

Birnbaum, Michael, and Deborah E. Halper. 2009. *Rethinking Service Delivery for High-Cost Patients*. New York: United Hospital Fund.

Blewett, Lynn A., Andrew Ward, and Timothy Beebe. 2006. "How Much Health Insurance Is Enough? Revisiting the Concept of Underinsurance." *Medical Care Research and Review* 63, no. 6: 663–700.

Blumberg, Linda J., Lisa Dubay, and Stephen A. Norton. 2000. "Did the Medicaid Expansions for Children Displace Private Insurance? An Analysis Using the SIPP." *Journal of Health Economics* 19:33–60.

Bolton, Jonathan R. 2003. "The Case of the Disappearing Statute: A Legal and Policy Critique of the Use of 1115 Waivers to Restructure the Medicaid Program." *Columbia Journal of Law and Social Problems* 37, no. 1: 91–179.

Boozang, Patricia, Melinda Dutton, and Julie Hudman. 2006. *Citizenship Documentation Requirements in the Deficit Reduction Act of 2005: Lessons from New York*. Washington, DC: Kaiser Commission on Medicaid and the Uninsured.

Bovbjerg, Randall R., Barbara A. Ormond, and Vicki Chen. 2011. *State Budgets under Federal Health Reform: The Extent and Causes of Variations in Estimated Impacts*. Washington, DC: Kaiser Commission on Medicaid and the Uninsured.

Brandon, William, and Patricia Alt. 2008. "The Elderly: Health Politics beyond Aging." In *Health Politics and Policy*, 4th ed., edited by J. A. Morone, T. J. Litman, and L. S. Robins. Clifton Park, NY: Delmar Cengage Learning.

Brodie, Mollyann, and Robert J. Blendon. 2008. "Public Opinion and Health Policy." In *Health Politics and Policy*, 4th ed., edited by J. A. Morone, T. J. Litman, and L. S. Robins. Clifton Park, NY: Delmar Cengage Learning.

Brodkin, Evelyn Z. 1986. *The False Promise of Administrative Reform*. Philadelphia: Temple University Press.

Brooks, Clem, and Jeff Manza. 2006. "Why Do Welfare States Persist?" *Journal of Politics* 68, no. 4: 816–27.

Brooks, David. 2011. "The New Normal." *New York Times*, March 1.

Brown, Lawrence D., and Michael S. Sparer. 2001. "Window Shopping: State Health Reform Politics in the 1990s." *Health Affairs* 20, no. 1: 50–67.

———. 2003. "Poor Program's Progress: The Unanticipated Politics of Medicaid Policy." *Health Affairs* 22, no. 1: 31–44.

Brownlee, W. Elliot. 2004. *Federal Taxation in America: A Short History*. New York: Cambridge University Press.

Buchanan, Will. 2010. "Who Is the Father of Health Care Reform: Obama or Mitt Romney?" *Christian Science Monitor*, March 31. www.csmonitor.com/USA/Politics/2010/0331/Who-is-the-father-of-healthcare-reform-Obama

Callahan, Daniel, and Sherwin B. Nuland. 2011. "The Quagmire." *New Republic*, June 9, 16–18.

Campbell, James E. 2010. "The Midterm Landslide of 2010: A Triple Wave Election." *The Forum* 8, no. 4. www.bepress.com/forum/vol8/iss4/art3.

Carey, Benedict. 2010. "Revising Book on Disorders of the Mind." *New York Times*, January 10.

Carlson, Barbara L., Stacy Dale, Leslie Foster, Randall Brown, Barbara Phillips, and Jennifer Schore. 2005. "Effect of Consumer Direction on Adults' Personal Care and Well-Being in Arkansas, New Jersey, and Florida." Mathematica Policy Research Institute. www.aspe.hhs.gov/daltcp/reports/adultpcw.htm.

Castellani, Paul J. 2005. *From Snake Pits to Cash Cows*. Albany: State University of New York Press.

Cauchi, Richard. 2011. *State Legislation and Actions Challenging Certain Health Reforms, 2010*. Denver: National Conference of State Legislatures.

CBO (US Congressional Budget Office). 2003. *How Many People Lack Health Insurance and for How Long?* Washington, DC: US Congress.

———. 2011. "Long-Term Analysis of a Budget Proposal by Chairman Ryan." April 5.

Center for Budget and Policy Priorities. 2011. *The United States Is a Low-Tax Country, Continued*. Washington, DC: Center for Budget and Policy Priorities. www.offthechartsblog.org/the-united-states-is-a-low-tax-country-cont/.

Chang, Debbie I., Alice Burton, John O'Brien, and Robert E. Hurley. 2003. "Honesty as Good Policy: Evaluating Maryland's Managed Care Program." *Milbank Quarterly* 81, no. 3: 389–414.

Clinton, Bill. 2004. *My Life*. New York: Alfred A. Knopf.

Confessore, Nicholas. 2007. "State to Fight U.S. Limits on Children's Health Plan." *New York Times*, August 22.

Congressional Quarterly. 1996. "Republicans Seek to Revamp Medicaid." In *1995 Congressional Quarterly Almanac*. Washington, DC: CQ Press.

Connolly, Ceci. 2003. "Governor's Effort to Revise Medicaid Stalls." *Washington Post*, February 13.

Cook, Fay Lomax, and Edith J. Barrett. 1992. *Support for the American Welfare State*. New York: Columbia University Press.

Coughlin, Brett. 2010. "CMS Issues Memo Allowing States to Expand 1915i HCBS Waiver Program." August 11. http://insidehealthreform.com/201008092048232/Health-Daily-News/Daily-News/cms-issues-me.

Coughlin, Theresa A., Sharon K. Long, Timothy Triplett, Samantha Artiga, Barbara Lyons, R. Paul Duncan, and Allyson G. Hall. 2008. "Florida's Medicaid Reform: Informed Consumer Choice?" *Health Affairs Web Exclusive* 27, no. 6: w523.

Coughlin, Theresa A., and Stephen Zuckerman. 2008. "State Responses to New Flexibility in Medicaid." *Milbank Quarterly* 86, no. 2: 209–40.

Courtot, Brigette, and Samantha Artiga. 2011. *Medicaid Enrollment and Expenditures by Federal Core Requirements and State Options*. Washington DC: Kaiser Commission on Medicaid and the Uninsured.

Cross-Call, Jesse, and Judith Solomon. 2011. *Rhode Island's Global Waiver Not a Model for How States Would Fare under a Medicaid Block Grant*. Washington, DC: Center on Budget and Policy Priorities.

Crowley, Jeffrey S. 2006. *Medicaid Long-Term Services Reform in the Deficit Reduction Act*. Washington, DC: Kaiser Commission on Medicaid and the Uninsured.

Crowley, Jeffrey S., and Molly O'Malley. 2006. *Profiles of Medicaid's High Cost Populations*. Washington, DC: Kaiser Commission on Medicaid and the Uninsured.

———. 2008. *Vermont's Choices for Care: Medicaid Long-Term Services Waiver: Progress and Challenges as the Program Concluded Its Third Year*. Washington, DC: Kaiser Commission on Medicaid and the Uninsured.

Cutler, David M., and Jonathan Gruber. 1997. "Medicaid and Private Insurance: Evidence and Implications." *Health Affairs* 16, no. 1: 194–201.

Dartmouth University. 2008. *Dartmouth Atlas of Health Care*. http://cccs.dartmouth.edu/atlas08/datatools/mce_s1.php.

Davis, Brittany. 2011. "100 Groups Fight Medicaid Waiver." July 2. www.healthnewsflorida.org/top_story/read/106_groups_oppose_medicaid_waiver.

Debt Reduction Task Force. 2010. *Restoring America's Future*. Washington, DC: Bipartisan Policy Center.

Derthick, Martha. 1979. *Policymaking for Social Security*. Washington, DC: Brookings Institution Press.

———. 1990. *Agency under Stress*. Washington, DC: Brookings Institution Press.

Dilger, Robert Jay. 2011. *Federal Grants-in-Aid: An Historical Perspective*. Washington, DC: Congressional Research Service.

Dixit, Rachana. 2011. "AARP Blasts Medicaid Block Grant Approach." April 27. http://insidehealthreform.com/201104282362272?Health-Blog/The-Vitals/aarp-blasts.

Dobson, Allen, Donald Moran, and Gary Young. 1992. "The Role of Federal Waivers in the Health Policy Process." *Health Affairs* 11, no. 4: 72–94.

Donahue, John D. 1997. *Disunited States*. New York: Basic Books.

Donelan, Karen, Craig A. Hill, Catherine Hoffman, Kimberly Scoles, Penny Hollander Feldman, Carol Levine, and David Gould. 2002. "Challenged to Care: Informal Caregivers in a Changing Health System." *Health Affairs* 21, no. 4: 222–31.

Dorn, Stan, and Matthew Buettgens. 2010. *Net Effects of the Affordable Care Act on State Budgets*. Washington, DC: Urban Institute Press.

Drew, Elizabeth. 1996. *Shutdown*. New York: Simon & Schuster.

Dutton, Melinda, William Bernstein, Kalpana Bahandarkar, and Susan Ingargiola. 2009. *The Role of Local Government in Administering Medicaid in New York*. New York: United Hospital Fund.

Edwards, Barbara Coulter, Susan P. Garcia, Aimee E. Lashbrook, and Lynda Flowers. 2007. *Let the Sunshine In: Assuring Public Involvement in State Medicaid Policy Making*. Washington, DC: AARP Public Policy Institute.

Edwards, Barbara Coulter, Vernon K. Smith, and Greg Moody. 2008. *Reforming New York State's Eligibility Process: Lessons from Other States*. New York: United Hospital Fund.

Engel, Jonathan. 2006. *Poor People's Medicine*. Durham, NC: Duke University Press.

Everstine, Brian. 2011. "House Panel Approves Medicaid MOE Repeal, Blocks Dem Efforts to Exempt Children, Elderly." May 12. http://insidehealthreform.com/201105122363806/Health-Daily-News/daily-News/housepanel-ap.

Fahrenthold, David A. 2006. "Mass. Marks Health Care Milestone: Insurance Required of All Residents, but Funding Isn't Final." *Washington Post*, April 13.

Feder, Judith, and Donald W. Moran. 2007. "Cost Containment and the Politics of Health Care Reform." In *Restoring Fiscal Sanity 2007: The Health Spending Challenge*, edited by A. M. Rivlin and J. R. Antos. Washington, DC: Brookings Institution Press.

Federman, Alex D., Bruce C. Vladeck, and Albert L. Siu. 2005. "Avoidance of Health Care Services Because of Cost: Impact of the Medicare Savings Program." *Health Affairs* 24, no. 1: 263–70.

Finkelstein, Amy, Sarah Taubman, Bill Wright, Mira Bernstein, Jonathan Gruber, Joseph P. Newhouse, Heidi Allen, and Katherine Becker. 2011. *The Oregon Health Insurance Experiment: Evidence from the First Year*. Cambridge, MA: National Bureau of Economic Research. www.nber.org/papers/w17190.

Fossett, James W. 1998. "Managed Care and Devolution." In *Medicaid and Devolution: A View from the States*, edited by F. J. Thompson and J. DiIulio Jr. Washington, DC: Brookings Institution Press.

Fossett, James, and Frank J. Thompson. 2006. "Administrative Responsiveness to the Disadvantaged: The Case of Children's Health Insurance." *Journal of Public Administration Research and Theory* 16, no. 3: 369–92.

Frakt, Austin. 2010. *How Much Do Hospitals Cost Shift? A Review of the Evidence*. Health Care Financing and Economics Working Paper 2011-01. Boston: Boston VA Healthcare System.

Frakt, Austin, Aaron E. Carroll, Harold A. Pollack, and Uwe Reinhardt. 2011. "Our Flawed but Beneficial Medicaid Program." *New England Journal of Medicine* 364, no. 31 (April 21). www.nejm.org/doi/ful/10.1056/NEJMp1103168.

Freund, Deborah A., Louis F. Rossiter, Peter D. Fox, Jack A. Meyer, Robert E. Hurley, Timothy S. Carey, and John E. Paul. 1989. "Evaluation of the Medicaid Comprehensive Demonstrations." *Health Care Financing Review* 11, no. 2: 81–97.

Friedman, Thomas.1993. "President Allows States Flexibility on Medicaid Funds." *New York Times*, February 2.

Gais, Thomas L. 2009. "Stretched Net: The Retrenchment of State and Local Social Welfare Spending before the Recession." *Publius: The Journal of Federalism* 39, no. 3: 557–79.

Gais, Thomas, and James Fossett. 2005. "Federalism and the Executive Branch." In *The Executive Branch*, edited by J. D. Aberbach and M. A. Peterson. New York: Oxford University Press.

GAO (US General Accounting Office until 2004; then US Government Accountability Office). 1989. *Health Care: Nine States' Experiences with Home Care Waivers*. Report GAO/HRD-89-95. Washington, DC: US Government Printing Office.

———. 1995a. *Medicaid: Tennessee's Program Broadens Coverage but Faces Uncertain Future*. Report GAO/HEHS-95-186. Washington, DC: US Government Printing Office.

———. 1995b. *Medicaid Spending Pressures Drive States toward Program Reinvention*. Report GAO/HEHS-95-122. Washington, DC: US Government Printing Office.

———. 1996. *Medicaid: Oversight of Institutions for the Mentally Retarded Should Be*

Strengthened. Report GAO/HEHS-96-131. Washington, DC: US Government Printing Office.

———. 1998. *Supplemental Security Income: SSA Needs a Uniform Standard for Assessing Childhood Disability*. Report GAO/T-HEHS-98-206. Washington, DC: US Government Printing Office.

———. 1999. *Supplemental Security Income: Additional Action Needed to Reduce Program Vulnerability to Fraud and Abuse*. Report : GAO/HEHS-99-151. Washington, DC: US Government Printing Office.

———. 2001. *Long-term Care: Implications of Supreme Court's Olmstead Decision Are Still Unfolding*. Report GAO-01-1167T. Washington, DC: US Government Printing Office.

———. 2002. *Medicaid and SCHIP: Recent HHS Approvals of Demonstration Waiver Projects Raise Concerns*. Report GAO-02-817. Washington, DC: US Government Printing Office.

———. 2003a. *Long-Term Care: Federal Oversight of Growing Medicaid Home and Community-Based Waivers Should Be Strengthened*. Report GAO-03-576. Washington, DC: US Government Printing Office.

———. 2003b. *Medicaid Formula: Differences in Funding Ability among States Often Are Widened*. Report GAO-03-620. Washington, DC: US Government Printing Office.

———. 2004a. *Forum on Health Care: Unsustainable Trends Necessitate Comprehensive and Fundamental Reforms to Control Spending and Improve Value*. Report GAO-04-793sp. Washington, DC: US Government Printing Office.

———. 2004b. *Medicaid Waivers: HHS Approvals of Pharmacy Plus Demonstrations Continue to Raise Cost and Oversight Concerns*. Report GAO-04-080. Washington, DC: US Government Printing Office.

———. 2004c. *Private Health Insurance: Coverage of Key Colorectal Screening Tests Is Common but Not Universal*. Report GAO-04-713. Washington, DC: US Government Printing Office.

———. 2004d. *SCHIP: HHS Continues to Approve Waivers That Are Inconsistent with Program Goals*. Report GAO-04166R. Washington, DC: US Government Printing Office.

———. 2007a. *Children's Health Insurance: State Experiences in Implementing SCHIP and Considerations for Reauthorization*. Report GAO-07-447T. Washington, DC: US Government Printing Office.

———. 2007b. *Employer-Sponsored Health and Retirement Benefits: Efforts to Control Employer Costs and the Implications for Workers*. Report GAO-07-355. Washington, DC: US Government Printing Office.

———. 2007c. *Medicaid: States Reported That Citizenship Documentation Requirement Resulted in Enrollment Declines for Eligible Citizens and Posed Administrative Burdens*. Report GAO-07-889. Washington, DC: US Government Printing Office.

———. 2007d. *Medicaid Demonstration Waivers: Lack of Opportunity for Federal Input during Federal Approval Process Still a Concern*. Report GAO-07-694R. Washington, DC: US Government Printing Office.

———. 2008a. *Congressional Review Act: Applicability to CMS Letter on State Children's Health Insurance Program*. Report GAO-08-785T. Washington, DC: US Government Printing Office.

———. 2008b. *Medicaid Home and Community-Based Waivers: CMS Should Encourage States to Conduct Mortality Reviews for Individuals with Developmental Disabilities*. Report GAO-08-529. Washington, DC: US Government Printing Office.

———. 2009a. *Health Resources and Services Administration: Many Underserved Areas Lack a Health Center Site, and Data Are Needed on Service Provision at Sites*. Report GAO-09-667T. Washington, DC: US Government Printing Office.

———. 2009b. *Nursing Homes: CMS's Special Focus Facility Methodology Should Better Target the Most Poorly Performing Homes, Which Tended to Be Chain Affiliated and For-Profit*. Report GAO-09-689. Washington, DC: US Government Printing Office.

———. 2009c. *Progress Made but Challenges Remain in Estimating and Reducing Improper Payments*. Report GAO-09-628T. Washington, DC: US Government Printing Office.

———. 2009d. *Recovery Act: As Initial Implementation Unfolds in States and Localities, Continued Attention to Accountability Issues Is Essential*. Report GAO-09-631T. Washington, DC: US Government Printing Office.

Geva-May, Iris. 2004. "Riding the Wave of Opportunity: Termination in Public Policy." *Journal of Public Administration Research and Theory* 14, no. 3: 309–33.

Gibson, Ginger. 2011. "Gov. Christie Travels to Chicago in Effort to Lure Business to N.J." February 5. www.nj.com/news/index.ssf/2011/02/gov_christie_travels_to_chicago.html.

Gibson, Mary Jo, Steven R. Gregory, and Sheel M. Pandya. 2003. *Long-Term Care in Developed Nations: A Brief Overview*. Washington, DC: AARP Public Policy Institute.

Gibson, Mary Jo, and Ari N. Houser. 2007. *Valuing the Invaluable: A New Look at the Economic Value of Family Caregiving*. Washington, DC: AARP Public Policy Institute.

Gifford, Kathleen, Vernon K. Smith, Dyke Snipes, and Julia Paradise. 2011. *A Profile of Medicaid Managed Care Programs in 2010: Findings from a 50-State Survey*. Washington, DC: Kaiser Commission on Medicaid and the Uninsured.

Gilman, Jean Donovan. 1998. *Medicaid and the Costs of Federalism, 1984–1992*. New York: Garland.

Goldman, Dana P., Baoping Shang, Jayanta Bhattacharya, Alan M. Garber, Michael Hurd, Geoffrey F. Joyce, Darius N. Lakdawalla, Constantijin Panis, and Paul G. Shekelle. 2005. "Consequences of Health Trends and Medical Innovation for the Future Elderly." *Health Affairs Web Exclusive* 24, Supplement 2: R5-R17.

Goldstein, Amy. 2003. "Governors Finalizing Proposal to Revamp Medicaid." *Washington Post*, June 3.

Goodnough, Abby. 2009. "Massachusetts Steps Back from Health Care for All." *New York Times*, July 15.

Gottlieb, Jane. 2010. "Name Change at Agency to Remove 'Retardation.'" *New York Times*, June 8.

Gottlieb, Scott. 2011. "Medicaid Is Worse Than No Coverage at All." *Wall Street Journal*, March 10. http://online.wsj.com/article/SB10001424052748704758904576188280858303612.html.

Gottschalk, Marie. 2000. *The Shadow Welfare State*. Ithaca, NY: ILR Press of Cornell University.

Grabowski, David C. 2006. "The Cost-Effectiveness of Noninstitutional Long-Term Care Services: Review and Synthesis of the Most Recent Evidence." *Medical Care Research and Review* 63, no. 1: 3–28.

———. 2009. "Special Needs Plans and the Coordination of Benefits and Services for Dual Eligibles." *Health Affairs* 28, no. 1: 136–46.

Grannemann, Thomas W., and Mark V. Pauly. 2009. *Reform Medicaid First*. Washington, DC: AEI Press.

———. 2010. *Medicaid Everyone Can Count On*. Washington, DC: AEI Press.

Griffen, Jane F., Joseph W. Hogan, Jay S. Buechner, and Tricia M. Leddy. 1999. "The Effect of a Medicaid Managed Care Program on the Adequacy of Prenatal Care Utilization in Rhode Island." *American Journal of Public Health* 89, no. 4: 497–501.

Grogan, Colleen M. 2008. "Medicaid: Health Care for You and Me?" In *Health Policy and Politics*, edited by J. A. Morone, T. J. Litman, and L. S. Robins. Clifton Park, NY: Delmar Cengage Learning.

Grogan, Colleen M., and Eric M. Patashnik. 2003. "Universalism within Targeting: Nursing Home Care, the Middle Class, and the Politics of the Medicaid Program." *Social Service Review* 77, no.1: 51–71.

Gruber, Jonathan. 2003. "Medicaid." In *Means-Tested Transfer Programs in the United States*, edited by R. A. Moffitt. Chicago: University of Chicago Press.

Guralnik, David B., ed. 1982. *Webster's New World Dictionary*. New York: Simon & Schuster.

Gusmano, Michael, Courtney Burke, and Frank J. Thompson. 2012. "Health Care Politics and Policy in New York State." In *Oxford Handbook of New York State Government*, edited by G. Benjamin. New York: Oxford University Press.

Gusmano, Michael, and Frank J. Thompson. 2012. "The Safety Net at the Crossroads? Whither Medicaid DSH?" In *The Health Care Safety-Net in a Post-Reform World*, edited by M. Hall and S. Rosenbaum. New Brunswick, NJ: Rutgers University Press.

Hacker, Jacob. S. 2002. *The Divided Welfare State*. New York: Cambridge University Press.

———. 2004. "Privatizing Risk without Privatizing the Welfare State: The Hidden Politics of Social Policy Retrenchment in the United States." *American Political Science Review* 98, no. 2: 243–60.

———. 2010. "The Road to Somewhere: Why Health Reform Happened, or Why Political Scientists Who Write about Public Policy Shouldn't Assume They Know How to Shape It." *Perspectives on Politics* 8, no.3: 861–76.

Hacker, Jacob S., and Paul Pierson. 2007. "Tax Politics and the Struggle over Activist Government." In *The Transformation of American Politics*, edited by P. Pierson and T. Skocpol. Princeton, NJ: Princeton University Press.

Hakim, Danny. 2011. "At State-Run Homes, Abuse and Impunity." *New York Times*, April 12. www.nytimes.com/2011/03/13/nyregion/13homes.html?_r=1.

Halpern, Michael T., Elizabeth M. Ward, Alexandre L. Pavluck, Nicole M. Schrag, John Bian, and Amy Y. Chen. 2008. "Association of Insurance Status and Ethnicity with Cancer Stage at Diagnosis for 12 Cancer Sites: A Retrospective Analysis." *Lancet Oncol* 9: 221–31.

Haskins, Ron. 2006. *Work over Welfare*. Washington, DC: Brookings Institution Press.

Havemann, Judith. 1995a. "House GOP Amends Medicaid Plan: Move Made to Bolster Support among Governors for Cutting Costs." *Washington Post*, September 19.

———. 1995b. "House Welfare Reform to Leave Medicaid Untouched, Governors Say." *Washington Post*, March 16.

———. 1995c. "Money Isn't the Deal-Breaker in Clinton Medicaid Proposal." *Washington Post*, December 8.

———. 1996. "Advocacy Groups Take on Governors' Reform Plan." *Washington Post*, February 20.

Havemann, Judith, and Amy Goldstein. 1995. "GOP Moves to End Medicaid Entitlement." *Washington Post*, September 20.

Havemann, Judith, and John F. Harris. 1996. "Governors' Welfare, Medicaid Deal Blows Up amid Charges of Partisanship." *Washington Post*, May 30.

Havemann, Judith, and Spencer Rich. 1995. "Senate Panel's Health Care Bill Draws Veto Vow." *Washington Post*, October 1.

HCFA (US Health Care Financing Administration). 1994. "Medicaid Program; Demonstration Proposals Pursuant to Section 1115(a) of the Social Security Act; Policy and Procedures." *Federal Register* 59: 23,960.

Heberlein, Martha, Tricia Brooks, Jocelyn Guyer, Samantha Artiga, and Jessica Stephens. 2011. *Holding Steady / Looking Ahead: Annual Findings of a 50-State Survey of Eligibility Rules, Enrollment and Renewal Procedures, and Cost-Sharing Practices in Medicaid and CHIP, 2010–2011*. Washington, DC: Kaiser Family Foundation.

Herszenhorn, David M. 2011. "Deficit Forecast Nears $1.5 Trillion, Fueling Partisan Battle on Federal Spending." *New York Times*, January 27.

Hetherington, Marc J. 2005. *Why Trust Matters*. Princeton, NJ: Princeton University Press.

Hetherington, Marc J., and Thomas J. Rudolph. 2008. "Priming, Performance, and the Dynamics of Political Trust." *Journal of Politics* 70, no. 2: 498–512.

Hoadley, Jack, and Joan Alker. 2011. *Proposed Medicaid Premiums Challenge Coverage for Florida's Children and Parents*. Jacksonville: Jessie Ball DuPont Fund and Winter Park Health Foundation.

Hoffman, Catherine, Anthony Damico, and Rachel Garfield. 2011. *Research Brief: Insurance and Access to Care in Primary Care Shortage Areas*. Washington, DC: Kaiser Commission on Medicaid and the Uninsured.

Holahan, John, Matthew Buettgens, Vicki Chen, Caitlin Carroll, and Emily Lawton. 2011. *House Republican Budget Plan: State-by-State Impact of Changes in Medicaid Financing*. Washington, DC: Kaiser Commission on Medicaid and the Uninsured.

Holahan, John, and Irene Headen. 2010. *Medicaid Coverage and Spending in Health Reform: National and State-by-State Results for Adults at or Below 133% FPL*. Washington, DC: Kaiser Commission on Medicaid and the Uninsured.

Holahan, John, Dawn M. Miller, and David Rousseau. 2009. *Dual Eligibles: Medicaid Enrollment and Spending for Medicare Beneficiaries in 2005*. Washington, DC: Kaiser Commission on Medicaid and the Uninsured.

Holahan, John, and Mary Beth Pohl. 2003. "Leaders and Laggards in State Coverage Expansions." In *Federalism & Health Policy*, edited by J. Holahan, A. Weil, and J. M. Weiner. Washington, DC: Urban Institute Press.

Horner, Dawn, Jocelyn Guyer, Cindy Mann, and Joan Alker. 2009. *The Children's Health Insurance Program Reauthorization Act of 2009*. Washington, DC: Georgetown University Health Policy Institute.

Howard, Jhamirah, Terence Ng, and Charlene Harrington. 2011. *Medicaid Home and Community-Based Services Programs: Data Update*. Washington, DC: Kaiser Commission on Medicaid and the Uninsured.

Howell, William G. 2003. *Power without Persuasion: The Politics of Direct Presidential Action*. Princeton, NJ: Princeton University Press.

Huber, John D., and Charles R. Shipan. 2003. *Deliberate Discretion? The Institutional Foundations of Bureaucratic Autonomy*. New York: Cambridge University Press.

Hudson, Julie L. 2009. "Families with Mixed Eligibility for Public Coverage: Navigating Medicaid, CHIP, and Uninsurance." *Health Affairs Web Exclusive* 28, no. 4: w697–709.

Huffington Post Chicago. 2011. "Indiana Governor Mitch Daniels: Illinois Tax Hike Good News for Indiana Business." January 11. www.huffingtonpost.com/2011/01/11/big-illinois-tax-increase_n_807269.html.

Hurley, Robert E. 2006. "TennCare: A Failure of Politics, Not Policy: A Conversation with Gordon Bonnyman." *Health Affairs Web Exclusive* 25, no. 20: w217–25.

Hurley, Robert E., and Stephen Zuckerman, 2003. "Medicaid Managed Care: State Flexibility in Action." In *Federalism & Health Policy*, edited by J. Holahan, A. Weil, and J. M. Wiener. Washington, DC: Urban Institute Press.

Inside CMS. 2006. "CMS Medicaid 'Proof-of-Citizenship' Guidance Eases House GOP Concerns." June 15.

Institute of Medicine. 2002. *Care without Coverage: Too Little, Too Late*. Washington, DC: National Academies Press.

———. 2003. *Hidden Costs, Value Lost: Uninsurance in America*. Washington, DC: National Academies Press.

Jacobs, Lawrence R., and Theda Skocpol. 2010. *Health Care Reform and American Politics: What Everyone Needs to Know*. New York: Oxford University Press.

Jha, Ashish K., E. John Arav, and Arnold M. Epstein. 2011. "Low-Quality, High-Cost Hospitals, Mainly in South, Care for Sharply Higher Shares of Elderly Black, Hispanic, and Medicaid Patients." *Health Affairs* 30, no. 10: 1904–12.

Jost, Timothy S. 2003. *Disentitlement?* New York: Oxford University Press.

———. 2010. "State Lawsuits Won't Succeed in Overturning the Individual Mandate." *Health Affairs* 29, no.6: 1225–28.

Kaestner, Robert, Lisa Dubay, and Genevieve Kenney. 2005. "Managed Care and Infant Health: An Evaluation of Medicaid in the US." *Social Science & Medicine* 60, no. 8: 1815–33.

Kaiser Commission on Medicaid and the Uninsured. 2009a. *American Recovery and Reinvestment Act (ARRA): Medicaid and Health Care Provisions*. Washington, DC: Kaiser Commission on Medicaid and the Uninsured.

———. 2009b. *CHIP Tips: CHIP Financing Structure*. Washington, DC: Kaiser Commission on Medicaid and the Uninsured.

———. 2009c. *CHIP Tips: Medicaid Performance Bonus*. Washington, DC: Kaiser Commission on Medicaid and the Uninsured.

———. 2009d. *CHIP Tips: Medicaid Performance Bonus "5 of 8" Requirements*. Washington, DC: Kaiser Commission on Medicaid and the Uninsured.

———. 2009e. *Federal Matching Rate (FMAP) for Medicaid and Multiplier*. Washington, DC: Kaiser Commission on Medicaid and the Uninsured. www.statehealthfacts.org/comparetable.jsp?ind=184&cat=4.

———. 2009f. *Medicaid Beneficiaries and Access to Care*. Washington, DC: Kaiser Commission on Medicaid and the Uninsured.

———. 2010. *Comparison of Medicaid Provisions in Deficit-Reduction Proposals*. Washington, DC: Kaiser Commission on Medicaid and the Uninsured.

———. 2011. *Federal Core Requirements and State Options in Medicaid: Current Policies and Key Issues*. Washington, DC: Kaiser Commission on Medicaid and the Uninsured.

Kaiser Family Foundation. 2008. *Employer Health Benefits, 2008 Annual Survey*. Washington DC: Available at http://ehbs.kff.org/.

———. 2010a. *Employer Health Benefits, 2010 Summary of Findings*. Washington, DC: Kaiser Family Foundation.

———. 2010b. *Kaiser Health Tracking Poll, November 2010*. Washington, DC: Kaiser Family Foundation.

———. 2010c. *Medicare Chart Book, Fourth Edition, 2010*. Washington, DC: Kaiser Family Foundation.

———. 2010d. *Side-by-Side Comparison of Major Health Care Reform Proposals*. Washington, DC: Kaiser Family Foundation.

———. 2011. *The Public, Health Care Reform, and Views on Repeal*. Kaiser Public Opinion Data Note. Washington, DC: Kaiser Family Foundation.

Karch, Andrew. 2007. *Democratic Laboratories: Policy Diffusion among the American States*. Ann Arbor: University of Michigan Press.

Kasper, Judith, Barbara Lyons, and Molly O'Malley. 2007. *Long-Term Services and Supports: The Future Role and Challenges for Medicaid*. Washington, DC: Kaiser Commission on Medicaid and the Uninsured.

Kaushal, Neeraj. 2010. "Elderly Immigrants' Labor Supply Response to Supplemental Security Income." *Journal of Policy Analysis and Management* 29, no. 1: 137–60.

Kaye, H. Stephen, Susan Chapman, Robert J. Newcomer, and Charlene Harrington. 2006. "The Personal Assistance Workforce: Trends in Supply and Demand." *Health Affairs* 25, no. 4: 1114–20.

Kaye, H. Stephen, Michael P. LaPlante, and Charlene Harrington. 2009. "Do Non-Institutional Long-Term Care Services Reduce Medicaid Spending?" *Health Affairs* 28, no.1: 262–72.

Kenney, Genevieve, Allison Cook, and Lisa Dubay. 2009. *Progress Enrolling Children in Medicaid/CHIP: Who Is Left and What Are the Prospects for Covering More Children?* Washington, DC: Urban Institute Press.

Kenney, Genevieve, Jennifer Haley, Jennifer E. Pelletier. 2009. *Health Care for the Uninsured: Low-Income Parents' Perceptions of Access and Quality*. Washington, DC: Urban Institute Press.

Kenney, Genevieve, and Justin Yee. 2007. "SCHIP at a Crossroads: Experiences to Date and Challenges Ahead." *Health Affairs* 26, no. 2: 356–69.

Kenyon, Daphne A. 1996. "Health Care Reform and Competition among the States." In *Health Policy, Federalism and the American States*, edited by R. F. Rich and W. D. White. Washington, DC: Urban Institute Press.

Kershaw, Sarah. 2007. "Eight States to Press Bush on Insurance Coverage of Children." *New York Times*, October 2.

Kingdon, John W. 1984. *Agendas, Alternatives, and Public Policies*. Boston: Little, Brown.

Kitchener, Martin, Terence Ng, Charlene Harrington, and Molly O'Malley. 2007. *Medicaid Home and Community-Based Services Program: Data Update*. Washington, DC: Kaiser Commission on Medicaid and the Uninsured.

Kitchener, Martin, Terence Ng, Nancy Miller, and Charlene Harrington. 2005. "Medicaid Home and Community-Based Services: National Program Trends." *Health Affairs* 24, no. 1: 206–12.

Kousser, Thad. 2005. *Term Limits and the Dismantling of State Legislative Professionalism*. New York: Cambridge University Press.

Kraemer, Richard H., Charldean Newell, and David F. Prindle. 2005. *Texas Politics*. Belmont, CA: Thomson Wadsworth.

Kronebusch, Karl, and Brian Elbel. 2004. "Enrolling Children in Public Insurance:

SCHIP, Medicaid, and State Implementation." *Journal of Health Politics, Policy, and Law* 29, no. 3: 451–90.

Kronick, Richard, and David Rousseau. 2007. "Is Medicaid Sustainable? Spending Projections for the Program's Second Forty Years." *Health Affairs Web Exclusive* 26, no. 2: w271–87.

Ku, Leighton, and Fouad Pervez. 2010. "Documenting Citizenship in Medicaid: The Struggle between Ideology and Evidence." *Journal of Health Politics, Policy, and Law* 35, no. 1: 5–28.

Lasswell, Harold. 1958. *Politics: Who Gets What, When, and How*. Cleveland: World Publishing.

Lav, Iris J., and Elizabeth McNichol. 2011. *Misunderstanding Regarding State Debt, Pensions, and Retiree Health Costs Create Unnecessary Alarm*. Washington, DC: Center on Budget and Policy Priorities.

Leibfried, Stephan, Francis G. Castles, and Herbert Obinger. 2005. "'Old' and 'New Politics' in Federal Welfare States." In *Federalism and the Welfare State*, edited by H. Obinger, S. Liebfried, and F. G. Castles. New York: Cambridge University Press.

Lemov, Penelope 2008. "Massachusetts Lite." *Governing* July 2008: 64.

Levinson, Arik, and Frank Ullman. 1998. "Medicaid Managed Care and Infant Health." *Journal of Health Economics* 17, no. 3 : 351–68.

Levitsky, Sandra R. 2008. "'What Rights?' The Construction of Political Claims to American Health Care Entitlements." *Law & Society Review* 48, no. 3: 551–89.

Light, Paul C. 1997. *The Tides of Reform*. New Haven, CT: Yale University Press.

Lindblom, Charles E., and David K. Cohen. 1979. *Usable Knowledge*. New Haven, CT: Yale University Press.

LoSasso, Anthony T., and Thomas C. Buchmueller. 2004. "The Effect of the State Children's Health Insurance Program on Health Insurance Coverage." *Journal of Health Economics* 23: 1059–82.

Lotven, Amy. 2010. "HHS Hikes State Matching Funds for Reform Law's Medicaid Eligibility Systems." *Inside Health Reform*, November 4. http://insidehealthreform.com/20101104234835/Health-Daily-News/Daily-News/hhs-hik . . .

Lowi, Theodore J. 1969. *The End of Liberalism*. New York: W. W. Norton.

Luo, Michael. 2005. "Taxi Fleet Owner Admits 26 Counts of Medicaid Fraud." *New York Times*, September 28.

Lykens, Kristine A., and Paul A. Jargowsky. 2002. "Medicaid Matters: Children's Health and Medicaid Eligibility Expansions." *Journal of Policy Analysis and Management* 21, no. 2: 219–38.

Mashaw, Jerry. 1983. *Bureaucratic Justice*. New Haven, CT: Yale University Press.

Martin, James. 2007. "The Impact of the Introduction of Premiums into a SCHIP Program." *Journal of Policy Analysis and Management* 26, no. 2: 237–56.

Matsusaka, John G. 2004. *For the Many or the Few*. Chicago: University of Chicago Press.

May, Peter J. 1992. "Policy Learning and Failure." *Journal of Public Policy* 12, no. 4: 331–54.

Mayhew, David R. 1991. *Divided We Govern*. New Haven, CT: Yale University Press.

McCarthy, Douglas, Sabrina How, Cathy Schoen, Joel Cantor, and Dina Beloff. 2009. *Aiming Higher: Results from a State Scorecard on Health System Performance, 2009*. New York: Commonwealth Fund Commission on a High Performance Health System.

McCarty, Nolan. 2007. "The Policy Effects of Political Polarization." In *The Transformation of American Politics*, edited by P. Pierson and T. Skocpol. Princeton NJ: Princeton University Press.

McCue, Michael J., and Michael H. Bailit. 2011. *Assessing the Financial Health of Medicaid Managed Care Plans and the Quality of Patient Care They Provide*. New York: Commonwealth Fund.

McDonough, John E. 2000. *Experiencing Politics*. Berkeley: University of California Press.

———. 2011. *Inside National Health Reform*. Berkeley: University of California Press.

McDonough, John E., Brian Rosman, Fawn Phelps, and Melissa Shannon. 2006. "The Third Wave of Massachusetts Access Reform." *Health Affairs Web Exclusive* 25 (September): w420–31.

Mechanic, David. 2006. *The Truth about Health Care*. New Brunswick, NJ: Rutgers University Press.

Mendeloff, John. 1977. "Welfare Procedures and Error Rates: An Alternative Perspective." *Policy Analysis* 3 (Summer): 357–74.

Miller, Edward A., and Vincent Mor. 2006. *Out of the Shadows: Envisioning a Brighter Future for Long-Term Care in America*. Providence: Brown University Press.

Miller, Nancy A. 1992. "Medicaid 2176 Home and Community-Based Care Waivers: The First Ten Years." *Health Affairs* 11, no. 4: 162–71.

Monheit, Alan C., and Joel C. Cantor, eds. 2004. *State Health Insurance Market Reform*. New York: Routledge.

Moon, Marilyn. 2006. *Medicare: A Policy Primer*. Washington, DC: Urban Institute Press.

Mor, Vincent, Jacqueline Zinn, Pedro Gozalo, Zhanlian Feng, Orna Intrater, and David C. Grabowski. 2007. "Prospects for Transferring Nursing Home Residents to the Community." *Health Affairs* 26, no. 6: 1762–71.

Morrow, Beth, and Julia Paradise. 2010. *Explaining Health Reform: Building Enrollment Systems That Meet the Expectations of the Affordable Care Act*. Washington, DC: Kaiser Family Foundation.

Murray, Shailagh. 2009. "States Resist Medicaid Growth." *Washington Post*, October 5.

Nathan, Richard P. 1981. *The Administrative Presidency*. New York: Macmillan.

———. 2000. *Social Science in Government*. Albany: Rockefeller Institute Press.

———. 2008. "Updating Theories of American Federalism." In *Intergovernmental Management for the 21st Century*, edited by T. J. Conlan and P. L. Posner. Washington, DC: Brookings Institution Press.

National Association of Community Health Centers. 2009. *A Sketch of Community Health Centers, Chart Book 2009*. Washington, DC: National Association of Community Health Centers.

National Association of State Budget Officers. 1993. *Fiscal 1992 State Expenditure Report*. Washington, DC: National Association of State Budget Officers.

———. 2009. *Fiscal 2008 Expenditure Report*. Washington, DC: National Association of State Budget Officers.

———. 2011. *Fiscal 2010 State Expenditures Report*. Washington, DC: National Association of State Budget Officers.

National Center for Health Statistics. 2009. *Health, United States, 2008*. Washington, DC: US Government Printing Office.

National Commission on Fiscal Responsibility and Reform. 2010. *The Moment of Truth*. Washington, DC: National Commission on Fiscal Responsibility and Reform.

Neustadt, Richard E. 1964. *Presidential Power*. New York: John Wiley & Sons.
New York State Health Policy Research Center. 2008. *Implementing Small Group Insurance Market Reforms: Lessons from the States*. Albany: Nelson A. Rockefeller Institute of Government.
Ng, Terence, Charlene Harrington, and Jhamirah Howard. 2011. *Medicaid Home and Community-Based Service Programs: Data Update*. Washington, DC. Kaiser Commission on Medicaid and the Uninsured.
Ng, Terence, Charlene Harrington, and Martin Kitchener. 2010. "Medicare and Medicaid in Long-Term Care." *Health Affairs* 29, no. 1: 22–28.
Ng, Terence, Charlene Harrington, and Molly O'Malley Watts. 2009. *Medicaid Home and Community-Based Service Programs: Data Update*. Washington, DC: Kaiser Commission on Medicaid and the Uninsured.
Nordlinger, Eric A. 1981. *On the Autonomy of the Democratic State*. Cambridge, MA: Harvard University Press.
Nugent, John D. 2009. *Safeguarding Federalism*. Norman: University of Oklahoma Press.
Oberlander, Jonathan. 2003. *The Political Life of Medicare*. Chicago: University of Chicago Press.
———. 2007. "Health Reform Interrupted: The Unraveling of the Oregon Health Plan." *Health Affairs Web Exclusive* 26, no. 1: w96–105.
Obinger, Herbert, Stephan Leibried, and Francis G. Castles, eds. 2005. *Federalism and the Welfare State*. New York: Cambridge University Press.
O'Brien, Ellen. 2005. *Medicaid's Coverage of Nursing Home Costs: Asset Shelter for the Wealthy or Essential Safety Net?* Washington, DC: Georgetown University Long-Term Care Financing Project.
Oliff, Phil. 2011. *Update on State Budgets*, Washington, DC: Center on Budget and Policy Priorities. www.ofsthechartsblog.org/update-on-state-budgets/.
Oliver, Thomas R. 2001. "State Health Politics and Policy: Rhetoric, Reality, and the Challenges Ahead." In *The New Politics of State Health Policy*, edited by R. B. Hackey and D. A. Rochefort. Lawrence: University of Kansas Press.
Olson, Laura Katz. 2010. *The Politics of Medicaid*. New York: Columbia University Press.
OMB (US Office of Management and Budget). 2008. *The Budget for Fiscal Year 2009, Historical Tables*. Washington, DC: US Government Printing Office.
———. 2010. *Budget of the United States Government, Fiscal Year 2011, Historical Tables*. Washington, DC: US Government Printing Office.
———. 2011. *The Budget for Fiscal Year 2012, Historical Tables*. www.whitehouse.gov/sites/default/files/omb/budget/fy2012/assets/hist.pdf.
Orszag, Peter. 2010. "A Health Care Plan for Colleges." *New York Times*, September 19.
Park, Edwin. 2005. *Failing to Deliver: Administration's Waiver Policy Excludes Many Katrina Survivors and Provides No Guarantee of Full Federal Financing*. Washington, DC: Center on Budget and Policy Priorities.
Parker, Suzanne L., and Terri L. Toner. 2008. "Political Culture and Political Attitudes in Florida." In *Government and Politics of Florida*, edited by J. E. Benton. Gainesville: University Press of Florida.
Patashnik, Eric M. 2008. *Reforms at Risk*. Princeton, NJ: Princeton University Press.
Pear, Robert. 1995a. "Congress Preparing a Major Overhaul of Medicaid." *New York Times*, June 12.

———. 1995b. "GAO Says White House Is Expanding Medicaid Coverage." *New York Times*, April 5.
———. 1995c. "Regions Fight over the Way Medicaid Is Distributed." *New York Times*, September 29.
———. 1997a. "Clinton Ordering Effort to Sign Up Medicaid Children." *New York Times*, December 29.
———. 1997b. "Hatch Joins Kennedy to Back a Health Program." *New York Times*, March 14.
———. 2003a. "All Governors to Be Asked to Back Bush on Medicaid." *New York Times*, February 20.
———. 2003b. "Governors Seek Aid from Congress and Decline to Back Medicaid Plan." *New York Times*, February 26.
———. 2003c. "Medicaid Proposal Would Give States More Say on Costs." *New York Times*, February 1.
———. 2006. "Medicaid Wants Citizenship Proof for Infant Care." *New York Times*, November 3.
———. 2007a. "Battle Takes Shape over Expansion of Children's Insurance." *New York Times*, July 9.
———. 2007b. "Children's Health Plan Focus of New Struggle." *New York Times*, August 1.
———. 2007c. "Rules May Limit Health Program Aiding Children." *New York Times*, August 21.
———. 2007d. "Senate Accord on Increasing Cigarette Tax to $1 a Pack." *New York Times*, July 14.
———. 2008. "U.S. Curtailing Bids to Expand Medicaid Rolls." *New York Times*, January 4.
———. 2009. "Senators Approve Health Bill for Children." *New York Times*, January 30.
———. 2011a. "Administration Opposes Challenges to Medicaid Cuts." *New York Times*, May 29.
———. 2011b. "Governors Fear Federal Cuts May Hobble Recovery." *New York Times*, February 27.
———. 2011c. "Rule Would Discourage States' Cutting Payment to Providers." *New York Times*, May 3.
Pear, Robert, and David M. Herszenhorn. 2009. "New Objections to Baucus Health Care Proposal." *New York Times*, September 15.
Peters, Christie Provost. 2008. *Medicaid Financing: How the FMAP Formula Works and Why It Falls Short*. Washington, DC: National Health Policy Forum.
Peterson, Mark A. 1999. "Introduction: Politics, Misperception, or Apropos?" *Journal of Health Politics, Policy, and Law* 24, no. 5: 873–86.
Peterson, Paul E. 1995. *The Price of Federalism*. Washington, DC: Brookings Institution Press.
Peterson, Paul E., and Mark C. Rom. 1990. *Welfare Magnets*. Washington, DC: Brookings Institution Press.
Pierson, Paul. ed. 2001. *The New Politics of the Welfare State*. New York: Oxford University Press.
———. 2004. *Politics in Time*. Princeton, NJ: Princeton University Press.
———. 2007. "The Rise of Activist Government." In *The Transformation of American Politics*, edited by P. Pierson and T. Skocpol. Princeton, NJ: Princeton University Press.

Posner, Paul L. 1998. *The Politics of Unfunded Mandates: Whither Federalism?* Washington, DC: Georgetown University Press.

Pressman, Jeffrey L., and Aaron Wildavsky. 1973. *Implementation*. Berkeley: University of California Press.

Provost, Colin. 2003. "State Attorneys General, Entrepreneurship, and Consumer Protection in the New Federalism." *Publius: The Journal of Federalism* 33, no.2: 37–53.

Pryor, Carol, and Andrew Cohen. 2009. *Consumers' Experience In Massachusetts: Lessons for National Health Reform*. Washington, DC: Kaiser Family Foundation.

Purdum, Todd S. 1996. "Governors Raise Hopes for Ending Budget Deadlock." *New York Times*, February 7.

Putnam, Robert D. 1993. *Making Democracy Work: Civic Traditions in Modern Italy*. Princeton, NJ: Princeton University Press.

Quirk, Paul J., and Sarah A. Binder. 2005. "Congress and American Democracy: Assessing Institutional Performance." In *The Legislative Branch*, edited by P. J. Quirk and S. A. Binder. New York: Oxford University Press.

Reinhard, Susan C. 2010. "Diversion, Transition Programs Target Nursing Homes' Status Quo." *Health Affairs* 29, no. 1: 44–48.

Republican Governors Policy Committee. 2011. *A New Medicaid: A Flexible, Innovative and Accountable Future*. www.scribed.com/embeds/63596104/content?startpage.

Roberts, Barbara. 1992. "Bush Blows It on Health Care." *New York Times*, August 11.

Rodden, Jonathan. 2003. "Revising Leviathan: Fiscal Federalism and the Growth of Government." *International Organization* 57 (Fall): 695–729.

———. 2006. *Hamilton's Paradox: The Promise and Peril of Fiscal Federalism*. New York: Cambridge University Press.

Rosenbaum, Sara. 2009. *Medicaid Payment Rates Lawsuits: Evolving Court Views Mean Uncertain Future for Medi-Cal*. Oakland: California Health Foundation.

———. 2010. "A 'Customary and Necessary' Program: Medicaid and Health Care Reform." *New England Journal of Medicine* 362, no. 21: 1952–55.

Rosenbaum, Sara, Emily Jones, Peter Shin, and Jennifer Tolbert. 2010. *Community Health Centers: Opportunities and Challenges of Health Reform*. Washington, DC: Kaiser Commission on Medicaid and the Uninsured.

Rosenbaum, Sara, and Joel Teitelbaum. 2004. *Olmstead at Five: Assessing the Impact*. Washington, DC: Kaiser Commission on Medicaid and the Uninsured.

Ross, Donna Cohen, and Caryn Marks. 2009. *Challenges of Providing Health Coverage for Children and Parents in a Recession: A 50-State Update on Eligibility Rules, Enrollment and Renewal Procedures, and Cost-Sharing Practices in Medicaid and SCHIP in 2009*. Washington, DC: Kaiser Commission on Medicaid and the Uninsured.

Rothkopf, Jennifer, Katie Brookler, Sandeep Wadhwa, and Michael Sajovetz. 2011. "Medicaid Patients Seen at Federally Qualified Health Centers Use Hospital Services Less Than Those Seen by Private Providers." *Health Affairs* 30, no. 7: 1335–41.

Ryan, Jennifer, and Safiya Mojerie. 2008. *Covering All Kids: States Setting the Pace*. Washington, DC: National Health Policy Forum.

Sack, Kevin. 2010a. "Arizona's Medicaid Cuts Are Seen as a Sign of the Financial Times." *New York Times*, December 5.

———. 2010b. "Florida Suit Rated Best as Challenge to Care Law." *New York Times*, May 11.

———. 2010c. "States Are Battling Health Law While Working to Follow It." *New York Times*, July 28.
———. 2011a. "Administration Seeks Clarity from Judge on Health Ruling." *New York Times*, February 18.
———. 2011b. "For Governors of Both Parties, Medicaid Looks Ripe to Slash." *New York Times*, January 29.
———. 2011c. "Opposing the Health Law, Florida Refuses Millions of Dollars." *New York Times*, August 1.
———. 2011d. "White House Clears the Way for Arizona to Shed Adults from Medicaid." *New York Times*, February 16.
Sack, Kevin, David Herszenhorn, and Robert Pear. 2011. "Along Party Lines, States Diverge on How to Deal with Health Care Ruling." *New York Times*, December 2.
Sack, Kevin, and Robert Pear. 2009. "Governors Fear Medicaid Costs in Health Plan." *New York Times*, July 20.
Salamon, Lester, ed. 2002. *The Tools of Government*. New York: Oxford University Press.
Sanford, Terry. 1967. *Storm over the States*. New York: McGraw-Hill.
Schneider, Anne, and Helen Ingram. 1993. "Social Construction of Target Populations: Implications for Politics and Policy." *American Political Science Review* 87, no. 2: 335–47.
Schoen, Cathy, Michelle M. Doty, Ruth H. Robertson, and Sara R. Collins. 2011. "Affordable Care Act Reforms Could Reduce the Number of Underinsured US Adults by 70 Percent." *Health Affairs* 30, no. 9: 1762–71.
Schwartz, Karyn, and Anthony Damico. 2010. *Expanding Medicaid under Health Reform: A Look at Adults At or Below 133% of Poverty*. Washington, DC: Kaiser Family Foundation.
Selden, Thomas M., and Bradley M. Gray. 2006. "Tax Subsidies for Employment-Related Health Insurance: Estimates for 2006." *Health Affairs* 25, no. 6: 1568–79.
Selden, Thomas M., Julie L. Hudson, and Jessica S. Banthin. 2004. "Tracking Changes in Eligibility and Coverage among Children, 1996–2002." *Health Affairs* 23, no. 5: 39–50.
Shapiro, Ilya. 2010. "State Suits against Health Reform Are Well Grounded in Law—and Pose Serious Challenges." *Health Affairs* 29, no. 6: 1229–33.
Shapiro, Robert Y., and Lawrence Jacobs. 2011. "Response to Quirk's 'Polarized Populism: Masses, Elites, and Partisan Conflict.'" *The Forum* 9, no. 2. www.bepress.com/forum/vol9/iss2/art11.
Shirk, Cynthia. 2006. *Rebalancing Long-Term Care: The Role of the Medicaid HCBS Waiver Program*. Washington, DC: National Health Policy Forum.
Sinclair, Upton. 1994. *I, Candidate for Governor—and How I Got Licked*. Berkeley: University of California Press. (Orig. pub. 1935.)
Skotch, Richard K. 1989. "Politics and Policy in the History of the Disability Rights Movement." *Milbank Quarterly* 67 (supplement 2, part 2): 380–400.
Smith, David Barton. 2006. "Organizing Care for Older Persons in New York: The Social Class Vulnerabilities of a World City." In *Growing Older in World Cities*, edited by V. G. Rodwin and M. K. Gusmano. Nashville: Vanderbilt University Press.
Smith, David Barton, and Zhanlian Feng. 2010. "The Accumulated Challenges of Long-Term Care." *Health Affairs* 29, no. 1: 29–43.
Smith, David G. 2002. *Entitlement Politics: Medicare and Medicaid, 1995–2001*. New York: Aldine de Gruyter.

Smith, David G., and Judith D. Moore. 2008. *Medicaid Politics and Policy, 1965–2007.* New Brunswick, NJ: Transaction.

Smith, Troy E. 1998. "When States Lobby." Ph.D. diss. in political science, State University of New York at Albany.

Smith, Vernon, Neva Kaye, Debbie Chang, Jennie Bonney, Carles Miligan, Dann Milne, Robert Mollica, and Cynthia Shirk. 2005. *Making Medicaid Work For the 21st Century.* Washington, DC: National Academy for State Health Policy.

Sommers, Benjamin D., and Sara Rosenbaum. 2011. "Issues In Health Reform: How Changes in Eligibility May Move Millions Back and Forth between Medicaid and Insurance Exchanges." *Health Affairs* 30, no. 2: 228–36.

Sorens, Jason. 2011. "The Institutions of Fiscal Federalism." *Publius: The Journal of Federalism* 41, no. 2: 207–31.

Soss, Joe, and Sanford F. Schram. 2007. "A Public Transformed? Welfare Reform as Policy Feedback." *American Political Science Review* 101, no. 1: 111–28.

Sparer, Michael. 2008. *Medicaid Managed Care Reexamined.* New York: United Hospital Fund.

———. 2009. "Medicaid and the US Path to National Health Insurance." *New England Journal of Medicine* 360, no. 4 (January 22): 323–25.

Sparer, Michael, and Lawrence D. Brown. 2002. "Nothing Exceeds Like Success: Managed Care Comes to Medicaid in New York City." *Milbank Quarterly* 77, no. 2: 205–23.

Sparer, Michael, George France, and Chelsea Clinton. 2011. "Inching toward Incrementalism: Federalism, Devolution, and Health Policy in the United States and the United Kingdom." *Journal of Health Politics, Policy, and Law* 36, no. 1: 33–58.

Starr, Paul. 2011. *Remedy and Reaction.* New Haven, CT: Yale University Press.

Stein, Sam. 2010. "Mitt Romney: Obama Health Care Plan NOT Like Massachusetts Plan." March 7. www.huffingtonpost.com(2010/03/07/mitt-romney-obama-health_n_489042.html.

Steinhauer, Jennifer. 2011. "Democrats Force a Medicare Vote Pressuring GOP." *New York Times*, May 26.

Stenberg, Carl W. 2008. "Block Grants and Evolution: A Future Tool?" In *Intergovernmental Management for the 21st Century*, edited by T. J. Conlan and P. L. Posner. Washington, DC: Brookings Institution Press.

Steuerle, C. Eugene. 2010. "America's Related Fiscal Problems." *Journal of Policy Analysis and Management* 29, no. 4: 883.

Stone, Deborah A. 1984. *The Disabled State.* Philadelphia: Temple University Press.

———. 1999. *Reframing Home Health-Care Policy.* Cambridge, MA: Radcliffe Public Policy Center.

———. 2002. *Policy Paradox.* New York: W. W. Norton.

Stuber, Jennifer, and Karl Kronebusch. 2004. "Stigma and Other Determinants of Participation in TANF and Medicaid." *Journal of Policy Analysis and Management* 23, no. 3: 509–30.

Swartz, Katherine. 2003. "Bush's Medicaid Proposal Puts States between a Rock and a Hard Place." *Inquiry* 40 (Spring): 3–5.

———. 2006. *Reinsuring Health.* New York: Russell Sage Foundation.

Switzer, Jacqueline V. 2003. *Disabled Rights.* Washington, DC: Georgetown University Press.

Tanner, Robert. 2003. "Governors Seek Solutions on Medicaid: Partisan Conflicts Threaten Consensus." *Washington Post*, February 24.

Texas Health and Human Services Commission and Texas Department of Insurance. 2010. *Impact on Texas if Medicaid Is Eliminated*. Austin: Texas Health and Human Services Commission and Texas Department of Insurance.

Thompson, Frank J. 1981. *Health Policy and the Bureaucracy*. Cambridge, MA: MIT Press.

———. 1987. "New Federalism and Health Care Policy: States and the Old Questions." In *Health Policy in Transition*, edited by L. D. Brown. Durham, NC: Duke University Press.

———. 1998. "Federalism and the Medicaid Challenge." In *Medicaid and Devolution: A View from the States*, edited by F. J. Thompson and J. J. DiIulio Jr. Washington, DC: Brookings Institution Press.

Thompson, Frank J., and Courtney Burke. 2007. "Executive Federalism and Medicaid Demonstration Waivers: Implications for Policy and Democratic Process." *Journal of Health Politics, Policy and Law* 32, no. 6: 971–1004.

———. 2009. "Federalism by Waiver: Medicaid and the Transformation of Long-Term Care." *Publius: The Journal of Federalism* 39, no. 1: 22–46.

Trent, James W., Jr. 1994. *Inventing the Feeble Mind*. Berkeley: University of California Press.

Turner, Grace-Marie. 2011. "Obamacare Can't Be Waived Away." *Galen Institute Newsletter*, September 9, 1–2.

US Census Bureau. 2005. *65+ in the United States: 2005*. Washington, DC: US Government Printing Office.

———. 2010. *Income, Poverty, and Health Insurance Coverage in the United States, 2009*. Washington, DC: US Government Printing Office.

———. 2011. *Current Population Survey, 2011 Annual Social and Economic Supplement*. Washington, DC: US Government Printing Office.

US Department of Health and Human Services. 2007a. "Medicaid Program: Citizenship Documentation Requirements; Final Rule." *Federal Register* 72, no. 134 (July 13): 38662–97.

———. 2007b. *2008 Budget in Brief*. www.hhs.gov/budget/08budget/2008budgetinbrief.pdf.

US House Committee on the Budget. 2011. *Concurrent Resolution on the Budget: Fiscal Year 2012 Report*. Washington, DC: US Government Printing Office.

———. 2012. *The Path to Prosperity, Fiscal Year 2013 Budget Resolution*. Washington, DC: US Government Printing Office.

US House Committee on Commerce. 1996a. *Transformation of the Medicaid Program: Part 1*. Washington, DC: US Government Printing Office.

———. 1996b. *Transformation of the Medicaid Program: Part 2*. Washington, DC: US Government Printing Office.

———. 1996c. *Transformation of the Medicaid Program: Part 3*. Washington, DC: US Government Printing Office.

———. 1996d. *The Unanimous Bipartisan National Governors Association Agreement on Medicaid*. Washington, DC: US Government Printing Office.

US House Committee on Energy and Commerce. 2003a. *Medicaid Today: The States' Perspective*. Washington, DC: US Government Printing Office.

———. 2003b. *A Review of the Administration's FY 2004 Health Care Priorities*. Washington, DC: US Government Printing Office.

———. 2005. *Long-term Care and Medicaid: Spiraling Costs and the Need for Reform.* Washington, DC: US Government Printing Office.

———. 2006. *Examining The Impact of Illegal Immigration on the Medicaid Program and Our Healthcare Delivery System.* Washington, DC: US Government Printing Office.

———. 2009a. "Comprehensive Health Reform Discussion Draft, Day 1." Hearings, Subcommittee on Health, Preliminary Transcript. http://energycommerce.house.gov/index.php?option=com_content&view=article&id=168.

———. 2009b. "Comprehensive Health Reform Discussion Draft, Day 2." Hearings. Subcommittee on Health, Preliminary Transcript. http://energycommerce.house.gov/index.php?option=com_content&view=article&id=169.

US House Committee on Ways and Means. 2008. *Background Material and Data on the Programs within the Jurisdiction of the Committee on Ways and Means.* Washington, DC: US Government Printing Office.

US Senate Committee on Finance. 1995. *Medicaid "1115" Waivers.* Washington, DC: US Government Printing Office.

———. 1996. *Governor's Proposal on Welfare and Medicaid.* Washington, DC: US Government Printing Office.

———. 1997a. *Governors' Perspective on Medicaid.* Washington, DC: US Government Printing Office.

———. 1997b. *Increasing Children's Access to Health Care.* Washington, DC: US Government Printing Office.

———. 1997c. *Welfare and Medicaid Reform.* Washington, DC: US Government Printing Office.

———. 2004. *Strategies to Improve Access to Medicaid Home and Community-Based Services.* Washington, DC: US Government Printing Office.

———. 2009. *Executive Committee Meeting to Consider Health Care Reform.* http://finance.senate.gov/hearings/hearing/id+d812a4e-bc6b-dc2c3-8b31-49ec4efd1824.

US Senate Special Committee on Aging. 2005. *Sound Policy, Smart Solutions: Saving Money in Medicaid.* Washington, DC: US Government Printing Office.

US Social Security Administration. 2009. *Annual Report of the Supplemental Security Income Program.* Baltimore: US Social Security Administration.

US Supreme Court. 1999. *Tommy Olmstead, Commissioner, Georgia Department of Human Resources et al. v. L.C., by Jonathan Zimring.* 527 US 581.

———. 2002a. *Gonzaga University et al. v. Doe.* (01-6679) 536 US 273.

———. 2012a. *Douglas, Director, California Department of Health Care Services v. Independent Living Center of Southern California.* 565 US ___ (2012).

———. 2012b. *National Federation of Independent Business et al. v. Sebelius, Secretary of Health and Human Services et al.* 567 US ___ (2012).

Vladeck, Bruce C. 1980. *Unloving Care: The Nursing Home Tragedy.* New York: Basic Books.

———. 1995. "Medicaid 1115 Demonstration Waivers: Progress through Partnership." *Health Affairs* 14, no. 1: 217–20.

———. 2003. "Where the Action Really Is: Medicaid and the Disabled." *Health Affairs* 22, no. 1: 90–100.

Vobejda, Barbara, and Judith Havemann. 1995. "GOP Plans Media Blitz on Reforms." *Washington Post*, December 3.

Volden, Craig. 2005. "Intergovernmental Political Competition in American Federalism." *American Journal of Political Science* 49, no 2: 327–42.

Wachino, Vikki, and Donna Cohen Ross. 2008. *Will the Payment Error Rate Measurement (PERM) Program Affect State Efforts to Facilitate Enrollment of Eligible Children and Parents in Medicaid and SCHIP?* Washington, DC: Kaiser Commission on Medicaid and the Uninsured.

Walker, Scott. 2011. "Our Obsolete Approach to Medicaid." *New York Times*, April 22.

Weaver, R. Kent, and Bert A. Rockman. 1993. "Assessing the Effects of Institutions." In *Do Institutions Matter?* edited by R. K. Weaver and B. A. Rockman. Washington, DC: Brookings Institution Press.

Weisman, Jonathan. 2009. "States Fight Medicaid Expansion." *Wall Street Journal*, June 23.

Weissert, Carol. S. and Daniel Scheller. 2008. "Learning from the States? Federalism and National Health Policy." *Public Administration Review* 68 (supplement): S162–S174.

Weissert, Carol. S., and William G. Weissert. 2008a. "Florida's Health Care Policy: Making Do on the Cheap." In *Government and Politics of Florida*, edited by J. E. Benton. Gainesville: University Press of Florida.

———. 2008b. "Medicaid Waivers: License to Shape the Future of Fiscal Federalism." In *Intergovernmental Management for the 21st Century*, edited by T. J. Conlan and P. L. Posner. Washington, DC: Brookings Institution Press.

White, Joseph. 2011. "Prices, Volume, and the Perverse Effects of the Variations Crusade." *Journal of Health Politics, Policy and Law* 36, no. 4: 775–90.

Wielawski, Irene M. 2009. "Enrolling Eligible People in Medicaid and the State Children's Health Insurance Program." In *To Improve Health and Health Care*, volume XII, edited by S. L. Isaacs and D. C. Colby. San Francisco: Jossey-Bass.

Wiener, Joshua M., and Jane Tilly. 2003. "Long-Term Care: Can States Be the Engine of Reform?" In *Federalism & Health Policy*, edited by J. Holahan, A. Weil, and J. M. Wiener. Washington, DC: Urban Institute Press.

Williamson, Vanessa, Theda Skocpol, and John Coggin. 2011. "The Tea Party and the Remaking of Republican Conservatism." *Perspectives on Politics* 9, no. 1: 25–44.

Wolfe, Barbara, and Scott Scrivner. 2005. "The Devil May Be in the Details: How the Characteristics of SCHIP Programs Affect Take-Up." *Journal of Policy Analysis and Management* 24, no. 3: 499–522.

Worden, Amy. 2006. "Many Wal-Mart Workers Use Medicaid." *Philadelphia Inquirer*, March 2.

Wright, Deil S. 1978. *Understanding Intergovernmental Relations*. Belmont, CA: Duxbury Press.

Yocom, Carolyn L. 2011. *Medicaid Program Integrity: Expanded Federal Role Presents Challenges to and Opportunities for Assisting States*. Report for US Government Accountability Office, GAO-12-288T. Washington, DC: US Government Printing Office.

Zaman, Obaid S., Linda C. Cummings, and Sari Siegel Spieler. 2010. *America's Public Hospitals and Health Systems, 2008*. Washington, DC: National Association of Public Hospitals and Health Systems.

Zeleny, Jeff, and Sheryl Gay Stolberg. 2010. "Chief of Staff Apologizes." *New York Times*, February 3.

Zelizer, Julian. 2007. "Seizing Power: Conservatives and Congress since the 1970s." In *The Transformation of American Politics*, edited by P. Pierson and T. Skocpol. Princeton, NJ: Princeton University Press, 105-134.

Zhu, Jane, Phyllis Brawarsky, Stuart Lipsitz, Haiden Huskamp, and Jennifer S. Haas. 2010. "Massachusetts Health Reform and Disparities in Coverage, Access and Health Status." *Journal of General Internal Medicine* 25, no. 12: 1356–62.

Zola, Irving K. 1989. "Toward the Necessary Universalizing of a Disability Policy." *Milbank Quarterly* 67 (supplement 2, part 2): 401–28.

Zuckerman, Stephen, Aimee F. Williams, and Karen E. Stockley. 2009. "Trends in Medicaid Physician Fees, 2003–2008." *Health Affairs Web Exclusive*, no. 3: w511–20.

Index